# Clinical Epilepsy

# Clinical Epilepsy

**John S. Duncan** MA DM FRCP

Reader in Clinical Neurology, Institute of Neurology and Consultant Neurologist, National Hospital for Neurology and Neurosurgery and National Society for Epilepsy, London, UK

**Simon D. Shorvon** MA MD FRCP

Professor in Clinical Neurology, Institute of Neurology, Consultant Neurologist, National Hospital for Neurology and Neurosurgery and Medical Director, National Society for Epilepsy, London, UK

**David R. Fish** MA MD FRCP

Senior Lecturer in Clinical Neurophysiology, Institute of Neurology and Consultant Neurophysiologist, National Hospital for Neurology and Neurosurgery and National Society for Epilepsy, London, UK

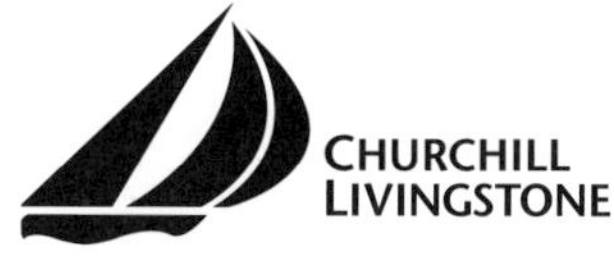


NEW YORK, EDINBURGH, LONDON, MADRID, MELBOURNE, SAN FRANCISCO, AND TOKYO 1995

CHURCHILL LIVINGSTONE
Medical Division of Pearson Professional Limited

Distributed in the United States of America by Churchill Livingstone Inc., 1560 Broadway, New York, NY10036, and by associated companies, branches and representatives throughout the world.



First published 1995

ISBN 0 443 04936 X



*For Churchill Livingstone*

*Publisher:* Lucy Gardner
*Design:* Sarah Cape
*Production:* Nora Cameron
*Page layout:* Janet Smith

The publisher's policy is to use paper manufactured from sustainable forests

Printed in Singapore

# Contents

# Contributors

**H. A. Ring** MD MRCPsych
Lecturer in Neuropsychiatry, Institute of Neurology, National Hospital for Neurology and Neurosurgery, London, UK

**J. W. A. S. Sander** MD PhD
Consultant in Epilepsy, National Society for Epilepsy and Senior Lecturer in Neurology, Institute of Neurology, London, UK

**Pamela J. Thompson** PhD DipPsych AFBPsS
Head of Psychology Service, National Society for Epilepsy, Chalfont St Peter, Buckinghamshire and Honorary Lecturer, Institute of Neurology, London, UK

**M. R. Trimble** MD FRCP FRCPsych
Raymond Way Professor in Behavioural Neurology and Consultant Physician in Psychological Medicine, Institute of Neurology, National Hospital for Neurology and Neurosurgery, London, UK

# Foreword

Much of the pioneering work in the field of clinical epilepsy was carried out in the United Kingdom and thereafter the National Hospital has remained an important resource for the development of neurology worldwide. In the last generation, however, epilepsy has not fired the enthusiasm of British neurologists and epileptologists in the UK have remained regrettably few. Recently, under the stewardship of Professor David Marsden, we have witnessed a renewal and a flowering of interest and expertise in epilepsy at the National Hospital. This was achieved through the recruitment of enthusiastic and committed epilepsy specialists: Drs John Duncan, Simon Shorvon and David Fish. This has led to increased activity which will undoubtedly affect the standard of care and investigation of people with epilepsy throughout the UK and beyond.

Recently, there have been many important contributions to the medical literature as well as educational activities which bode well both for teaching and clinical care. The Queen Square Group of epileptologists have been in the forefront of these activities and have now summarized current knowledge and experience in this volume. Clear, readable and eminently practical the information is up-to-date, abundantly referenced and, above all, stimulating and critical. The excitement, coupled with sound clinical judgement, which permeates this book is characteristic of all three authors. One may hope that it will kindle interest and enthusiasm for a previously stagnant area of medical practice. The views and approaches of this new Queen Square school should lead to improved management and treatment of epilepsy which deserves to be disseminated and made available to students and physicians who treat epilepsy worldwide. Hopefully, the authors will continue to screen and evaluate new developments, and in due course, prepare a second edition to this useful and easily readable book.

Montreal, 1995

Frederick Andermann,
M.D., FRCP(C).

# Preface

The last decade has seen dramatic developments in the understanding and treatment of epilepsy. Much of this information is hidden in journals and weighty reference texts and has not been disseminated to the physicians who treat the generality of patients. The idea for this book arose from the International League against Epilepsy teaching weekends for senior registrars/residents and consultants that we have organized over the last 10 years, at which we were struck by delegates saying how difficult it was to obtain ready access to practical and modern epileptology. The aim of this book is to present current thinking about epilepsy and the management of the patient with epilepsy in a readable and accessible format, highlighting recent advances and points of practical clinical relevance.

We have all had a hand in all the chapters, which we have written ourselves or with colleagues in our group. We have deliberately based much of what is written on our own clinical practice, so that there is a consistent approach and one which gives the book a 'Queen Square approach to epilepsy' flavour.

J.S.D.
S.D.S.
D.R.F.

London, 1995

# Acknowledgements

We are very grateful to our colleagues in the Epilepsy Group of the National Hospital for Neurology and Neurosurgery and the National Society for Epilepsy for their collaboration and for writing and reviewing parts of this book, in particular: Dr Pamela Thompson, consultant clinical psychologist; Dr Ley Sander, consultant in epilepsy; Professor Michael Trimble and Dr Howard Ring, neuro-psychiatrists; Dr Philip Patsalos, pharmacologist; Professor David Thomas and Mr William Harkness, consultant neurosurgeons. We are also very grateful to Lucy Gardner and Michael Parkinson at Churchill Livingstone for working with us and seeing this project through from conception to completion.

# 1 Diagnosis: is it epilepsy?

## 1.1 INTRODUCTION

When a patient presents with an event that has been thought to possibly be an epileptic seizure, it is the history from the patient and any witnesses to the attack that is the most crucial part of the evaluation. Complete reliance should never be placed on the history related by the patient alone. Often he or she will have only a limited recall of events and can only summarize what was passed on by witnesses. Phrases such as 'you were having a fit' can lead to a lifelong misdiagnosis unless a detailed first-hand account of what actually happened is obtained. A videotape record made on a hand-held video recorder often provides invaluable objective data on the nature and sequence of events in a seizure (Samuel & Duncan 1994).

The differential diagnosis of seizures varies with the pre-dominant clinical features of the presenting symptomatology (Table 1.1). Often these present in combination, with one or other being the differentiating feature (e.g. loss of awareness with either drop attacks or psychic phenomena). In this chapter we will consider these presenting symptoms in turn, and the differential diagnosis of their causation.

**Table 1.1** Main categories of episodic symptoms that may be caused by epilepsy

- Loss of awareness
- Generalized convulsive movements
- Drop attacks
- Transient focal motor attacks
- Transient focal sensory attacks
- Facial muscle and eye movements
- Psychic experiences
- Aggressive or vocal outbursts
- Episodic phenomena in sleep
- Prolonged confusional or fugue states

## 1.2 LOSS OF AWARENESS

In clinical practice patients often present with 'blackouts' and there may be little information available. Whatever the cause the patient may have amnesia for both the event and its exact circumstances. The three main causes are syncope, epilepsy and cardiac arrhythmias. Transient cerebral ischaemia due to vascular abnormalities is less common. Microsleeps (very short daytime naps) may occur with any cause of severe sleep deprivation or disruption. Other causes of diagnostic confusion are much rarer and include hypoglycaemia or other intermittent metabolic disorders, structural anomalies of the skull base affecting the brainstem, and lesions affecting the CSF circulation.

### 1.2.1 Syncope

Syncope is the commonest cause of episodes of loss of awareness. Correct diagnosis is crucial to avoid mis-labelling and/or over-investigation (Lempert et al 1994).

Simple faints or vasovagal syncopal attacks can usually be related to identifiable precipitants. Most often they occur on getting up quickly, or standing for prolonged periods, particularly if associated with peripheral vasodilation (e.g. during hot, stuffy weather, in crowded trains or rooms, or related to drug or alcohol use). Frightening, emotional or unpleasant scenes and painful stimuli may also be triggers, due to increased vagal activity, as may Valsalva procedures. A popular misconception is that such attacks cannot occur when lying or sitting.

Syncopal attacks are often preceded by a feeling of lightheadedness, dizziness or nausea, ringing in the ears and the vision 'going black' (Table 1.2). This latter feature is very rare in epilepsy. Although occipital seizures may present with elementary visual hallucinations these are often restricted to a part of the visual field, and on the very rare occasions when bilateral loss of vision is reported in epilepsy it is usually as a postictal phenomenon rather than as an aura (Ch. 2, 2.4.4).

**Table 1.2** Key features of syncopal attacks

- Evidence of precipitant factors
- Lightheadedness, dizziness, nausea
- Pallor
- Ringing in the ears
- Bilateral loss of vision
- Collapse
- Some twitching movements may occur
- Rapid recovery when supine
- Sweating, subsequent flushing

Following a syncopal attack, pallor may be replaced by flushing and sweating. Consciousness is regained within a minute or two if the patient is allowed to lie flat, but may be delayed if this is prevented. Although usually isolated, flurries of attacks may occur if the patient gets up quickly or remains exposed to the relevant precipitant. Incontinence is rare in simple faints unless there is secondary anoxia with convulsions, but is more common if the patient has a full bladder at the time. Irregular and myoclonic jerking is common in syncope and is often mistaken for epilepsy. However, such jerking is sporadic, uncoordinated, lasts for a few seconds and is not associated with tonic stiffening. These features should differentiate syncope from the motor phenomena of a tonic-clonic seizure.

There are various other causes of syncopal attacks, and classification is somewhat dependent upon terminology. Cough and micturition syncope are well recognized. The latter most often occurs in older subjects who have difficulty micturating (e.g. prostatic hypertrophy) and get up out of bed to do so during the night. Straining leads to a Valsalva manoeuvre. In this setting the attacks are unlikely to be witnessed, and falls in a restricted space may prevent the patient from lying flat, leading to prolonged or complex episodes. Other family members may hear the fall and then come to investigate. At this stage there may be little to see or, if present, jerking movements may lead to the erroneous assumption that a seizure has occurred. Changes in intrathoracic pressure (cough syncope), impaired baroreceptors due to atheroma of the carotid (carotid sinus syncope), cardiac arrhythmias and autonomic disturbances may also lead to cerebral hypoperfusion and fainting. As these may not be due to vasovagal reflex changes, the typical aura of a vasovagal syncope may not be present.

In children, voluntary so-called 'breath-holding' attacks may cause syncope, cyanosis and sometimes secondary anoxic seizures. The onset of these episodes is usually before 18 months of age. The frequency commonly increases over the next year and then decreases, to cease spontaneously. So-called pallid attacks often occur a few seconds after an unpleasant, unexpected or frightening experience. The child becomes floppy and unresponsive, stops breathing and may have a few clonic limb twitches, and then returns to normal.

Cyanotic attacks are generally a response to a greater stimulus, such as pain or frustration. The apnoea is longer-lasting than in a pallid attack and the child becomes cyanosed and may be incontinent and then sleep for some hours.

### 1.2.2 Epilepsy

Several types of seizure may present with loss of awareness as the sole reported manifestation. These include absences, complex partial, tonic or atonic seizures (Ch. 2, 2.2). Typical absences involve arrest of activity, reduced or lost awareness, eyelid blinking or twitching, and sometimes small myoclonic facial or limb jerks, or brief facial automatisms such as lip-smacking or chewing. They occur in the idiopathic generalized epilepsies (Ch. 2, 2.7). Typical absences are usually brief but frequent, often occurring many times per day. There may be other associated seizure types, and a careful history should include specific enquiry about isolated myoclonic jerks, especially on waking (these may be reported as clumsiness rather than involuntary movements). The EEG changes are characteristic (Ch. 3, 3.2.4). 'Atypical absences' are usually associated with mental retardation and other seizure types, and are often more prolonged. Atonic seizures usually give rise to drop attacks (see below, 1.4.1) but may appear to cause blank spells if the patient is sitting or lying down and so cannot fall. Complex partial seizures have many forms depending upon the cerebral structures that are involved and may cause loss of awareness with few if any other features. Detailed enquiry must always be made for any associated psychic or motor phenomena that may raise the possibility of a seizure disorder. In addition, partial seizures that predominantly involve loss of speech or memory may also be referred to as 'blackouts'.

### 1.2.3 Cardiac disorders

Transient cardiac arrhythmias may cause episodes of abrupt loss of awareness mimicking epileptic seizures. There are often prodromal features similar to those seen with simple syncope, as well as palpitations, chest pain, shortness of breath or other features of cardiovascular insufficiency. Attacks may vary in duration and severity according to the arrhythmia. For example, Stokes–Adams attacks due to transient complete heart block are abrupt and short with rapid loss of consciousness. Stokes–Adams attacks are especially prone to cause confusion. In these episodes there is complete heart block with profound bradycardia or asystole. Apparently syncopal features are followed by rapid collapse and sometimes secondary anoxic seizures. Usually the attacks last for less than 1 min. Sometimes the lack of cardiac output is due to short episodes of ventricular tachycardia or fibrillation. Prolongation of the QT interval may lead to such events (Pacia et al 1994). Attacks may be preceded by palpitations, extreme fatigue or presyncopal features. There is a high risk of sudden death. The resting ECG often shows some evidence of heart block or bundle branch block. In contrast, supraventricular tachycardias are usually well tolerated unless there is other cardiovascular disease, and may persist for hours or days.

Occasionally cardiac disorders may present with impaired awareness and focal neurological features, presumably due to critical hypoperfusion of specific brain regions. Cardiac valve disease, especially mitral valve prolapse and aortic stenosis, may also present with episodic loss of awareness due to fluctuating cardiac output or associated arrhythmias. Aortic stenosis with hypertrophic cardiomyopathy is especially prone to present with episodes of sudden collapse with loss of awareness during exercise. In consequence, patients with unexplained blackouts will require detailed cardiac evaluation, with ECG, 24-h ECG tape, chest radiograph and an echocardiogram, especially if there are no abnormal neurological features.

### 1.2.4 Transient cerebral ischaemia

Transient cerebral ischaemia may occur due to impaired cardiac output (see above), or occlusion of vessels due to thrombosis or emboli. Global cerebral ischaemia that causes a loss of awareness is rare and supratentorial transient ischaemic attacks seldom cause loss of consciousness. Cerebrovascular disease usually manifests with focal neurological deficits that are primarily negative, such as paralysis or loss of sensation, although positive phenomena such as paraesthesiae may occur (see below, 1.5.3). Vertebrobasilar ischaemia is overdiagnosed; in this condition there is usually other evidence of brainstem dysfunction during the attacks (such as diplopia, nausea, unsteadiness and limb and facial motor and sensory deficits). Transient ischaemic attacks tend to occur abruptly and then rapidly improve and do not develop over the same time course as is common in epilepsy.

### 1.2.5 Microsleeps

Any cause of sleep deprivation may lead to brief daytime naps, sometimes lasting for only a few seconds. The history of this is usually clear from the patient. Impaired quality of sleep due to other disorders, however, may be less apparent. The most important of these is obstructive sleep apnoea. This occurs most commonly in obese males with short fat necks, reduced oropharyngeal space or other upper respiratory tract problems, and may be exacerbated by alcohol. There may be a long history of severe snoring. Airflow may cease during sleep many times for 10–30 s while respiratory efforts continue, to be terminated with a grunt. Such episodes cause numerous arousals during sleep and may prevent sustained periods of deeper sleep. This results in chronic daytime hypersomnolence that may be manifest as short or prolonged daytime naps. Similar disruption can occur in shift workers. Rarely, narcolepsy can present with short periods of suddenly falling asleep during the daytime that are misinterpreted as brief epileptic attacks of loss of awareness.

### 1.2.6 Panic attacks

Panic attacks usually present with feelings of fear and anxiety, associated with autonomic changes and hyperventilation (see below). This leads to dizziness or lightheadedness, orofacial and/or peripheral paraesthesia (which may be asymmetric), carpopedal spasm, twitching of the peripheries, blurred vision, or nausea. Occasionally these preludes may be forgotten, and attacks present with loss of awareness. Often, but not always, there is a clear precipitant, such as a particular situation (e.g. being in a confined space, on public transport, in a busy shop etc), or the recall of a previous distressing experience. None of these features are consistent, however, and differentiation from epilepsy can sometimes be difficult.

### 1.2.7 Hypoglycaemia

Hypoglycaemic attacks causing loss of consciousness are extremely rare except in patients with treated diabetes mellitus. Very occasional cases may be seen due to insulin-secreting tumours. In such cases there may be a history of a missed meal prior to the attack and previous weight gain due to increased appetite. The attacks are usually preceded by autonomic features (tachycardia, sweating) and lightheadedness and may include features such as mood change, irrational behaviour or involuntary movements (Winer et al 1990).

### 1.2.8 Other neurological disorders

If a head injury causes loss of consciousness, there is amnesia. In accidental head injury, particularly road traffic accidents, it may be difficult to distinguish amnesia caused by the injury from cases in which there was a loss of consciousness that caused the accident. If there was no known external cause for the accident the patient should be fully evaluated and consideration should be given to the causes described above. Isolated episodes of loss of awareness may also be caused by abuse of psychotropic drugs or other substances.

Occasionally, structural CNS abnormalities may present with episodes of loss of awareness. Such disorders include Arnold–Chiari malformation causing distortion of the brainstem (Fish et al 1988), or conditions such as tumours of the third ventricle, which may give rise to acute obstructive hydrocephalus.

### 1.2.9 Non-epileptic attack disorder

The diagnosis of non-epileptic attack disorder (NEAD), previously known as pseudoseizures, involves both the exclusion of organic causes and the elucidation of positive phenomena suggestive of this entity (Meierkord et al 1991). Although the manifestations may be varied, episodes of NEAD typically fall into two broad types:

1. Attacks involving motor phenomena
2. Attacks of lying motionless

The latter are often prolonged, continuing for several minutes or sometimes hours. Such behaviour is very rare in epileptic seizures: there will nearly always be other positive phenomena in epileptic attacks that last for more than a few minutes. In addition attacks are often triggered by external events or stress.

The sequence of events of NEAD is usually different to that of epileptic attacks (Table 1.3). They may build up slowly and wax and wane. There is often excess salivation but cyanosis is extremely rare. During attacks patients may resist examination, and screw up their eyes if attempts are made to open them; and, if their own hand is held above their face and then released, the hand deviates to one side, missing the face. If the patients are examined they may show semi-purposeful movements or directed violence. Urinary incontinence is uncommon, but may occur, as may self-injury, particularly if episodes have been recurring over many months or years. Recovery is variable and may be much quicker than expected from the duration of the attack. Patients may respond, often claiming to have some recall of things that were said to them during the attacks, and may become tearful after the attacks. The longer the duration of such episodes the less likely they are to be epileptic.

Patients with NEAD often have a history of abnormal illness behaviour (e.g. recurrent unexplained abdominal pains, or operations without clearly abnormal findings). Non-epileptic attack disorder is much commoner in females than males, and usually commences in adolescence or early adulthood. Occasionally there is an obvious secondary gain, but usually the psychological basis is more complex (Ch. 9, 9.1). A history of sexual abuse is common, but of course this may be coincidental and is not that rare in patients with epileptic seizures. Similarly, there may be previous overt psychiatric illness. Attacks are usually resistant to antiepileptic drug treatment and this may lead to escalating dosages and severe iatrogenic complications. The diagnosis should always be

**Table 1.3** Differentiation of epileptic seizures and non-epileptic attack disorder (NEAD)

| | Epileptic attack | NEAD |
|---|---|---|
| Precipitating cause | Rare | Common, emotional and stress related |
| When alone or asleep | Common | May be reported |
| Onset | Usually short | May be short or over several minutes |
| Aura | Various, usually stereotyped | Fear, panic, altered mental state |
| Speech | Cry, grunt at onset; muttering, words in automatisms | Semi-voluntary, often unintelligible |
| Movement | Atonic, tonic; if clonic synchronous small-amplitude jerks | Asynchronous flailing of limbs; pelvic thrusting; opisthotonous |
| Injury | Tongue-biting, fall; directed violence rare | May bite tongue, cheeks, lip, hands, throw self to ground. Directed violence not uncommon |
| Consciousness | Complete loss in generalized tonic-clonic; may be incomplete in complex partial | Variable, often inconsistent with seizure type |
| Response to stimulation | None in generalized tonic-clonic; may respond in complex partial and postictally | Often reacts and this may terminate episode |
| Incontinence | Common | Sometimes |
| Duration | Few minutes | Few minutes, may be prolonged |
| Recovery | Depends on seizure type. Few minutes and more prolonged confusion | May be rapid or very prolonged |

considered (even if then excluded) in anyone with prolonged drug-resistant attacks. The most useful test is to record an attack with simultaneous EEG and video (Ch. 3, 3.2.2), but this depends upon their frequency and reproducibility. Videotapes of seizures obtained using a hand-held video recorder may provide useful diagnostic data and can be combined with 24-h ambulatory EEG recordings (Samuel & Duncan 1994). Some patients have both epileptic and non-epileptic attacks, but usually one of these types clearly predominates.

## 1.3 GENERALIZED CONVULSIVE MOVEMENTS

### 1.3.1 Epilepsy

A generalized convulsion is generally the most readily diagnosed epileptic phenomenon. Classically, there is a cry, generalized stiffening of body and limbs, followed by rhythmic jerking of all four limbs, associated with loss of awareness, eyes staring blankly, tongue-biting and urinary incontinence (Ch. 2, 2.2). The generalized convulsive movements usually last for a minute or so and, as the attack proceeds, the jerking slows in frequency and increases in amplitude. There is often cyanosis and afterwards irregular breathing followed by confusion, headache and sleepiness. When all or most of these features are present there is little room for diagnostic confusion.

### 1.3.2 Syncope with secondary jerking movements.

People who faint often have small, brief myoclonic twitches of the extremities, and this feature is often under-recognized by physicians (Lempert et al 1994). With more prolonged cerebral hypoperfusion (e.g. due to something preventing the subject lying flat) these may be more prominent and become reported as 'a convulsion'. The myoclonic jerking is usually irregular, short-lived and does not have a pattern which evolves in the same way as do the convulsive movements of a tonic-clonic seizure. These features should differentiate syncope from the motor phenomena of a tonic-clonic seizure.

Every effort must be made to obtain an accurate picture of the extent of the jerking movements and any associated features suggestive of syncope, particularly the circumstances and prodromal symptoms (see above, 1.2.1).

### 1.3.3 Primary cardiac or respiratory abnormalities presenting with secondary anoxic seizures

In any patient presenting with a convulsion, the possibility of primary cardiorespiratory disease that may manifest with secondary anoxic seizures should be considered. This is especially important when the preceding history is uncertain, for example attacks occurring in sleep or when no neurological abnormalities are evident on examination or investigation. Stokes–Adams attacks are especially prone to cause confusion. In these episodes there is complete heart block with profound bradycardia or asystole. Apparently syncopal features are followed by rapid collapse and sometimes secondary anoxic seizures. Usually the attacks last for less than 1 min. The resting ECG often shows some evidence of heart block or bundle branch block. In cases of uncertainty further cardiac investigation is appropriate (see above, 1.2.3).

### 1.3.4 Involuntary movement disorders and other neurological conditions

Episodic involuntary movement disorders are rare, and often familial, although both sporadic and symptomatic cases are well described (Fahn 1994). There is no alteration in consciousness. The best known is paroxysmal kinesogenic choreoathetosis. Attacks are usually precipitated by sudden specific movements. They are of short duration (a few seconds to minutes), but may occur in clusters. The movements may be unilateral or bilateral, and their nature varies considerably from case to case, although for an individual may be stereotyped. Males are more often affected than females. Presentation is usually in late childhood or adolescence. Other forms of paroxysmal movement disorder may be more prolonged. Paroxysmal dystonia presents with attacks lasting for minutes to hours. Precipitants include caffeine, alcohol and prolonged exercise.

Sometimes patients with known involuntary movement disorders such as idiopathic torsion dystonia or Wilson's disease may show severe acute exacerbations mimicking convulsive movements.

It is rare for epileptic seizures to be provoked by movements, but such cases are sometimes seen, especially in extratemporal epilepsies (Fish & Marsden 1994). Patients with metabolic disorders causing hypocalcaemia or hypomagnesaemia may present with seizures or peripheral twitching (tetany).

Tetanus is a very rare condition caused by infection with *Clostridium tetani*. The incubation period is about 1 week, after which there is general lethargy and spasms of the face, neck or whole body, followed by generalized rigidity.

Patients with mental retardation often have stereotyped or repetitive movements, which may include head banging or body rocking, either in the daytime or occasionally in sleep, and more subtle movements which can be difficult to differentiate from complex partial seizures on clinical grounds.

### 1.3.5 Hyperekplexia

This is a rare, usually familial condition (Andermann & Andermann 1986). There may be a history of hypertonia in infancy. Attacks are characterized by excessive startle, and may cause stiffening and collapse with a sudden jerk of all four limbs. Urinary incontinence may occur, presumably due to changes in intrathoracic and abdominal pressure. Although uncommon, respiratory arrest may cause cyanosis and secondary anoxic seizures. All attacks are provoked by sudden unexpected stimuli, usually auditory.

Hyperekplexia needs to be distinguished from seizures induced by startle (startle epilepsy). Startle epilepsy is a rare form of reflex epilepsy which is often but not always associated with a severe congenital deficit such as a hemiplegia (Ch. 2, 2.5.11). Patients may have a variety of seizures, although it is most often seen in frontal lobe epilepsy and spontaneous seizures are common in addition to the reflex events. In many patients the reflex nature of the seizures is transient, in spite of persistence of the spontaneous attacks.

### 1.3.6 Non-epileptic attack disorder

Non-epileptic attacks involving prominent motor phenomena are commoner than those with arrest of activity (see above, 1.2.9). Movements are varied but often involve semi-purposeful thrashing of all four limbs, waxing and waning over many minutes, distractibility or interaction with the environment, prominent pelvic movements and back-arching (see Table 1.3). The patients often share similar clinical features to those with NEAD that predominantly involve arrest of activity and collapse without convulsive movements, although it has been suggested that there is an even higher evidence of previous sexual abuse in the category with flailing movements.

Non-epileptic attacks may be especially difficult to differentiate from complex partial seizures of frontal lobe origin, which can present with very bizarre motor attacks, with some retained awareness and with quick recovery and which may not be associated with scalp EEG changes (Ch. 2, 2.4.2).

## 1.4 DROP ATTACKS

Any cause of loss of awareness may proceed to a sudden collapse or drop attack. Epilepsy, syncope and other cardiovascular disorders are the commonest causes of drop attacks (Table 1.4).

**Table 1.4** Causes of drop attacks

*Epilepsies*

- Secondary generalized tonic or atonic seizures (including startle induced seizures and Lennox–Gastaut syndrome)

*Cardiovascular*

- Syncope
- Stokes–Adams attacks
- Transient brainstem ischaemia (vertebro-basilar insufficiency)

*Movement disorders*

- Hyperekplexia
- Steele–Richardson–Olszewki syndrome
- Parkinson's disease
- Multisystem atrophy
- Paroxysmal kinesogenic choreoathetosis
- Subcortical myoclonus

*Other*

- Brainstem, spinal or lower limb abnormalities (e.g. Arnold–Chiari malformation, cervical disc disease, spinal angioma, cauda equina disease)
- Third ventricle tumours
- Vestibular
- Cataplexy
- Metabolic (e.g. periodic hypokalaemia)
- Non-epileptic attack disorder
- Idiopathic drop attacks

### 1.4.1 Epilepsies

Sudden drop attacks are common in patients with mental retardation and secondary generalized epilepsies. The falls may be tonic or atonic, and are especially prominent in the Lennox–Gastaut syndrome (Ch. 2, 2.6.8). Such seizure types may also occur in patients with other extratemporal epilepsies, especially those involving the frontal lobes. Drop attacks are less common in temporal lobe epilepsy, although they may occur as a consequence of rapid seizure propagation, usually developing several years after the onset of the epilepsy (Gambardella et al 1994). Generalized tonic-clonic seizures may be modified in patients receiving antiepileptic drugs to take the form of drop attacks.

### 1.4.2 Cardiovascular

If cerebral hypoperfusion is sufficient to cause sudden collapse there is usually loss of awareness (see above, 1.2).

### 1.4.3 Movement disorders

Most movement disorders that cause drop attacks have other more prominent features that make the diagnosis clear (e.g. Parkinson's disease). Hyperekplexia may present with such attacks (see above, 1.3.5), and precipitating factors should be sought. Paroxysmal kinesogenic choreoathetosis may cause drop attacks if there is lower limb involvement.

### 1.4.5 Brainstem, spinal or lower limb abnormalities

There are usually fixed neurological signs, which are exacerbated by movement or exertion. In the Arnold–Chiari malformation there is descent of the cerebellar tonsils through the foramen magnum and this may lead to distortion of the brainstem. Often it is asymptomatic and noted only as a coincidental finding on MRI but it may be associated with pain or motor and sensory deficits in the limbs. Rarely, sudden exacerbations may occur due to movement or mild trauma causing acute distortion of the upper cervical cord or brainstem. Sudden falls may be associated with ataxia, other brainstem symptoms or cardiorespiratory disturbances (Fish et al 1988). Care should be taken to look for nystagmus (especially downbeating), other brainstem signs or clinical features to suggest an associated syrinx. An MRI scan, including views of the foramen magnum is required if the diagnosis is suspected.

Tumours of the third ventricle are very rare, but may present with sudden episodes of collapse and associated headache, presumably due to acute changes in CSF pressure. Spinal cord vascular abnormalities or cauda equina lesions may present with lower limb weakness leading to falls, often on exertion, and without impairment of awareness.

### 1.4.6 Cataplexy

Cataplexy usually occurs in association with narcolepsy, although it may be the presenting clinical feature. There is no loss of consciousness with attacks. Attacks may be precipitated by emotion, especially laughter. Although cataplectic attacks are often thought to involve buckling of the knees with collapse to the ground they are usually more subtle: often there is only loss of tone in the neck muscles with slumping of the head rather than complete falls. A careful history should be taken to look for such minor events, which are often frequent in affected individuals.

### 1.4.7 Metabolic disorders

Periodic paralysis due to sudden changes in serum potassium is rare. The condition may be familial or associated with other endocrine disorders (hyperthyroidism, hyperaldosteronism) or drugs. Attacks may be precipitated by carbohydrate loads, emotion, or rest after exertion. Usually there is a gradual onset and the attacks last for hours. There should not be any difficulty differentiating this condition from epilepsy.

Hyponatraemia may lead to hypovolaemic syncope, which could, superficially, appear to present as a drop attack.

### 1.4.8 Idiopathic drop attacks

These attacks are most common in middle-aged females. They take the form of a sudden fall without loss of consciousness. Characteristically the patients remember falling and hitting the ground. Recovery is instantaneous, but injury may occur. The pathophysiological explanation for these episodes is not clear, and they may be due to abnormalities of spinal reflexes affecting the lower limbs.

### 1.4.9 Vertebrobasilar ischaemia

This condition is overdiagnosed and probably accounts for very few drop attacks. Typically, the attacks occur in the elderly, with evidence of vascular disease and cervical spondylosis. The attacks may be precipitated by head turning or neck extension, resulting in distortion of the vertebral arteries, and are of sudden onset, with features of brainstem ischaemia such as diplopia, vertigo and bilateral facial and limb sensory and motor deficits.

## 1.5 TRANSIENT FOCAL MOTOR ATTACKS

The commonest cause of transient focal motor attacks is epilepsy. In children and adolescents consideration should be given to tics and associated syndromes. Paroxysmal movement disorders are rare, although unilateral paroxysmal kinesogenic choreoathetosis may mimic motor seizures (see above, 1.3.4). Transient cerebral ischaemia usually presents with negative phenomena. Tonic spasms of multiple sclerosis are usually seen once other features of the illness have become apparent, but may be a presenting feature.

### 1.5.1 Focal motor seizures

Focal motor seizures represent one of the most readily recognized localization-related partial epilepsies (Manford et al 1992). Classical Jacksonian seizures reflect the sequential spread of epileptic activity along the primary motor cortex. Other patients present with attacks showing little clinical evidence of spread to adjacent structures. The closeness of the primary sensory cortex frequently leads to an overlap of symptomatology, with not only jerking but also paraesthesia. There may be localized transient weakness following the attack for seconds or minutes, sometimes longer (Todd's paresis). Seizures arising in many different brain regions may cause dystonic posturing, possibly by subsequent spread to the supplementary motor area or basal ganglia.

Benign rolandic epilepsy usually presents in late childhood, and is characterized by relatively infrequent attacks involving jerking of one side (often restricted to the face) or occasional secondary generalized seizures, especially during sleep (Ch. 2, 2.6.5).

Epilepsia partialis continua is a rare form of epilepsy that often presents with diagnostic confusion (Ch. 5, 5.2.2). There is very frequent focal motor activity such as jerking of the hand. This can persist for hours or days, continuing into sleep, and may go on relentlessly for years. The movements often become slow and pendulous, with some associated dystonic posturing leading to the erroneous diagnosis of a movement disorder or hysteria.

### 1.5.2 Tics

Tics usually present with stereotyped movements in childhood or adolescence, sometimes restricted to one particular action (e.g. eyeblink) but sometimes multiple in nature. Gilles de la Tourette syndrome is characterized by associated vocalization, sleep disturbance and obsessive–compulsive behaviour. Tics may be confused with myoclonic jerks. They can be suppressed voluntarily, although to do so leads to a rise in psychological tension and anxiety that is then relieved by the patient allowing the tics to occur. Repetitive tics and stereotypies are particularly common in the mentally retarded.

### 1.5.3 Transient cerebral ischaemia

Transient ischaemic attacks (TIAs) usually present with negative phenomena, i.e. loss of use of a limb, hemiplegia or other deficits, although positive phenomena such as paraesthesiae may occur. Involuntary movements can be seen occasionally, for example with basal ganglia ischaemia. Transient ischaemic attacks may last for a few minutes, but may persist for up to 24 h. The terminology is generally inappropriate: the neurological signs and symptoms may be transient but an MRI scan often reveals areas of infarction. TIAs are not usually stereotyped or repeated with the frequency of epileptic seizures, and there are usually associated features to suggest vascular disease. In suspected cases risk factors for vascular disease should be evaluated, and evidence should always be sought of a source of emboli.

### 1.5.4 Tonic spasms of multiple sclerosis

These spasms usually occur in the setting of known multiple sclerosis, but rarely they may be the presenting feature (Twomey & Espir 1980, Rose et al 1993), although other evidence of multiple sclerosis may be found on examination and investigation. The spasms may last for several seconds, sometimes longer than 1 min, and often respond to low doses of an AED.

### 1.5.5 Paroxysmal movement disorders

Paroxysmal kinesogenic choreoathetosis may present with focal motor attacks that are very similar to epileptic events (Fish & Marsden 1994). Even the occurrence of a trigger is not of absolute diagnostic significance: there are well described patients in the literature with focal motor seizures provoked by movement. Paroxysmal kinesogenic choreoathetosis is usually an autosomal dominant condition, and there are no interictal or ictal epileptiform EEG abnormalities on scalp recordings. Tremor may occur in a variety of movement disorders and is usually sufficiently persistent to elucidate the non-epileptic nature, but may be difficult to distinguish from certain forms of epilepsia partialis continua (see above, 1.5.1, and Ch. 5, 5.2.2). Myoclonus of subcortical origin may be suspected from the distribution of involved muscles (e.g. spinal myoclonus may be restricted to specific segments, either unilateral or bilateral). Peripheral nerve entrapment usually presents with weakness but occasionally can present with episodic jerks or twitches, presumably due to nerve irritation.

## 1.6 TRANSIENT FOCAL SENSORY ATTACKS

### 1.6.1 Somatosensory attacks

Epileptic seizures involving the primary sensory cortex are less common than motor seizures, and may have similar modes of propagation to Jacksonian motor seizures, with spreading paraesthesia. Seizures involving the second sensory areas or mesial frontal cortex may cause sensory illusions, but usually have less well defined qualitative and anatomical features. There are usually other epileptic features due to involvement of adjacent or related brain structures. Transient sensory phenomena may also be seen in peripheral nerve compression or other abnormalities of the ascending sensory pathways, hyperventilation or panic attacks and in TIAs. TIAs are not usually stereotyped or repeated with the frequency of epileptic seizures, and there are usually associated features to suggest vascular disease.

Lesions of sensory pathways cause persistent symptoms, but diagnostic confusion may arise in the early natural history when complaints are intermittent or if they are posture-related. Hyperventilation may be associated with localized areas of paraesthesia (e.g. one arm). Intermittent sensory illusions may be experienced in relation to amputated or anaesthetic limbs. Migrainous episodes may also cause localized areas of paraesthesia, but usually have the distinction of a gradual evolution of sensory phenomena, both positive and negative, and associated features of migraine.

### 1.6.2 Transient vestibular symptoms

Acute attacks of vertigo may occasionally be due to a seizure in parietal or temporal lobes (Sveinbjornsdóttir & Duncan 1993). In these cases there are generally associated features that point to cerebral involvement, such as focal somatosensory symptoms, déjà vu or disordered perception. Peripheral vestibular disease, however, is a much more common cause and may give rise to paroxysmal rotational vertigo and perception of linear motion. Other symptoms of auditory and vestibular disease should be sought, principally: deafness, tinnitus, pressure in the ear and relation to head position. If these features are present there is usually little diagnostic uncertainty that the pathology is vestibular in origin.

## 1.7 FACIAL MUSCLE AND EYE MOVEMENTS

Changes in facial movements may occur in various neurological conditions including focal motor seizures, complex partial seizures with automatisms (e.g. chewing, lip-smacking, grimacing), tics, dystonias or other paroxysmal movement disorders, especially drug-induced dyskinesias and hemifacial spasm, as well as psychological disorders. Intermittent eye deviation may be a particular problem in patients with neurological abnormalities due to nystagmus or other problems with eye movement control (Donat & Wright 1990).

### 1.7.1 Partial seizures

Benign rolandic epilepsy usually presents with seizures in childhood affecting the face, often with unilateral grimacing, hemicorporeal sensory and motor phenomena, or secondarily generalized seizures occurring in sleep. Focal motor seizures may cause twitching of one side of the face (although it should be noted that this may occasionally be bilateral due to the bilateral representation of the face in the primary motor cortex) that may be restricted to specific areas (e.g. eyes, perioral). Eye deviation is often seen with seizures arising in frontal parietal or occipital cortex. Diagnostic problems arise if focal motor activity is the predominant feature of epilepsia partialis continua, although there is usually a history of some seizures spreading, with more widespread jerking.

Complex partial seizures may cause automatisms with lip-smacking, chewing, swallowing, sniffing or grimacing, with amnesia and impaired awareness. Occasionally, however, such automatisms are the main semiology, or it is not possible to obtain further information (e.g. in patients with mental retardation). If these features are due to seizure activity the attacks are usually relatively infrequent, whereas with dystonia or other movement disorders episodes are likely to occur many times per day.

### 1.7.2 Movement disorders

Hemifacial spasm typically presents in the elderly or middle-aged with clusters of attacks that initially involve the eye but subsequently spread to the rest of that side of the face. Facial weakness may develop that persists between attacks.

Bruxism may occur either during the day or in sleep, especially in children with mental retardation. Episodes are usually more prolonged than with the automatisms of complex partial seizures, and there are no associated features to suggest an epileptic basis.

Tics usually present in childhood or adolescence, especially if they are part of Gilles de la Tourette syndrome and are usually stereotyped (see above, 1.5.2). As with dyßstonia and other movement disorders affecting the face there may be evidence of involvement elsewhere, and attacks are usually more frequent than is seen with isolated seizures.

### 1.7.3 Other neurological disorders

Defects of eye movement control are common in patients with a wide range of neurological disorders. There are usually associated features that indicate a non-epileptic basis. Bizarre eye movements also occur in blindness and may be mistaken for epileptic activity. Careful examination is required to ascertain the precise features of the eye movement disorder, and in particular any precipitating factors or features of cerebellar or brainstem disease.

## 1.8 PSYCHIC EXPERIENCES

Intermittent psychic phenomena can be seen in partial seizures (especially of temporal lobe origin), migraine, panic attacks, transient cerebral ischaemia, drug-induced flashbacks, or with illusions associated with loss of a sensory modality as well as psychotic illnesses.

### 1.8.1 Epilepsy

Partial seizures of temporal lobe origin are especially likely to manifest themselves with auras involving psychic phenomena. The most common are fear, déjà vu, memory flashbacks, visual, olfactory or auditory hallucinations (Palmini & Gloor 1992, Fish et al 1993). Other manifestations include: altered perception of the environment with a distancing from reality or change in size or shape of objects; altered language function; and emotions such as sadness, elation, and sexual arousal.

Psychic experiences are often individualized and may have some relation to past experiences. Structured hallucinations or illusions may have a compelling quality and be associated with emotional experiences. They are usually recalled as brief scenes, sometimes strung together but rarely evolving in the manner of a cinema film. They usually lack clarity: for example a patient may describe an illusion of someone standing in front of them whom they know, but they cannot name them or describe them in detail. A rising epigastric sensation may occur alone or in association with such experiences. Elemental visual phenomena, such as flashing lights, are more often seen in occipital lobe epilepsy. Altered thought patterns may be seen in both temporal and frontal lobe seizures. The bizarre nature of many auras needs to be understood during the evaluation of the history. Patients may be reluctant to discuss such feelings, being afraid that they will be considered insane. It is often helpful to ask a patient if they ever think that they are going to have an attack and then do not, as a way to elicit the presence of an aura.

### 1.8.2 Migraine

Migrainous psychic phenomena may involve an initial heightening of awareness. The principal features are usually visual illusions that may be elemental or complex. They rarely have the same intense emotional components of temporal lobe illusions or hallucinations. The time course is usually more prolonged than with partial seizures, and there are associated features of a pounding headache, photophobia and nausea or vomiting. There may be recognized precipitants, and there is often a relevant family history.

### 1.8.3 Panic attacks

These are usually associated with feelings of fear and anxiety. Hyperventilation may lead to dizziness and lightheadedness. There are often unpleasant abdominal sensations similar to the epigastric aura of partial seizures. The evolution, associated increases in heart rate and respiration, longer time course and history of precipitating factors generally make the diagnosis clear.

### 1.8.4 Drug-induced flashbacks

These share many of the qualities of psychic temporal lobe seizures. They are individualized, often brief hallucinations usually related to the circumstances of the drug abuse, often with emotional content of fear or anxiety. A careful history should be taken for substance abuse, especially LSD and mescaline. The episodes may cease spontaneously over time.

### 1.8.5 Hallucinations or illusions caused by loss of a primary sense

Hallucinations and illusions of an absent limb are well recognized in amputees. Similarly, people who lose sight either in the whole or part field may experience visual hallucinations or illusions in the blind field. Such phenomena can be elemental or complex and include evolving scenes. Similar experiences can occur with deafness. Olfactory hallucinations, however are rare in patients with anosmia.

Such experiences due to the loss of a primary sense present particular diagnostic difficulty when they occur in the setting of a structural lesion that could also result in epilepsy. An occipital glioma or infarction, for example, could cause visual loss and could also give rise to epileptic seizures. Often the hallucinations due to sensory loss are more prolonged, lasting for minutes or hours, but they can be brief. Scalp EEG studies may not be helpful, as this test may show little change with simple partial seizures (Ch. 3, 3.2.4). Complex hallucinations have similarly been reported in patients with peduncular lesions, although their basis remains uncertain.

### 1.8.6 Psychotic hallucinations and delusions

Hallucinations and delusions are the hallmark of psychotic illnesses. The following features would suggest a psychiatric rather than epileptic basis: complex nature with an evolving or argued theme, auditory nature involving instructions or third-person language, paranoid content and associated thought disorder. Psychotic episodes are usually more long-lasting than isolated epileptic seizures, although intermittent psychosis may have a similar time course to non-convulsive status epilepticus (see below, 1.11.2, and Ch. 5, 5.2.3). Persistent mood changes may be a helpful guide, but even short temporal lobe seizures may be followed by mood changes lasting for hours or days. Furthermore, flurries of epileptic attacks may themselves cause an organic psychosis lasting for several days. Ruminations and pseudohallucinations, in which the patient retains some insight, may occur in affective disorders.

### 1.8.7 Non-epileptic attack disorder

Non-epileptic attack disorder may be associated with reports of hallucinations and illusions. These often evolve out of previous questioning by members of the medical profession. Initially the symptoms may seem plausible but they should be suspected if they are florid and multiple in type (e.g. auditory, olfactory and visual at different times) with evolving stories or patterns of expression.

## 1.9 AGGRESSIVE OR VOCAL OUTBURSTS

These are rarely epileptic in nature if they occur in isolation. They are especially common in adults and children with mental retardation (Donat & Wright 1990). In this setting there is of course organic brain disease, which could lower the overall seizure threshold. Great care should be given to attempting to elicit other clinical features of epilepsy; these are usually absent and most cases do not have their basis in epilepsy. It must be remembered that EEG studies are often abnormal because of the underlying brain disorder and that, unless striking, interictal changes are not in themselves strong support for a diagnosis of epilepsy in this setting.

A not infrequent forensic issue is the occurrence of violent, or other, crimes in patients with epilepsy in which it is a defence claim that the crime was committed in a state of automatism. Certain features are strong evidence against an epileptic basis to the attack (Table 1.5).

**Table 1.5** Features against there being epileptic basis to an aggressive attack

- Absence of a prior history of epilepsy with automatisms
- Premeditation and evidence of planning or preparation
- Directed violence
- Evidence of complicated and organized activity during the episode
- Recall of events during the episode
- Witness accounts not indicative of a disturbance of consciousness
- Subsequent attempts at escape or concealment of evidence

## 1.10 EPISODIC PHENOMENA IN SLEEP

Attacks occurring during sleep (Table 1.6) present particular diagnostic difficulties because they are often poorly witnessed and the patient may have little, if any, recall of the event or the preceding circumstances.

### 1.10.1 Normal physiological movements

Whole-body (hypnic) jerks commonly occur in normal subjects on falling asleep. Fragmentary physiological myoclonus usually involves the peripheries or the face, and occurs during stages 1 and 2 and REM sleep. Periodic movements of sleep may be an age-related phenomenon, being seen in less than 1% of young adults, but occurring with increasing frequency during middle and old age such that they are present in perhaps half the elderly population. The movements involve a triple flexion of the lower limb with dorsiflexion of the ankle and great toe, flexion of the knee and hip. The movements are not myoclonic but usually more sustained, lasting for a few seconds. Sometimes they have a beating quality with several briefer movements

**Table 1.6** Episodic phenomena in sleep

*Normal physiological activity*

- Whole body jerks (hypnic jerks)
- Fragmentary myoclonus
- Periodic movements of sleep

*Epilepsies*

- Frontal lobe seizures
- Other partial epilepsies
- Generalized convulsions

*Sleep disorders*

- Pathological fragmentary myoclonus
- Restless leg syndrome
- Non-REM parasomnias
- REM parasomnias
- Sleep apnoea

within a few seconds. Rarely they involve the upper limbs as well. Typically these movements occur at regular intervals of 10–60 s, and this is the characteristic hallmark to elicit in the history from a witness. In normal subjects such activity usually occurs in light sleep, and periodic movements may occur in clusters over many minutes.

### 1.10.2 Frontal lobe epilepsy

Frontal lobe seizures may display specific sleep-related characteristics causing diagnostic confusion. Such attacks are often frequent, brief, bizarre and may be restricted to sleep. Earlier workers referred to such attacks as 'nocturnal paroxysmal dystonia', although they appear to have an epileptic basis. Careful observation of such attacks often reveals apnoea, dystonic, myoclonic, or choreiform movements that may be unilateral or bilateral, and some retention of awareness. The attacks are scattered throughout the night, and usually arise from non-REM sleep. Frequency is highly variable, but some patients have very many (> 20) attacks in a single night. An important clue to the diagnosis is the occurrence of additional secondary generalized seizures and seizures occurring in wakefulness (Meierkord et al 1992).

### 1.10.3 Other epilepsies

Seizures arising in other brain regions may also present with nocturnal attacks, although they usually lack the frequency of frontal lobe seizures. Rarely patients may be aroused by an aura, although often this is not recalled by patients when attacks arise from sleep. Complex automatisms, in which patients get out of bed and wander around the house, are rare and may cause confusion with parasomnias. With nocturnal seizures of any type the partner is frequently awoken by particular components, such as vocalization, and does not witness the onset. It is noteworthy that screams often occur in seizures, and their occurrence does not imply a night terror (see below, 1.10.6).

Generalized tonic-clonic seizures (GTCS) on awakening form a subgroup of the idiopathic generalized epilepsies, while patients with juvenile myoclonic epilepsy (JME) often have more pronounced myoclonus and GTCS during the hours immediately after awakening (Ch. 2, 2.7).

### 1.10.4 Pathological fragmentary myoclonus

Excessive fragmentary myoclonus persisting into sleep stages 3 and 4 may be seen with any cause of disrupted nocturnal sleep (Broughton et al 1985).

### 1.10.5 Restless leg syndrome

The restless leg syndrome is characterized by an urge to move the legs, especially in the evening when lying or sitting. It may be associated with various unpleasant paraesthesiae. Occasionally the condition is familial with onset in adolescence or early adulthood. More often onset is in middle or old age. All patients with restless legs have periodic movements of sleep (Krueger 1990). These may be severe and can also occur during wakefulness. In addition there may be a variety of brief daytime dyskinesias (Hening et al 1986). Investigations usually give negative results, although the possibility of associated iron deficiency anaemia, peripheral or spinal abnormalities should be considered.

### 1.10.6 Non-REM parasomnias

These involve night terrors or sleep walking (Broughton 1968). They usually present in childhood or adolescence, and are often familial. The attacks arise from slow-wave sleep. In consequence they typically occur at least 30 min, but not more than 4 h, after going to sleep and the timing is often stereotyped (early sleep is predominantly stage 1 and 2, while prior to awakening REM sleep and light sleep predominate). The episodes are infrequent. Sometimes attacks may be spaced out by months or years: they rarely occur more than once per week, and usually no more than one attack occurs in a single night. They may represent a disorder of arousal, and in consequence appear more likely after stressful events, or when sleeping in a strange bed (e.g. on holiday).

Night terrors involve intense autonomic features (sweating, flushing, palpitations) and a look of fear. Patients may recall a frightening scene or experience, but do not usually recount a vivid dream prior to the attacks. They may be difficult to arouse, and confused for several minutes. Vocalizations are common. Sleep-walking may involve getting out of bed and performing complex tasks. Sometimes it is possible to lead the patient back to bed without awakening. They may respond if spoken to, but their speech is usually slow or monosyllabic. Brief, abortive episodes are commoner, involving sitting up in bed with fidgeting and shuffling (mimicking a complex partial seizure). Non-REM parasomnias may cause self-injury but rarely directed aggression. They are associated with enuresis. Treatment with suppression of slow-wave sleep (e.g. using benzodiazepines) rarely produces a lasting benefit. Most patients grow out of the tendency.

### 1.10.7 REM parasomnias

REM parasomnias usually occur in middle age or the elderly, and show a marked male predominance. They are due to a lack of the normal atonia of REM sleep (Schenck et al 1987). In consequence they more often occur in the later portion of sleep. During REM sleep patients may have an increase in the frequency or severity of fragmentary myoclonus, thrash about, call out, display directed violence, or appear to enact vivid dreams. Attacks may last from seconds to minutes. If awoken patients may recall part of these dreams. Although REM sleep behaviour disorders may occur in healthy elderly subjects they are also seen in association with drugs (e.g. tricyclics) or alcohol, or central nervous system diseases affecting the pathways controlling REM atonia, such as multisystem atrophy. The possibility of REM sleep disorders needs to be considered both at initial presentation and also in patients known to have central nervous system disorders, and are often misdiagnosed as epilepsy. It is of note that REM sleep disorders respond well to clonazepam.

### 1.10.8 Sleep apnoea

Patients with sleep apnoea usually present with daytime hypersomnolence. However, the apnoeic episodes may cause episodic grunting, flailing about or other restless activity that appears to mimic nocturnal epilepsy. Occasionally the resultant hypoxia leads itself to secondary seizures.

### 1.10.9 Other movements in sleep

Nocturnal body rocking may occur in patients with mental retardation, or following head injuries. In patients with many different forms of daytime dyskinesia, similar movements may occasionally occur during overnight sleep, usually in the setting of brief arousals (Fish et al 1991).

## 1.11 PROLONGED CONFUSIONAL OR FUGUE STATES

Epileptic seizures usually last for seconds or minutes. After generalized convulsions (or less often complex partial seizures) there may be confusion lasting for many minutes, but rarely more than an hour. Such episodes only present diagnostic difficulty if the initial seizure is unwitnessed or forgotten. Nevertheless, epileptic states can last for longer periods of time, as can other types of cerebral disorder, and the differential diagnosis of prolonged epileptic confusional states (non-convulsive status, Ch. 5, 5.2.3) should include:

- Acute encephalopathy
- Non-convulsive status epilepticus
- Transient global amnesia
- Intermittent psychosis
- Hysterical fugue (NEAD).

### 1.11.1 Acute encephalopathy

Virtually any severe metabolic disturbance may cause an acute encephalopathy (e.g. diabetic ketoacidosis, hypoglycaemia, respiratory, renal or hepatic failure, drug ingestion, hyperpyrexia, sepsis). Transient metabolic disturbances are most often seen in treated diabetes mellitus due to insulin induced hypoglycaemia. Occasionally metabolic disorders may present with exacerbations, with symptomatology lasting for hours or days, that give the appearance of an episodic condition. These include porphyria, urea cycle enzyme defects and cerebral lupus erythematosus.

Acute neurological conditions also need to be considered, particularly: encephalitis, meningitis, other intracranial infection, head injury, cerebral infarction or haemorrhage. Screening of patients with such episodic confusional states should include appropriate laboratory tests for these conditions (urine, faecal and serum porphyrins, post-prandial serum ammonia, plasma amino acids, urine organic acid screen and autoimmune studies). Drug abuse may cause isolated episodes or recurrent bouts, related to intoxications.

### 1.11.2 Non-convulsive status epilepticus

Patients with complex partial seizures, typical or atypical absences may present with prolonged confusional states due to complex partial epilepticus or absence status (Ch. 5, 5.2). Such attacks may be the first manifestation of the seizure disorder, or occur in the setting of known epilepsy.

### 1.11.3 Intermittent psychosis

Although usually more sustained, psychiatric disorders may present with episodes of delusions, hallucinations or apparent confusion, lasting for hours or days.

### 1.11.4 Transient global amnesia

These episodes typically commence acutely, last for minutes or hours and involve both retrograde and anterograde amnesia. Patients may perform complex activities but afterwards have no recall of them. There is a lack of other neurological features to the attacks, and consciousness appears to be preserved. There is often some evidence of cerebrovascular disease. Although the basis of the attacks remains uncertain they may involve bilateral medial temporal dysfunction, which in some patients may be on the basis of ischaemia while others may have an epileptic basis.

### 1.11.5 Hysterical fugue

A fugue state may arise without an organic physical cause, as a conversion symptom. These episodes may be brief or very prolonged, lasting for days or even weeks. If seen at the time of an episode inconsistencies are often found on examination of the mental state, and an EEG will be unremarkable. In some cases, the question of malingering arises, most commonly in a situation in which the person's state prevents questioning by law, customs or immigration officers.

The diagnosis is more difficult if the patient is only seen after the event. The matching of witness accounts and the apparent sequence of events is essential, but it may remain difficult to come to a firm conclusion. In this situation there is sometimes a forensic aspect, typically when the person is alleged to have committed a crime and professes to have no memory of the events.

## REFERENCES


Andermann F, Andermann E 1986 Excessive startle syndromes: startle disease, jumping and startle epilepsy. Adv Neurol 43: 321–328

Broughton R 1968 Sleep disorders: disorders of arousal. Science 159: 1070–1078

Broughton R, Tolentino MA, Krelina M 1985 Excessive fragmentary myoclonus in non-REM sleep: a report of 38 cases. Electroenceph Clin Neurophysiol 61: 123–133

Donat JF, Wright FS 1990 Episodic symptoms mistaken for seizures in the neurologically impaired child. Neurology 40: 156–157

Fahn S 1994 Paroxysmal dyskinesias. In: Marsden CD, Fahn S (eds) Movement disorders 3. Butterworth Scientific, London, pp 310–345

Fish DR, Marsden CD 1994 Epilepsy masquerading as a movement disorder. In: Marsden CD, Fahn S (eds) Movement disorders 3. Butterworth Scientific, London, pp 346–358

Fish DR, Howard RS, Symon L, Wiles CM 1988 Respiratory arrest: a complication of cerebellar ectopia. J Neurol Neurosurg Psychiat 51: 714–716

Fish DR, Sawyer D, Allen PJ, Lees A, Marsden CD 1991 The effect of sleep on the dyskinesias of Parkinson's disease, Huntington's chorea, Gilles de la Tourette syndrome and torsion dystonia. Arch Neurol 48: 210–214

Fish DR, Gloor P, Quesney LF, Olivier A 1993 Clinical responses elicited by electrical brain stimulation in patients with temporal and frontal lobe epilepsy: pathophysiological implications. Brain 116: 397–414

Gambardella A, Reutens DC, Andermann F et al 1994 Late onset drop attacks in temporal lobe epilepsy: a reevaluation of the concept of temporal lobe syncope. Neurology 44: 1074–1078

Hening WA, Walters A, Kavey N et al 1986 Dyskinesia while awake and periodic movements in sleep in restless leg syndrome; treatment with opioids. Neurology 36: 1363–1366

Krueger BR 1990 Restless legs and periodic movements of sleep. Mayo Clin Proc 65: 999–1006

Lempert T, Bauer M, Schmidt D 1994 Syncope: a videometric analysis of 56 episodes of transient cerebral hypoxia. Ann Neurol 36: 233–237

Manford M, Hart YM, Sander JWAS, Shorvon SD 1992 National General Practice Study of Epilepsy (NGPSE): the syndromic classification of the ILAE applied to epilepsy in a general population. Archives of Neurology 49: 801–809

Meierkord H, Will R, Fish DR, Shorvon SD 1991 The clinical features and prognosis of pseudoseizures diagnosed using video-EEG telemetry. Neurology 41: 1643–1646

Meierkord H, Fish DR, Smith SJM, Scott CA, Shorvon SD, Marsden CD 1992 Is nocturnal paroxysmal dystonia a form of frontal lobe epilepsy? Movement Disorders 7: 38–42

Pacia SV, Devinsky O, Luciano DJ, Vasquez B 1994 The prolonged QT syndrome presenting as epilepsy. Neurology 44: 1408–1410

Palmini A, Gloor P 1992 The localizing value of auras in partial seizures. A prospective and retrospective study. Neurology 42: 801–808

Rose MR, Ball JA, Thompson PD 1993 Magnetic resonance imaging in tonic spasms of multiple sclerosis. J Neurol 241: 115–117

Samuel M, Duncan JS 1994 The use of the hand-held video camcorder in the evaluation of seizures. J Neurol Neurosurg Psychiat 57: 1417–1418

Schenck CH, Bundlie SR, Patterson AI, Mahowald MW 1987 Rapid eye movement sleep behaviour disorder. JAMA 257: 1786–1789

Sveinbjornsdóttir S, Duncan JS 1993 Parietal and occipital lobe epilepsy: a review. Epilepsia 34: 493–521.

Twomey JA, Espir ME 1980 Paroxysmal symptoms as the first manifestations of multiple sclerosis. J Neurol Neurosurg Psychiat 43: 296–304.

Winer JB, Fish DR, Sawyers D, Marsden CD 1990 A movement disorder as a presenting feature of recurrent hypoglycaemia. Movement Disorders 5: 176–177

# 2 The spectrum of epileptic seizures and syndromes

## 2.1 INTRODUCTION

Epilepsy is best viewed, not as a single condition, but rather as a symptom of neurological disorder. The clinical manifestations depend upon the cause of the epilepsy, the anatomical location within the brain of the epileptic focus, the pattern of spread of epileptic discharges through the brain, and also on the age and the level of cerebral maturity of the patient. It is not surprising therefore that attempts at classification have been fraught with difficulty. In the 19th century, epilepsy was usually classified into three broad categories, based upon presumed mechanisms and causes: idiopathic, symptomatic and sympathetic epilepsy. Idiopathic epilepsy was construed as a functional disturbance of the brain (a neurosis). In symptomatic epilepsy, the epileptic seizures were seen as effects of an underlying brain disorder. Sympathetic epilepsy included those conditions in which seizures were postulated to arise from lower brain centres, the spinal cord or the peripheral nervous system. This approach was not universally accepted even then, yet elements of this classification exist to this day.

A second approach to classification was based upon the clinical manifestations of the epileptic seizure, the forerunner of today's classification of seizure types. Hughlings Jackson (Taylor 1931) divided seizures into attacks which were generalized and attacks starting unilaterally. Sociological and psychological classifications were also attempted, based both upon aspects of the ethno-psychological constitution of the epileptic patient, moral status and degeneracy, and also the effects of epilepsy upon psychological health. Thus, terminology became increasingly disordered.

The introduction of the electro-encephalogram (EEG) in the 1930s had a major impact on classification, providing, it was hoped, a method of measuring and visualizing the physiological correlates of the clinical seizure. EEG data was enthusiastically incorporated into classification schemes, often in a complex and idiosyncratic manner, obscuring rather than enlightening matters. By the middle of the 20th century, the classification of epilepsy had become highly confusing and had not in any fundamental sense improved upon the schemes devised a century earlier.

Today, epilepsy might be classified in one of a number of ways (Table 2.1) (Parsonage 1983). Each criterion has advantages and drawbacks and, for a classification to be useful in general clinical circumstances, compound systems must be used, which recognize the multitude of influences in the production of epilepsy. The issue of classification was taken up by the International League Against Epilepsy (ILAE) in the 1960s and in the past 20 years the ILAE has formulated systems of classification that have become widely accepted. It should be remembered, however, that in the absence of any comprehensive understanding of the pathophysiology of epilepsy, or indeed its aetiology, all schemes are to a large extent arbitrary. A good system can provide a framework only, necessarily mutable as knowledge advances, to provide a common basis for communication, and sufficiently pragmatic to be usable in the clinical setting. In this chapter the clinical spectrum of epilepsy will be considered within two such frameworks, the ILAE classification of seizure type, and the ILAE classification of the epilepsies and epileptic syndromes.

**Table 2.1** Criteria that could be used for classifying epilepsy

- Aetiology
- Anatomical basis
- Ictal EEG
- Interictal EEG
- Age
- Clinical phenomenology (seizure type)
- Physiological basis of seizures
- Neurochemical basis of epilepsy
- Response to specific treatment
- Prognosis

## 2.2 THE ILAE CLASSIFICATION OF SEIZURE TYPE

The method of classification which is now most widely used is a descriptive scheme based on the clinical and EEG manifestations of the seizures, devised by the International League Against Epilepsy (ILAE). This was first proposed in 1970 (Gastaut 1970) using six criteria for classification: clinical form; interictal EEG; ictal EEG; anatomical substrate; age; and aetiology. The scheme dropped Gastaut's original proposal to also include interictal neuro-psychiatric changes, response to treatment and pathophysiology. Three main categories of seizure type were identified, based on clinical and EEG features: partial, subdivided into simple and complex; generalized, subdivided into convulsive and non-convulsive; and unilateral, the features of which were similar in character to generalized seizures but their expression was confined 'principally' to one half of the body. The criteria used to classify individual cases were ill-defined and, although a major step in the history of classification, the scheme lacked pragmatic usefulness. In 1981, a revision was proposed, and officially adopted in 1982 (Commission on Classification and Terminology of the International

**Table 2.2** The International League Against Epilepsy (ILAE) classification of seizure type (Commission on Classification and Terminology of the International League Against Epilepsy 1981) – criteria used for classification are seizure phenomenology and EEG findings

**I. Partial (focal, local) seizures**

*A. Simple partial seizures*
1. With motor signs: focal motor with or without march, versive, postural, phonatory
2. With somatosensory or special sensory symptoms: somatosensory, visual, auditory, olfactory, gustatory, vertiginous, simple hallucinations (e.g. tingling, light flashing, buzzing)
3. With autonomic symptoms or signs, including epigastric aura
4. With psychic symptoms (disturbances of higher mental function): dysphasic, dysmnestic, cognitive, affective; illusions, structured hallucinations

*B. Complex partial seizures*
1. Simple partial onset followed by impairment of consciousness
   a. With simple partial features (A1 to A4) followed by impaired consciousness
   b. With automatisms
2. With impairment of consciousness at onset
   a. With impairment of consciousness only
   b. With automatisms

*C. Partial seizures evolving to secondarily generalized seizures (tonic-clonic, tonic, or clonic)*
1. Simple partial seizures evolving to generalized seizures
2. Complex partial seizures evolving to generalized seizures
3. Simple partial seizures evolving to complex partial seizures evolving to generalized seizures

**II. Generalized seizures (convulsive and non-convulsive)**

*A. Absence seizures*
1. Absence seizures with impairment of consciousness only, mild clonic components, atonic components, tonic components, automatisms, autonomic components
2. Atypical absence seizures with changes in tone more pronounced than in A1 and with onset and/or cessation that is not abrupt

*B. Myoclonic seizures*

*C. Clonic seizures*

*D. Tonic seizures*

*E. Tonic-clonic seizures*

*F. Atonic seizures*

(Combinations may occur, such as B and F or B and D)

**III. Unclassified epileptic seizures**

League Against Epilepsy 1981). The original scheme was preserved, but partial seizures were subdivided into 'simple' and 'complex' according to whether or not consciousness was retained or lost, the unilateral category was abolished and a category of 'unclassified epileptic seizures' was introduced. Of the original six taxonomic criteria, three – anatomical substrate, aetiology, age – were deleted. Seizure type was defined solely on the basis of clinical and EEG signs, ictal and interictal (Table 2.2). The classification is highly empirical, based simply upon the visible manifestations of the seizure and its EEG correlate; pathology, anatomy, cause and underlying physiology are entirely ignored.

Problems of definition exist in the classification, worth touching upon to emphasize its incomplete nature. First, there is the difficulty of dividing simple and complex partial seizures on the basis of impaired consciousness. Consciousness is defined operationally as the inability to respond normally to exogenous stimuli by virtue of altered awareness and/or responsiveness. This is a problematic definition at both philosophical and practical levels. Furthermore, in the same patient, a seizure may on one occasion cause alteration in consciousness and on another not. A second problem is the large number of seizures which cross the boundaries of the clinical classification, especially seizures modified by treatment. How, for instance, should one classify a seizure in which the patient blanks out and falls to the ground without any convulsions or other specific motor feature and in whom the EEG shows non-specific changes? This could be included in the atonic, tonic, atypical absence, atypical tonic-clonic or complex partial seizure categories. A third problem is that of defining focality. There are many seizures with highly focal underlying aetiologies in which clinical or

**Table 2.3** Seizure type and aetiology in a population-based series of 564 incident cases of newly diagnosed epilepsy in the United Kingdom (Sander et al 1990)

| | | Percentages |
|---|---|---|
| **Seizure type** | | |
| *Partial* | Simple partial | 2 |
| | Complex partial | 11 |
| | Secondarily generalized | 28 |
| | Mixed partial | 16 |
| | Total partial | 57 |
| *Generalized* | Tonic-clonic | 29 |
| | Absence | 1 |
| | Myoclonic | <1 |
| | Other generalized | <1 |
| | Mixed generalized | 3 |
| | Total generalized | 34 |
| *Unclassifiable* | | 9 |
| **Aetiology** | | |
| No aetiology determined | | 62 |
| Cerebrovascular | | 15 |
| Alcohol-related seizures | | 6 |
| Cerebral tumour | | 6 |
| Cerebral infection | | 2 |
| Cerebral trauma | | 2 |
| Others | | 6 |
| **Aetiological category** | | |
| Cryptogenic | | 62 |
| Acute symptomatic | | 15 |
| Remote symptomatic | | 21 |
| Neurological deficit since birth | | 3 |

EEG evidence of a local onset is missing, and others in which whole regions are involved in the focal onset. Finally, there is the problem of incorporating EEG data into the classification. The wide variation of EEG in the same patient on different occasions and in the same seizure type in different patients is a confounding factor that is not clearly addressed.

Although, criteria are still ill-defined, this scheme is now widely used, and has the virtue of simplicity and clinical utility. The incident frequencies of the differing seizure types in a population-based survey are shown in Table 2.3. (See Ch. 3, 3.2 for details of EEG investigations.)

## 2.2.1 Partial seizures

Partial seizures are those in which electrographic activity commences in a part (focus) of the cerebrum. The clinical characteristics of the seizure reflect the part of the brain affected, and a wide variety of symptoms may thus occur. Partial seizures are divided into three main categories:

- Simple partial seizures, in which there is no alteration of consciousness
- Complex partial seizures, in which consciousness is altered or lost
- Partial seizures evolving to secondarily generalized seizures

Simple partial seizures may progress to become complex partial seizures (i.e. consciousness, although originally preserved, may be lost as the seizure evolves), the aura of the complex partial seizure being in effect the simple partial seizure. Both simple and complex partial seizures may develop into a secondarily generalized seizure (usually a tonic-clonic seizure).

*Simple partial seizures*

Most simple partial seizures are short-lived, lasting a few seconds or so. Prolonged simple partial motor seizures tend to be confined to a limited anatomical region, and take the form of epilepsia partialis continua (Ch. 5, 5.2.2). Less commonly, non-convulsive simple partial seizures are also prolonged (Manford & Shorvon 1992). Simple partial seizures (including those evolving to complex partial seizures) may have the manifestations shown in Table 2.4.

*Motor manifestations:* The most common motor signs are jerking (clonus) or spasm. These most commonly occur in epilepsies arising in frontal or central regions (see below, 2.4.2, 2.4.3).

**Table 2.4** Clinical features of simple partial seizures

- No alteration of consciousness
- No amnesia
- Focal symptoms or signs:
  Motor
  Sensory or special sensory
  Psychic (dysphasic, dysmnestic, cognitive, affective, illusions, hallucinations)
- Sudden onset and cessation
- Due to focal cortical pathology
- The focal symptoms/signs reflect the anatomical origin of the seizure, and are thus useful in localizing the underlying pathology

*Somatosensory or special sensory manifestations (simple hallucinations):* Tingling or numbness (or less commonly an electric-shock-like feeling, burning, pain or a feeling of heat) can occur. These symptoms are most common in epileptic foci in central or parietal regions, although they may occur with spread to postrolandic areas from other epileptic foci. Simple visual phenomena such as flashing lights and colours occur if the calcarine cortex is affected. The cephalic aura is a common manifestation of an epileptic discharge in many cortical areas.

*Autonomic manifestations:* Autonomic symptoms such as changes in skin colour, blood pressure, heart rate, pupil size and piloerection usually occur as a component of generalized or complex partial seizures of frontal or temporal origin. An epigastric sensation (often described as nausea, an empty or sick feeling), which may rise up to the throat, is the most common manifestation of a partial seizure arising in the temporal lobe and is frequently associated with psychic symptoms or alterations in consciousness as the attack evolves into a complex partial seizure.

*Psychic manifestations:* Psychic 'auras' can occur with very discrete discharges, and patients may retain normal awareness. Although there are recognized patterns, auras are not of reliable localizing value as discharges may activate widely distributed neuronal circuits. There are six principal categories.

- *Dysphasic symptoms* occur if cortical speech areas (frontal or temporoparietal) are affected. Speech usually ceases or is severely reduced. Repetitive vocalization with formed words may occur if a discharge originates in the non-dominant temporal lobe.
- *Dysmnestic symptoms* (disturbance of memory) may take the form of flashbacks, déjà vu, jamais vu or panoramic experiences (recollections of previous experiences, former life or childhood), and occur with temporal lobe seizure discharges.
- *Cognitive symptoms* include dreamy states and sensations of unreality or depersonalization and occur primarily in temporal lobe seizures.
- *Affective symptoms* include fear (the commonest symptom, which is sometimes very intense), depression, anger and irritability, and may be accompanied by autonomic effects. Elation, erotic thoughts, serenity or exhilaration may occur. Affective symptomatology is most commonly seen with mesiobasal temporal lobe foci.
- *Illusions* of size (macropsia, micropsia), shape, weight, distance, or sound occur, progressing as the seizure evolves. These symptoms are characteristic of temporal or parieto-occipital epileptic foci.
- *Structured hallucinations* of visual, auditory, gustatory, or olfactory forms, which can be crude or elaborate, are usually due to epileptic discharges in the temporal or parieto-occipital association areas.

The scalp EEG during a localized simple partial seizure is often normal, presumably because the discharge is too small and circumscribed to be picked up by the scalp electrodes. In a temporal lobe simple partial seizure the commonest finding on a scalp EEG is rhythmic theta activity.

Other seizure patterns are a run of fast activity (13–30 Hz) that progressively increases in amplitude and decreases in frequency and is followed by slow activity, or slow spike and wave activity (Ch. 3, 3.2.4). The interictal EEG may be normal or show spikes, sharp waves, focal slow activity, suppression of normal rhythms and other signs. Before the seizure, the interictal EEG may show a sudden reduction in the frequency of interictal spike or sharp waves.

Simple partial seizures occur at any age and imply localized cerebral disease. Any cortical region may be affected, the most common sites being the frontal and temporal lobes. The symptoms are useful in the anatomical localization of the seizures, but the form of the seizures has no pathological specificity.

*Complex partial seizures*

Complex partial seizures have three components (Table 2.5) (Delgado-Escueta et al 1982, Kotagal et al 1988).

*Aura*: These are simple partial seizures and can take any of the forms described above. The aura is usually short-lived, lasting a few seconds or

**Table 2.5** Cinical features of complex partial seizures (see Tables 2.16–2.20 for summaries of features of partial seizures in different cerebral regions)

- Aura (focal symptoms/signs as in simple partial seizure)
- Absence (altered consciousness)
- Amnesia
- Automatism (oro-alimentary, mimicry, gestural, ambulatory verbal, responsive)
- Sudden onset and gradual recovery
- Due to focal cortical pathology
- Complex partial seizures arise most commonly in the temporal lobe, but can also occur in extratemporal, especially frontal, cortex
- Some complex partial seizures consist simply of altered consciousness, some the aura and altered consciousness, some the altered consciousness and automatism and some all three components

so, although in rare cases a prolonged aura persists for minutes, hours or even days. Patients often describe the same features occurring in isolation as self-limited simple partial seizures. The occurrence of an aura prior to complex partial seizures may be noticed by an alert witness, but not subsequently recalled by the patient.

*Altered consciousness:* This may follow the aura or evolve simultaneously. The altered consciousness takes the form of an absence and motor arrest, during which the patient is motionless and inaccessible. There is sometimes no outward sign; the patient's eyes may appear vacant or glazed, though sometimes minor motor signs, posturing or tone changes occur. Unilateral dystonic posturing of the limbs is common in temporal lobe complex partial seizures, and is reliably contralateral to the side of seizure onset.

*Automatism:* Automatisms occur during or after the impairment of consciousness. An automatism is defined as 'a more or less coordinated involuntary motor activity occurring during the state of clouding of consciousness either in the course of, or after, an epileptic seizure, usually followed by amnesia of the event' (Delgado-Escueta et al 1982). Automatisms (in distinction to aura) are of no localizing value and should be distinguished from simple post-ictal confusion, hysterical fugues, acute confusional states and somnambulism. Automatisms are usually divided into:

- *Oro-alimentary:* orofacial movements such as chewing, lip smacking, swallowing, or drooling
- *Mimicry:* with emotional expressions, including displays of laughter or fear, anger or excitement
- *Gestural:* Common movements include fiddling movements with the hands, tapping, patting, or rubbing, ordering and tidying movements; complex actions such as undressing; and genitally directed actions
- *Ambulatory automatisms:* include walking, circling, running; sometimes the patient may wander around carrying out more or less purposeful movements, and quite complex activity may be performed
- *Verbal automatisms:* sometimes these are meaningless sounds, humming, whistling, grunting, and sometimes words which may be repeated, or formed sentences
- *Responsive automatisms:* in which there is quasi-purposeful behaviour, seemingly responsive to environmental stimuli

Violent behaviour sometimes occurs in an automatism, as it might in any acute confusional state, and is especially likely if the patient is restrained. The violent actions of an epileptic automatism are never premeditated, never remembered, never highly coordinated or skilful and seldom goal-directed; these are useful diagnostic features in a forensic context. There is generally total amnesia for the events of the automatism, although a patient may not recognize that consciousness was fully lost.

Complex partial seizures arise from the temporal lobe in about 60% of cases and the frontal lobe in about 30%. Automatisms may occur as part of a complex partial seizure arising from any brain location, although they are most common in temporal and frontal lobe seizures (see below, 2.4.1, 2.4.2).

Complex partial seizures vary considerably in duration. In one series the ictal phase lasted between 3 and 343 s (mean, 54 s), the postictal phase 3–767 s and the total seizure duration 5–998 s (mean, 128 s) (Theodore et al 1983). Clinical events lasting for up to 28 min were recorded in another series (Delgado-Escueta et al 1982).

In about 10–30% of seizures, the scalp EEG is unchanged and in the rest, runs of fast activity, localized spike and wave complexes, spikes or sharp waves or slow activity may occur, or the EEG may simply show flattening (desynchronization). The patterns can be focal (indicating the site or origin of the seizure), lateralized, bilateral or diffuse (Ch. 3, 3.2.4).

*Partial seizures evolving to secondarily generalized seizures*

Partial seizures (simple, complex, or simple evolving to complex) may spread to become generalized. The partial seizure is often experienced as an aura in the seconds before the generalized seizure. The generalized seizure is usually tonic-clonic, tonic or atonic.

## 2.2.2 Generalized seizures

A generalized seizure is defined as an attack in which the epileptic disturbance involves wide areas of both cerebral hemispheres simultaneously from the onset of the attack, with no evidence of an anatomic or functional focus.

Consciousness is almost invariably impaired from the onset of the attack (owing to the extensive cortical and subcortical involvement), motor changes are bilateral and more or less symmetric and the EEG patterns are bilateral and grossly synchronous and symmetrical over both hemispheres. Generalized seizures are divided into several clinical types, but atypical forms are not uncommon (especially in patients receiving treatment).

*Typical absence seizures*

The ILAE classification divides absence seizures into typical and atypical forms. The typical absence seizure was once known as the petit mal seizure (Duncan & Panayiotopoulos 1995) (Table 2.6). There is no warning or aura, the seizure comprises an abrupt sudden loss of consciousness (the absence) and cessation of motor activity (e.g. speaking, eating, walking). Tone is usually preserved and falling does not occur. The patient is unaware, inaccessible and motionless. The eyes appear glazed, usually staring ahead. The attack ends as abruptly as it started and previous activity is resumed as if nothing had happened (Table 2.6). There is no confusion, but the patient is often unaware that an attack has occurred.

**Table 2.6** Clinical features of typical absence seizures

- Absence (blank stare)
- Consciousness lost (with total amnesia)
- Other signs (usually slight; including minor tone changes, blinking, eyes rolling, jerking)*
- Sudden onset and cessation, usually short lived
- Occur as part of the syndrome of idiopathic generalized epilepsy

*see Table 2.7

Other clinical phenomena can occur with the absence, including slight clonic movements, eyelid fluttering, alterations in tone and brief automatisms. These extra features are more common than was previously recognized and are more frequent and more obvious the longer the attack continues. In one study, for instance, automatisms occurred in 22% of attacks lasting 3 s or less and in 95% of attacks that lasted 18 s or longer (Penry et al 1975) (Table 2.7). More than 80% of absence seizures last less than 10 s and many hundreds of attacks may occur in a single day. The attacks often cluster and are often worse when the patient is awakening or drifting off to sleep. Absences may be precipitated by a number of factors

**Table 2.7** Clinical manifestations of typical absence seizures – a total of 374 seizures in a selected group of 48 severe cases documented by simultaneous video and EEG recording; the frequency of motor manifestations, changes in tone and automatism increase with increasing duration of the absence seizure (Penry et al 1975)

| Manifestation | % |
|---|---|
| Simple absence | 9 |
| Clonic components | 45 |
| Decreased postural tone | 22 |
| Increased postural tone | 4 |
| Automatism | 63 |

such as drowsiness, relaxation, photic stimulation and hyperventilation.

The classic EEG pattern during a typical absence is a regular, symmetric, and synchronous 3 Hz spike and wave paroxysm (see Fig. 3.9). In fact, not all paroxysms are entirely regular and frequencies vary between 2 and 4 Hz. Polyspike and wave complexes also occur, and are usually more or less symmetric and synchronous. The interictal EEG has normal background activity. Brief generalized spike and wave or spike activity occur intermittently; such paroxysms have a variation in pattern and are more likely to occur in the hour or so after awakening. Spike and wave paroxysms can frequently be induced by hyperventilation and less commonly by photic stimulation. The features useful in differentiating a complex partial seizure and a typical absence are shown in Table 2.8.

Typical absence seizures most often develop in childhood or adolescence and are encountered almost exclusively in idiopathic generalized epilepsy (see below, 2.7) (Lugaresi et al 1973, Gloor 1979, Duncan & Panayiotopoulos 1995).

*Atypical absence seizures*

Atypical absence seizures are a form of generalized absence that differ from typical absences in clinical form, EEG, aetiology and clinical context (Table 2.9). The duration is longer, loss of awareness is often incomplete, associated tone changes are more severe than in typical absence seizures and the onset and cessation of the attacks are not so abrupt (Lennox & Davis 1950, Gastaut et al 1966, Chevrie & Aicardi 1972). The subject may be able to answer questions and remember events occurring during the attack. Atonic, clonic or tonic phenomena are often present and autonomic disturbance and automatisms frequently occur. The attacks can wax and wane and may be of long duration.

The ictal EEG shows usually diffuse but often asymmetric and irregular spike and wave bursts at 2–2.5 Hz (not the classical 3 Hz of the typical absence) and sometimes fast activity or bursts of spikes and sharp waves (Blume et al 1973, Gastaut et al 1966). The background interictal EEG is usually abnormal, with continuous slowing, spikes or irregular spike and wave activity, and the ictal and interictal EEGs may be similar. The seizures are often not induced by hyperventilation or photic stimulation.

Atypical absences occur in the symptomatic epilepsies and are associated with mental retardation, other neurological abnormalities and

**Table 2.8** Differentiation between typical absences and complex partial seizures

| | Typical absence | Complex partial seizure |
|---|---|---|
| Age of onset | Childhood or early adult | Any age |
| Aetiology | Idiopathic generalized epilepsy | Any focal pathology or cryptogenic |
| Underlying focal anatomical lesion | None | Archicortex (hippocampus, amygdala)<br>Neocortex |
| Duration of attack | Short (usually < 30 s) | Longer, usually several minutes |
| Awareness that attack has occurred | Often not, if brief | Usually |
| Other clinical features | Slight (tone changes or motor phenomena) | May be marked; including aura, automatism |
| Postictal | None | Confusion, headache, emotional disturbance |
| Frequency | May be numerous and cluster | Usually less frequent |
| EEG | 3 Hz spike/wave | Variable focal disturbance |
| Photosensitivity | 10–30% | None |
| Effect of hyperventilation | Often marked increase | None, modest increase |

multiple seizure types. They form part of the Lennox–Gastaut syndrome and they may occur at any age.

*Myoclonic seizures*

Myoclonus is a brief contraction of a muscle, muscle group or several muscle groups (Table 2.10). It can be single or repetitive, varying in severity from an almost imperceptible twitch to a severe jerking, resulting, for instance, in a sudden fall or the propulsion of hand-held objects (the 'flying saucer' syndrome). Recovery is immediate and the patient often maintains that consciousness was not lost. During a myoclonic jerk, the electromyogram shows biphasic or polyphasic potentials of 20–120 ms in duration followed

**Table 2.9** Clinical features of atypical absence seizures

- Absence (blank stare)
- Consciousness may be only partially impaired, and there may be partial responsiveness
- Focal signs are more prominent than in a typical absence seizure and include tone changes, clonic jerking, motor spasm, automatism
- Onset and cessation often gradual, and seizure may be prolonged
- Occurs in patients with diffuse cerebral damage, usually with mental retardation, other seizure types and other neurological deficit

**Table 2.10** Clinical features of myoclonic seizures

- Brief jerk, singly or in series, may be induced by stimulus
- Intensity varies from slight tremor to massive jerk
- Distribution varies, from single muscle to generalized jerking
- Consciousness usually not altered
- Rapid onset and cessation
- Associated features depend on the clinical context of the myoclonus
- Occurs as part of: the syndrome of idiopathic generalized epilepsy; the syndrome of the progressive myoclonus epilepsy; or as a reflection of diffuse cerebral damage associated with mental retardation, other seizure types and neurological handicap

by tonic contraction or hypotonia (Niedermeyer et al 1979). When part of the syndrome of idiopathic generalized epilepsy (see below, 2.7), myoclonus is often noticeable on waking or when dropping off to sleep and may be exacerbated by movement. It may be mild and insignificant or it can constitute a major clinical problem, and it can precede a tonic-clonic seizure.

The ictal EEG usually shows a generalized spike, spike and wave or polyspike and wave discharge, which is often asymmetric or irregular and frequently has a frontal predominance. In certain types of epilepsy, there may be desynchronization only or no change on the scalp EEG. The interictal EEG varies with the cause, usually being normal in idiopathic generalized epilepsy and abnormal in other types of myoclonic epilepsy, showing generalized changes.

Myoclonus can develop at any age. It occurs in idiopathic generalized epilepsy (Asconape & Penry 1984, Lugaresi et al 1973), in the Lennox–Gastaut syndrome and other forms of epilepsy in patients with mental retardation, and in the progressive myoclonic epilepsies (see below 2.8) (Berkovic et al 1989, So et al 1989, Marseilles Consensus Group 1990).

*Clonic seizures*

Generalized clonic movements can occur without a preceding tonic phase (Table 2.11). The jerking is often asymmetric and irregular; the postictal state is often but not always short. Clonic seizures are most frequent in neonates, infants or young children and are always symptomatic (Lombroso 1983). The EEG may show fast activity (10 Hz); fast activity mixed with larger amplitude slow waves; or, more rarely, polyspike and wave or spike and wave discharges. The interictal EEG is usually abnormal, showing generalized changes. Bilateral clonic jerking (with or without loss of consciousness, even if involving all four limbs) may be the only feature of a partial seizure arising in the frontal lobe, and this should not be confused with the generalized clonic seizure.

**Table 2.11** Clinical features of clonic seizures

- Asymmetrical and irregular rhythmic jerking
- Rapid onset and cessation
- Associated features depend on clinical context

*Tonic seizures*

Tonic seizures take the form of a tonic muscle contraction with altered consciousness without a clonic phase (Table 2.12) and can be divided into three types: axial, axorhizomelic and global. Axial tonic seizures comprise a sequence of: extension of the neck; contraction of the facial muscles, with the eyes opening widely; upturning of the eyeballs; contraction of the muscles of mastication; and contraction of the muscles of respiration, causing a cry and apnoea.

**Table 2.12** Clinical features of tonic seizures

- Tonic muscle spasm, which can take three forms: axial, axorhizomelic, global
- Fall (commonly with injury)
- Can be brief, or prolonged with fluctuating motor signs
- Postictal phase short
- Sudden onset and cessation
- Usually occur in patients with diffuse cerebral damage associated with mental retardation, other seizure types and neurological handicap

In axorhizomelic tonic seizures this pattern is followed by tonic contraction of the proximal upper limb muscles, causing the abduction and elevation of the semiflexed arms and the shoulders. In global tonic seizures the tonic contractions spread distally and the arms rise up and are held as if defending the head against a blow. The lower limbs may be affected and may become forcibly extended or contracted in triple flexion. Variations on these patterns are seen, perhaps reflecting a continuum which has been arbitrarily subdivided. The spasm may fluctuate during the seizure, causing head nodding or slight alterations in the posture of the extended limbs, and autonomic changes can be marked. Tonic seizures are invariably brief, lasting less than 60 s.

The ictal EEG may show flattening (desynchronization), fast activity (15–25 Hz) with increasing amplitude (to about 100 μV) as the attack progresses, or a rhythmic 10 Hz discharge similar to that seen in the tonic phase of the tonic-clonic seizure. On a scalp recording, however, the ictal EEG changes are often obscured by artefact from muscle activity and movement. The interictal EEG is seldom normal, usually showing generalized changes. Tonic seizures occur at all ages, are usually caused by diffuse cerebral damage and are associated with other seizure types, neurological damage and mental retardation. Generalized tonic seizures should not be confused with partial motor seizures, which can also show predominately tonic features.

*Tonic-clonic seizures*

Tonic-clonic seizures (Table 2.13) may or may not be preceded by a prodromal period during which an attack is anticipated, often by an ill-defined vague feeling or sometimes more specifically, for instance, by the occurrence of increasing myoclonic jerking. An aura (in fact a simple or complex partial seizure) may occur in the seconds before the attack, and is indicative of a secondarily generalized tonic-clonic seizure.

The tonic-clonic seizure is initiated by loss of consciousness, and

**Table 2.13** Clinical features of tonic-clonic seizures

- Loss of consciousness
- Fall (often with injury)
- Tonic phase (stiffening)
- Clonic phase (generalized jerking, amplitude increasing and frequency slowing as seizure continues)
- Tongue biting, incontinence, cyanosis, vocalization, autonomic features
- Postictal confusion, drowsiness, sleep, headache, muscle pain
- Sudden onset and gradual recovery
- An aura may precede the tonic-clonic seizure, indicating a partial onset (i.e. a secondarily generalized tonic-clonic seizure)
- Diurnal pattern common when part of idiopathic generalized epilepsy
- Occurs in cryptogenic and symptomatic epilepsy with a wide variety of underlying pathologies, with diffuse cerebral damage, and also in idiopathic generalized epilepsy

sometimes the epileptic cry, 'a wild harsh screaming sound' (Gowers 1881). The patient may fall; there is a brief period of tonic flexion and then a longer phase of rigidity and axial extension, with the eyes rolled up, the jaw clamped shut, the limbs stiff, adducted and extended and the fists either clenched or held in the *main d'accoucheur* position. Respiration ceases and cyanosis is common.

The tonic stage lasts on average 10–30 s and is succeeded by the clonic phase, during which convulsive movements, usually of all four limbs, jaw and facial muscles, occur; breathing may be stertorous and saliva (sometimes bloodstained owing to tongue-biting) may froth from the mouth. The convulsive movements of the limbs decrease in frequency (eventually to about four clonic jerks per second) and increase in amplitude as the attack progresses. Autonomic features such as flushing, changes in blood pressure, changes in pulse rate and increased salivation are common. The clonic phase lasts between 30 and 60 s and is followed by a further brief tonic contraction of all muscles, sometimes with incontinence.

The final phase lasts between 2 and 30 min and is characterized by flaccidity of the muscles. Consciousness is slowly regained. The plantar responses are usually extensor at this time and the tendon jerks are diminished. Confusion is invariable in the postictal phase and the patient then often lapses into deep sleep, awakening minutes or hours later with no symptoms other than muscle soreness and headache. Tonic-clonic seizures occur commonly in non-REM sleep (Janz 1969) and numerous other precipitating factors have been reported (Gastaut & Tassinari 1966). In partially treated patients, the tonic-clonic seizure may be modified to take a form more like a tonic, clonic or atonic attack. Tonic-clonic seizures can occur at any age and are encountered in many varieties of epilepsy, and have no pathological specificity.

During the tonic phase, the ictal EEG begins with generalized EEG flattening (desynchronization) for a few seconds or with low voltage fast activity and then 10 Hz rhythms appear and increase in amplitude (recruiting rhythms). These are followed some seconds later by slow waves increasing in amplitude and decreasing in frequency from 3–1 Hz. During the clonic phase, the slow waves are interrupted by bursts of faster activity (at about 10 Hz) corresponding to the clonic jerks and, as the phase progresses, the slow waves widen and these bursts become less frequent. With scalp recordings, however, these EEG patterns will often be obscured by artefact from muscle and movement.

As the jerks cease, the EEG becomes silent for several seconds and then slow delta activity develops. This persists for a variable period and the EEG background rhythms then slowly increase in frequency. Minutes or hours may elapse before the EEG activity returns to normal. In patients with idiopathic generalized epilepsy (see below, 2.7) the EEG in the pre-ictal period may show increasing abnormalities with spike and wave or spike paroxysms. The interictal EEG has a variable appearance, depending on the cause of the tonic-clonic seizures.

*Atonic seizures*

Atonic seizures may take several forms (Table 2.14). The classic drop attack (astatic seizure) is an atonic seizure in which postural tone is suddenly lost, the patient collapsing to the ground like a rag doll. The sudden loss of tone may be more restricted and less severe, resulting for instance in nodding of the head, a bowing movement or sagging at the knee. These seizures are brief, occur without warning and are followed by immediate recovery. Longer (inhibitory) atonic attacks can develop in a stepwise fashion with progressively increasing nodding, sagging or folding. Serial atonic attacks may occur, and atonic seizures are often associated with myoclonic jerks. The seizures denote diffuse brain dysfunction, occur usually in the setting of mental retardation and are common in severe symptomatic epilepsies (Gastaut et al 1966). Also, in some instances where treatment is only partially effective, a tonic-clonic seizure can take an atonic form.

**Table 2.14** Clinical features of atonic seizures

- Atonia with fall (astatic or drop attack)
- Atonia may be more limited (e.g. head nodding, bending)
- Attack may progress in a stepwise fashion with increasing atonia (inhibitory atonic attack)
- Usually occur in diffuse cerebral damage associated with mental retardation, other seizure types and neurological handicap

The ictal EEG is variable, showing irregular spike and wave, polyspike and wave, slow wave or low-amplitude fast activity, or a mixture of these, and may be obscured by movement artefact. The interictal EEG is usually abnormal. Atonic seizures may occur at any age.

### 2.2.3 Unclassifiable seizures

Up to one-third of seizures in many clinical series are considered unclassifiable using the current ILAE classification scheme, taking forms which do not conform to the typical clinical and EEG patterns described above.

## 2.3 THE ILAE CLASSIFICATION OF THE EPILEPSIES AND EPILEPSY SYNDROMES

In recognition of the limitations of a seizure type classification, the ILAE Commission on Classification and Terminology proposed a new compound scheme (Commission on Classification and Terminology of the International League Against Epilepsy 1989). This was a more ambitious attempt to classify the epilepsies, not simply on the basis of seizure type, but also to incorporate anatomical, EEG, aetiological, seizure type and precipitation and syndromic features. In spite of unsatisfactory features, outlined below, the classification is an important step in developing a comprehensive epilepsy classification.

As with the classification of seizure type, the epilepsies are divided into two major groupings according to whether or not there is a generalized or focal (localization-related) origin to the seizures. A third category of epilepsies or syndromes which are undetermined whether generalized or focal is also included, and there is a fourth category of special syndromes (Table 2.15).

*Idiopathic generalized epilepsies and syndromes*

The idiopathic generalized epilepsies comprise several age-related syndromes. Other categories have been proposed and no doubt this list will increase as knowledge increases. Controversy exists, however, about the utility and validity of such subdivision, and nowhere is the debate between 'splitters and lumpers' more fierce. These conditions are considered in more detail under the heading of idiopathic generalized epilepsy (see below 2.7).

*Cryptogenic or symptomatic generalized epilepsies*

This category includes West's syndrome, Lennox–Gastaut syndrome and forms of myoclonic epilepsy. The nosological position of Lennox–Gastaut syndrome and of the myoclonic epilepsies is unclear and there is considerable overlap between the core conditions and other symptomatic epileptic encephalopathies. See below (2.6) for details.

*Symptomatic generalized epilepsies*

This category poses other problems for classification. The epilepsies are divided into those with a non-specific aetiology and those with a specific identifiable cause. The non-specific category are a poorly defined group of epileptic encephalopathies, often with underlying focal aetiologies and whether or not these are best categorized as generalized is doubtful. The specific group include patients with malformations, inborn errors of metabolism and hereditary or congenital disorders including those underlying the progressive myoclonus epilepsies (see below, 2.8). Again, some conditions have identifiable focal or multifocal lesions, and their inclusion in a category of generalized epilepsy is contentious.

*Idiopathic localization-related epilepsies and syndromes*

Three conditions are included here, including benign childhood epilepsy with centrotemporal spikes (see below, 2.6.5) which is said to account for up to 15% of childhood epilepsies, and two much less common syndromes, childhood epilepsy with occipital paroxysms and primary reading epilepsy. Other genetic and idiopathic syndromes will no doubt be added as knowledge advances, such as the recently described syndrome of dominantly inherited nocturnal frontal lobe epilepsy.

**Table 2.15** The ILAE classification of the epilepsies and epilepsy syndromes

*1. Generalized*

Idiopathic generalized epilepsies with age-related onset (in order of age)
Benign neonatal familial convulsions
Benign neonatal convulsions
Benign myoclonic epilepsy in infancy
Childhood absence epilepsy
Juvenile absence epilepsy
Juvenile myoclonic epilepsy
Epilepsy with generalized tonic-clonic seizures on awakening
Other idiopathic generalized epilepsies not defined above
Epilepsies with seizures precipitated by specific modes of activation

Cryptogenic or symptomatic generalized epilepsies (in order of age)
West's syndrome
Lennox–Gastaut syndrome
Epilepsy with myoclonic–astatic seizures
Epilepsy with myoclonic absences

Symptomatic generalized epilepsies
Non-specific aetiology
Early myoclonic encephalopathies
Early infantile encephalopathy with burst suppression
Other symptomatic epilepsies not defined above
Specific syndromes
Epilepsies in other disease states

*2. Localization-related*

Localization-related epilepsies – idiopathic with age related onset
Benign epilepsy with centrotemporal spikes
Childhood epilepsy with occipital paroxysms
Primary reading epilepsy

Localization-related epilepsies – symptomatic
Epilepsia partialis continua
Syndromes characterized by specific modes of precipitation
Temporal lobe epilepsies
Frontal lobe epilepsies
Parietal lobe epilepsies
Occipital lobe epilepsies

Localization-related epilepsies – idiopathic

*3. Epilepsies and syndromes undetermined as to whether focal or generalized*

With both generalized and focal seizures
Neonatal seizures
Severe myoclonic epilepsy in infancy
Electrical status epilepticus in slow wave sleep
Acquired epileptic aphasia

Other undetermined epilepsies (not defined above) with unequivocal generalized or focal features

*4. Special syndromes*

Febrile convulsions
Isolated seizures or isolated status epilepticus
Seizures occurring only when there is an acute metabolic or toxic event due to factors such as alcohol, drugs, eclampsia, non-ketotic hyperglycinaemia

*Symptomatic localization-related epilepsies and syndromes*

This syndrome includes epilepsia partialis continua (Ch. 5, 5.2.2), in spite of the fact that this can be caused by various aetiologies, and the symptomatic reflex epilepsies (see below, 2.5.11). To these rare conditions are added all other symptomatic partial epilepsies that can be categorized according to the anatomical location of the lesion (frontal, temporal etc), seizure type (simple partial, complex partial or secondarily generalized seizures) or aetiology (cardiovascular, tumour, infection etc). These conditions are considered elsewhere in this chapter.

*Cryptogenic localization-related epilepsies and syndromes*

This category has been created to include symptomatic focal epilepsies in which the aetiology is unknown. With increasingly sophisticated neuroimaging techniques, this category is a lot smaller than it was 10 years ago (Ch. 3, 3.3).

*Epilepsies and syndromes undetermined as to whether they are focal or generalized*

The existence of this category is an acknowledgement that the differentiation between focal and generalized epilepsy is not always easy to make. The category is divided into those syndromes with both focal and generalized seizures and those without unequivocal generalized or focal features. Included in the first subdivision are a rag-bag of 'syndromes', including: neonatal seizures, which have a variety of forms that overlap with other categories; infantile myoclonic epilepsy, which would usually be grouped with other myoclonic epilepsies; and ESES and the Landau–Kleffner syndrome, which are epileptic encephalopathies of unknown pathophysiology. In the second subdivision are those epilepsies with tonic-clonic seizures in which clinical and EEG features do not allow categorization into focal or generalized groups.

*Special syndromes*

This category includes the 'situational-related syndromes', a category that is quite impossible to define or clearly differentiate from other overlapping categories. It includes febrile seizures (see below, 2.6.3), isolated seizures (including single seizures and isolated status epilepticus), and the epilepsies precipitated by acute toxic or metabolic events (see below, 2.5.5).

The advantages of the classification are its flexibility, the potential for change and expansion, the acknowledgement of the complex interplay of factors underlying epilepsy and (an advantage over the seizure type classification) it avoids the problems of defining consciousness. There are, however, a number of profound disadvantages. First, it is a highly complex system with a very clumsy terminology, and for this reason alone it is unlikely ever to gain widespread clinical usage, especially in non-specialist settings. A second problem is the maintenance of the distinction between focal and generalized epilepsies, which in many types of epilepsy is difficult to justify and presumes an unrealistic knowledge of the underlying physiological processes. It is perhaps in recognition of this problem that the third category is introduced, although it might have been better to avoid this distinction altogether. A third problem is that, in the attempt to be all-inclusive, this classification becomes unwieldy. Common syndromes are mixed in with those that are extremely rare and syndromes whose identity is contentious are also included. In normal clinical practice, a large proportion of patients with epilepsy seen will fall into categories 1.2, 2.3 and 4.1,'non-specific' categories that are poorly defined. In one population-based survey of 594 newly diagnosed patients, 66.4% of the patients fell into these non-specific categories (Manford et al 1992a). Also, the arbitrary nature of some categories (notably 3 and 4) results in the grouping of epilepsies that have little else in common. Finally, there is the difficulty of justifying the full sobriquet of 'syndrome' for some of the idiopathic conditions listed. Some prefer to see the idiopathic generalized epilepsies, for instance, as a 'neurobiological continuum' while others have split the conditions into at least 10 subdivisions; and there is no general agreement whatsoever about the criteria required to constitute a syndrome.

## 2.4 FEATURES OF PARTIAL EPILEPSY ARISING IN DIFFERENT ANATOMICAL REGIONS

Partial seizures arising in different anatomical locations take different forms. About 60% of complex partial seizures have their origin in the temporal lobe and about 40% are extratemporal (Manford et al 1992b), and simple partial seizures are more commonly extratemporal. Simple and complex partial seizures arising from any cortical area can spread to other regions (and also evolve into secondarily generalized epileptic attacks) and this spread blurs distinctions between seizure types, with the clinical and EEG features of epilepsy from frontal, temporal or parieto-occipital regions overlapping. Nevertheless, characteristic clinical and EEG features exist for epilepsy in each cortical region, and a knowledge of these is important when attempting to localize seizures clinically.

### 2.4.1 Partial seizures arising in the temporal lobe

A number of subclassifications exist. The most complex is that of Wieser (1983) who has divided temporal lobe seizures into opercular, temporal polar and basal or limbic types; whether such detailed classification schemes are valid or useful is debatable. The distinction into mesio-basal and lateral neocortical types, however, is widely accepted and, even though symptomatology overlaps and spread from lateral to mesial cortex (and vice versa) is common, this remains a useful distinction.

*Epilepsy arising in the mesial temporal lobe (limbic epilepsy)* (Table 2.16)

The commonest pathology underlying this type of epilepsy is hippocampal sclerosis (or Ammons Horn sclerosis, mesial temporal sclerosis – terms which, in clinical practice are largely synonymous) (Margerison & Corsellis 1966, Gloor 1991). This pathology is associated with febrile convulsions in young children (particularly complex febrile convulsions), possibly predisposing the child to febrile seizures or possibly as the result of a complex febrile convulsion. Other pathologies include dysembryoplastic neuroepithelioma and other benign tumours, arteriovenous malformations, glioma, neuronal migration defects and gliotic damage as a result of encephalitis.

The seizures take the form of simple partial seizures (aura alone with clear consciousness) or more commonly complex partial seizures

**Table 2.16** Features of partial seizures of mesial temporal lobe origin (This table includes those clinical features that are particularly characteristic of temporal lobe epilepsy. In many cases, however, these features do not occur)

*Clinical features*

- Past history of febrile convulsions (in those with mesial temporal sclerosis)
- Seizures longer than frontal lobe seizures (typically > 2 min), with a slower evolution and more gradual onset/offset
- Auras are common. Typical of mesial temporal (rather than lateral temporal origin) are visceral, cephalic, gustatory, dysmnestic, affective, perceptual or autonomic auras
- Partial awareness commonly preserved, especially in early stages, and slow evolution of seizure
- Prominent motor arrest or absence (the 'motionless stare')
- Postictal confusion and dysphasia common
- Autonomic changes (e.g. pallor, redness, and tachycardia)
- Automatisms: less violent than in frontal lobe epilepsy and usually take the form of oro-alimentary (lip-smacking, chewing, swallowing) or gestural (e.g. fumbling, fidgeting, repetitive motor actions, undressing, walking, sexually-directed actions, walking, running) and sometimes prolonged; vocalization also common, and other motor automatisms can occur

*EEG*

- Anterior or mid-temporal spikes (best shown on sphenoidal electrodes)
- Other focal discharges in temporal lobe regions (EEG signs can be unilateral or bilateral)

*Imaging*

- Hippocampal sclerosis (demonstrable by unilateral decrease in hippocampal volume and increase in signal on T2-weighted MRI scan)
- Structural lesion (most commonly: hamartoma, other benign tumours, glioma, angioma, dysplasia)

(Delgado-Escueta et al 1982, Duncan & Sagar 1987, Wieser & Kauser 1987, Malonado et al 1987, Kotagal et al 1988). The complex partial seizure typically has a relatively gradual evolution (compared to extra-temporal seizures), develops over 1–2 min, has an indistinct onset with partial awareness at the onset and lasts longer than most extratemporal complex partial seizures (2–10 min). The typical complex partial seizure of temporal lobe origin has three components.

*Aura:* An aura can occur in isolation as a simple partial seizure or the initial manifestation of a complex partial seizure. It typically comprises visceral, cephalic, gustatory, dysmnestic, or affective symptoms (see above, Simple partial seizure, 2.2.1). The rising epigastric sensation is the commonest aura, and other auras include perceptual or autonomic aura. Autonomic symptoms include changes in skin colour, blood pressure, heart rate, pupil size and piloerection. Speech usually ceases or is severely reduced, but occasionally repetitive vocalization may occur. Simple auditory phenomena such as humming, buzzing, hissing and roaring may occur if the discharges occur in the superior temporal gyrus; and olfactory sensations, which are usually unpleasant and difficult to define, with seizures in the Sylvian region. More complex hallucinatory or illusionary states are produced with seizure discharges in association areas (e.g. structured visual hallucinations, complex visual patterns and musical sounds, and speech). A cephalic aura can also occur in focal temporal lobe seizures, although it is more typical of a frontal lobe focus.

*Absence:* Motor arrest or absence (the so-called 'motionless stare') is prominent, especially in the early stages of seizures arising in mesial temporal structures, and usually more so than in extratemporal lobe epilepsy.

*Automatism:* The automatisms of mesio-basal temporal lobe epilepsy are typically less violent than in frontal lobe seizures, and are usually oroalimentary (lip-smacking, chewing, swallowing), or gestural (e.g. fumbling, fidgeting, repetitive motor actions, undressing, walking, running, sexually directed actions), and sometimes prolonged. Limb automatisms are usually ipsilateral to the focus, with contralateral dystonic posturing. Vocalization is also common and other motor automatisms can occur. Generally, vocalization of identifiable words suggests a non-dominant seizure focus.

Postictal confusion and headache are common after a temporal lobe complex partial seizure, and if dysphasia occurs this is a useful lateralizing sign indicating seizure origin in the dominant temporal lobe. Amnesia is the rule for the absence and the automatism. Secondary generalization is much less common than in extratemporal lobe epilepsy. Psychiatric or behavioural disturbances often accompany the epilepsy (Ch. 9, 9.4).

The EEG in mesiobasal temporal lobe epilepsy can show anterior or mid-temporal spikes. Superficial sphenoidal or zygomatic electrodes may occasionally be necessary for their detection. Other changes include intermittent or persisting slow activity over the temporal lobes. The EEG signs can be unilateral or bilateral. Modern MRI will frequently reveal the abnormality underlying the epilepsy (Ch. 3, 3.3).

*Epilepsy arising in the lateral temporal neocortex* (Table 2.17)

There is considerable overlap between the clinical and EEG features of mesio-basal and lateral temporal lobe epilepsy (Wieser & Muller 1987, Williams et al 1987). There is usually a detectable underlying structural pathology, the commonest being a glioma, angioma, hamartoma, dysembryoplastic neuroepithelial tumour, other benign tumour, neuronal migration defect and post-traumatic change. There is no association with a history of febrile convulsions. Consciousness may be preserved for longer than in a typical mesial temporal seizure. The typical aura includes hallucinations that are often structured and of visual, auditory, gustatory or olfactory forms, which can be crude or elaborate, or illusions of size (macropsia, micropsia), shape, weight, distance or sound. Affective, visceral or psychic auras occur but are less common than in mesio-basal temporal lobe epilepsy. The automatisms can be unilateral and have more prominent motor manifestations than in mesio-basal temporal lobe epilepsy. Postictal phenomena, amnesia for the attack and the psychiatric accompaniments are probably equally common in this form of temporal lobe epilepsy as in the mesio-basal form.

The interictal EEG often shows spikes over the temporal region, maximal over the lateral convexity rather than inferomesial electrodes. Hippocampal volumes and T2 measures on MRI scanning are usually normal, in contrast to mesial temporal epilepsy, and MRI will reliably demonstrate the other structural lesions responsible for the epilepsy (Ch. 3, 3.3).

**Table 2.17** Features of partial seizures of lateral temporal lobe origin (This table includes those clinical features that are particularly characteristic of temporal lobe epilepsy. In many cases, however, these features do not occur)

*Clinical features*

- Typically no history of febrile seizure
- Auras are common; hallucinations (especially auditory) or illusions more suggestive of lateral rather than mesial temporal origin, but any other temporal lobe aura may occur
- The motionless stare and the automatisms are similar to those in mesial temporal lobe epilepsy

*EEG*

- Spikes and focal discharges from the temporal region
- Spikes often shorter than in mesial temporal lobe epilepsy and are not prominent at the sphenoidal electrodes

*Imaging*

- Structural changes (especially dysplasia, benign tumour, glioma, post-traumatic changes, angioma)

## 2.4.2 Epilepsy arising in the frontal lobe

Seizures of frontal lobe origin can take the form of complex partial seizures, simple partial seizures, and secondarily generalized attacks (Table 2.18) (Williamson et al 1985, Chauvel et al 1992a).

The clinical and EEG features overlap with complex partial seizures of temporal lobe origin, not least because of the rapid spread from seizure foci in the frontal lobe to other cortical areas and to the mesial temporal lobe, but there are nevertheless a number of core features that are strongly suggestive of a frontal lobe origin. Typically the seizures are frequent with a marked tendency to cluster. The attacks are brief, with a sudden onset and offset, without the gradual evolution of the temporal lobe seizure. Some types of frontal lobe seizure occur largely during sleep, and in some patients the epilepsy comprises frequent short nocturnal attacks (paroxysmal nocturnal dystonia).

A brief, non-specific 'cephalic aura' may occur, which is a vague sensation of dizziness, strangeness, headache or the feeling that an attack is coming on, but not the rich range of auras of temporal lobe epilepsy, unless seizure activity spreads to limbic or temporal lobe structures. The absence (motor arrest) is usually short, and may be obscured by the prominent motor signs of the automatisms.

There are qualitative differences between frontal and temporal lobe automatisms, although seldom are these specific enough to be reliably of diagnostic value. Temporal lobe automatisms are typically of the oro-alimentary type or gestural, with coordinated automatic movements of the upper as opposed to lower limbs. Automatisms with mimicry are also common, as is ambulation. Frontal lobe

**Table 2.18** Features of partial seizures of frontal lobe origin (This table includes those clinical features that are particularly characteristic of frontal lobe epilepsy. In many cases, however, these features do not occur)

*Clinical features*

- Frequent attacks with clustering
- Brief stereotyped seizures (< 30 s)
- Nocturnal attacks
- Sudden onset and cessation
- Absence of psychic aura
- Absence of postictal confusion
- Rapid evolution with awareness lost at onset
- Prominent complex bilateral motor automatisms involving lower limbs
- Prominent ictal posturing and tonic spasms
- Bizarre automatisms (often diagnosed as non-epileptic seizures)
- Frequent secondary generalization
- History of status epilepticus

*EEG*

- May show no focal abnormality ictally or interictally
- May show bilateral spike wave
- May show focal changes, often widespread

*Imaging*

- May show structural lesions of cortex (commonly: hamartoma, other benign tumours, glioma, angioma, dysplasia, post-traumatic lesions, atrophy)
- Absence of hippocampal changes

automatisms are typically gestural, especially comprising bilateral leg movements (e.g. cycling, stepping, kicking). The automatisms are often highly excited, violent or bizarre and this leads, not infrequently, to a misdiagnosis of non-epileptic attacks (pseudoseizures); a misdiagnosis which is all the more common as there may be no marked EEG changes in frontal lobe complex partial seizures. In other frontal seizures, posturing or muscle spasms predominate. Vocalization is common in frontal lobe automatisms. This can be a cry, sometimes very shrill and loud, other sounds or speech fragments. Postictal recovery is usually rapid, with a shorter period of postictal confusion than is common in temporal lobe epilepsy.

Frontal lobe partial seizures have a more marked tendency to secondarily generalize than partial seizures of temporal lobe origin, and there is also commonly a history of status epilepticus, of both the tonic-clonic and non-convulsive types.

Although the typical pattern of aura/absence/automatism is sometimes seen in frontal lobe complex partial seizures, it is seldom as well defined as in temporal lobe epilepsy. Other partial seizure patterns (simple and complex) are commonly encountered, of which the following forms are common: seizures comprising clonic jerking of the contralateral limbs, with or without loss of consciousness; seizures with bilateral motor activity (jerking or posturing) with retained (or at least only mildly impaired) consciousness, and without the typical evolution or rhythmical pattern of a true tonic-clonic seizure. Because consciousness is retained in the presence of bilateral limb jerking, these attacks are commonly misdiagnosed as non-epileptic attacks. Apparently generalized tonic-clonic seizures, without lateralizing features, are particularly characteristic of seizures arising in the cingulate or dorsolateral cortex, but can occur from other frontal lobe sites also. Blank spells, sometimes called pseudo-absence seizures, occur with mesial frontal lobe epilepsy and are sometimes indistinguishable from typical absences on clinical grounds. Secondarily generalized atonic or tonic seizures indistinguishable on clinical grounds from their generalized equivalents may also occur. Seizures arising in the dorsolateral convexity sometimes take the form of a sudden assumption of an abnormal posture (usually bilateral and asymmetrical) with or without loss of consciousness, lasting a second or two only and which cluster, with numerous attacks over a few minutes.

Version of the head and eyes is also common in many types of frontal lobe (and less frequently temporal lobe) epilepsy, and is sometimes the only seizure manifestation (versive seizures). When version occurs in full consciousness at the onset of a seizure, this is useful evidence of a focus in the contralateral frontal dorsolateral convexity, but in other situations the direction of version is of little lateralizing value (Ochs et al 1984). Occasionally, seizures with adversion of the head and the body occur, in which the patient circles. Autonomic features are common in frontal lobe epilepsy and may occasionally be an isolated manifestation of an epileptic focus, usually in the orbitofrontal cortex. Dysphasia in frontal seizures is often accompanied by adversive or clonic movements, and in epileptic discharges in Sylvian areas the aphasia is often preceded by numbness in the mouth and throat.

The scalp EEG in frontal lobe epilepsy is often rather disappointing, partly because of the large area of frontal cortex covered by the relatively few scalp electrodes and the inaccessibility of scalp electrodes to the medial and inferior frontal lobe surfaces. Many frontal lobe seizures fail to show a focus, and where focal disturbances are seen they are often widespread and poorly localized. Apparently generalized irregular or bilateral and synchronous spike and wave or polyspike discharges with anterior predominance can occur. Sometimes, the interictal and ictal EEGs show non-specific generalized slow activity only.

### 2.4.3 Epilepsy arising in the central region

These seizures can occur in clear consciousness (i.e. simple partial seizures) or with impairment or loss of consciousness (i.e. complex partial seizures) (Mauguiere & Courjon 1978, Chauvel et al 1992b). The primary manifestations are jerking, dystonic spasm and posturing (Table 2.19). The jerking can affect any muscle group, usually unilaterally, the exact site depending on the part of the precentral gyrus involved in the seizure, and the jerks may 'march' (the Jacksonian march) from one part of the body to another as the discharge spreads over the motor cortex. The seizure discharge may remain limited to one small segment for long

**Table 2.19** Features of partial seizures of central origin (This table includes those clinical features that are particularly characteristic of central epilepsy. In many cases, however, these features do not occur)

*Clinical features*

- No loss of consciousness (simple partial seizure)
- Contralateral jerking (which may or may not march)
- Contralateral tonic spasm or dystonia
- Posturing, which is often bilateral
- Speech arrest and paralysis of bulbar musculature
- Contralateral sensory symptoms

*EEG*

- Often normal, even during an attack
- May show focal central discharges

*Imaging*

- May show structural changes (commonly: hamartoma, other benign tumours, glioma, angioma, dysplasia, post-traumatic lesions, atrophy)

periods of time, and when it does spread it is typically very slow. The clonic jerks appear in the parts of the body represented in the rolandic homunculus and usually consist of brief tetanic contractions of all the muscles that cooperate in a single movement. Thus, for instance, if flexion of the elbows is involved, the brachialis, the supinator and the long flexors of the wrists and fingers contract as well as the biceps, and antagonist muscles relax. The seizures spread through the cortex, producing clonic movements according to the sequence of cortical representation. A seizure which begins in the hand usually passes up the arm and down the leg and if it begins in the foot it passes up the leg and down the arm. A seizure beginning in the face is most apt to originate in the mouth because of the correspondingly large area of cortical representation. Head or eye turning can occur as an initial seizure manifestation (the adversive seizure).

If the seizure is initiated in or evolves to affect supplementary motor areas, posturing of the arms may develop, classically with adversial head and eye deviation, abduction and external rotation of the contralateral arm and flexion at the elbows, often combined with posturing of the legs, and speech arrest or stereotyped vocalizations. Consciousness is usually maintained unless secondary generalization occurs. There is often an aura in these seizures, consisting of a very brief jolt, shock or emotional sensation. The classical posture is named by Penfield the 'fencing posture' (resembling as it does the *en garde* position). Other forms of tonic posturing are common, including ipsiversive tonic postures. The pos-turing is often bilateral and asymmetric. The fencing posture or fragments of it can also occur in seizures originating in various other frontal and temporal brain regions, presumably due to spread of the seizure discharge to pre-motor cortex. In contrast to Jacksonian seizures, supple-mentary motor area seizures are often very brief, occur frequently and in clusters, sometimes hundreds each day and are sometimes also pre-cipitated by startle.

Head and eye version is common, and nystagmus may also occur

(Furman et al 1990). Arrest of speech (anarthria) may occur if the motor area of the muscles of articulation is affected (phonatory seizures) and is usually associated with spasm or clonic movements of the jaw. After focal seizure activity, there may be localized paralysis in the affected limbs (Todd's paralysis), which is usually short-lived although, as Todd (1854) noted, this can occasionally persist for several days. Recognizable vocalizations, sounds, grunts or a long-drawn-out cry occur, most commonly in seizures involving the anterior frontal or supplementary motor areas.

If the seizure discharge originates in or spreads to the post-central region, somatosensory or special sensory manifestations (simple hallucinations) occur, typically tingling, numbness, an electric-shock-like feeling, a tickling or crawling feeling, burning, pain, or a feeling of heat). These symptoms are usually accompanied by jerking, posturing or spasms as the epileptic discharges usually spread anteriorly. The sensory symptoms may remain localized or march in a Jacksonian manner. Ictal pain is occasionally a prominent symptom and can be severe and poorly localized.

Interictal and ictal scalp EEGs in focal epilepsy in central regions are often normal as the focus may be small and buried within the central gyri.

### 2.4.4 Epilepsy arising in the parietal and occipital lobes

Focal seizures arise from foci in these locations less commonly than from frontal, central or temporal lobe regions (Table 2.20). The typical manifestations of the seizures are subjective sensory and visual disturbances (Sveinbjornsdóttir & Duncan 1993). The seizures tend to spread widely, however, and additional features are common, because of activation of adjacent cortical regions.

Parietal lobe seizures typically comprise sensory manifestations, which include the sensory illusions described above (probably due to spread to the postcentral gyrus). Illusions of bodily distortion include a feeling of swelling or shrinking (macrosomatognosia, microsomatognosia), or lengthening or shortening (hyperschematica or hyposchematica), particularly affecting the tongue, mouth or extremities. Ictal apraxia, alexia and agnosia have been reported. Gustatory seizures have their origin in the suprasylvian region (adjacent to the mouth and throat primary sensory region). Occasionally, there is a sensation of an absence of the limb or a phantom limb. Ictal vertigo also originates in the suprasylvian region. Sexual feelings occur in central or parietal lobe seizures, and may be accompanied by erection, ejaculation and other sexual sensations. A feeling of ictal paralysis can occur with seizures involving the suprasylvian region, and if the epileptic discharge spreads anteriorly this can be followed by clonic jerking in the affected body part.

Seizures from the occipital, parieto-occipital, and temporo-occipital cortex are characterized by visual symptoms. Elementary visual hallucinations are most common , including sensations of colours, shapes, flashes and patterns. These are intermittent, and can be stationary or appear to move. More complex hallucinations can be experienced which are usually stereotyped. The visual hallucinations can take the form of scenes, animals, people (including self-images – autoscopia). Illusions of

**Table 2.20** Features of parietal and occipital lobe epilepsy (This table includes those clinical features that are particularly characteristic of occipital or parietal epilepsy. In many cases, however, these features do not occur)

*Clinical features*

- Somatosensory symptoms (e.g. tingling, numbness or more complex sensations – may or may not march)
- Sensation of inability to move
- Sexual sensations
- Illusions of change in body size/shape
- Vertigo
- Gustatory seizures
- Elementary visual hallucinations (e.g. flashes, colours, shapes, patterns)
- Complex visual hallucinations (e.g. objects, scenes, autoscopia – often moving)
- Head turning (usually adversive, with sensation of following or looking at the visual hallucinations)
- Visual-spatial distortions (e.g. of size (micropsia, macropsia), shape, position)
- Loss or dulling of vision (amaurosis)
- Eyelid fluttering, blinking, nystagmus

*EEG*

- Focal spikes or slow wave discharges which are often not well localized, and often are maximal in temporal or even frontal regions

*Imaging*

- May show structural changes (especially dysplasia, tumour, post-traumatic changes, angioma)

topographical or spatial orientation can occur (e.g. teleopsia), alterations of size and shape (micropsia, macropsia), perseveration or repetition of objects (palinopsia), break-up of visual objects or movement. Forced head and eye turning are a common accompaniment, with the patient believing that the visual hallucination is being tracked voluntarily. Rapid blinking or eyelid flutter are common features of occipital cortical seizures and contraversive epileptic nystagmus is occasionally a feature of parieto-occipital epilepsy.

The EEG in occipital or parietal epilepsy may show appropriate focal discharges, although often the epileptic disturbance is poorly localized without correlation to the ictal symptoms. This may be due partly to the rapid spread of the epileptic discharge to temporal or frontal regions.

## 2.5 THE CAUSES OF EPILEPSY

Almost all grey matter conditions can result in epilepsy, and the range of causes is strongly age-dependent. In children, congenital and genetic causes are most common, in young adults tumours and drug and alcohol abuse, and in the elderly cerebrovascular disease. In a population-based survey in the United Kingdom of 784 patients developing seizures, 220 (28%) were febrile convulsions, 87 (11%) due to overt cerebrovascular disease, 35 (4%) caused by alcohol, 34 (4%) by cerebral tumour, 14 (2%)

post-traumatic and 9 (1%) postinfective (Sander et al 1990). There is marked geographic variation in aetiology, and in many parts of South America, Asia and Africa, for instance, infective causes are much more common (Shorvon & Bharucha 1992). Epilepsy is also commonly multifactorial, and this complicates the assessment of cause. After mild head injury, for instance, the rate of seizures is three times higher in those with first-degree family members with epilepsy (Majkowski 1990), although other studies have not found the family history to be a significant factor in the development of post-traumatic epilepsy (Jennett 1975, Salazar et al 1985).

### 2.5.1 Post-traumatic epilepsy

Seizures are common after severe head injuries. In a community study, head injury was the attributed cause of epilepsy in 2% of cases (Sander et al 1990). It is usual to divide post traumatic epilepsy into early (seizures occurring in the first week after injury) and late categories. Late post-traumatic epilepsy is defined as seizures occurring after the first week. Early seizures are more common than late seizures, occurring in between 2–5% of cases admitted to hospital with head injury in civilian practice (Jennett 1975, Annegers et al 1980).

The community-based Mayo Clinic study (Annegers et al 1980) divided head injuries into mild, moderate and severe categories, as follows:

*Severe*: intracranial haematoma, cerebral contusion or post-traumatic amnesia for more than 24 h.

*Moderate*: skull fracture or post-traumatic amnesia for more than 30 min, but less than 24 h.

*Mild*: no skull fracture and less than 30 min post-traumatic amnesia.

After severe head injuries, the risk of early seizures was 30% in children and 10% in adults. The risk of late seizures was 7% at 1 year and 11% at 5 years.

After moderate head injuries the risk of late seizures was 0.7% at 1 year and 1.6% at 5 years.

After mild head injuries the risk of late seizures was 0.1% at 1 year and 0.6% at 5 years, which was not different from the risks in the general population.

#### *Closed head injury*

Jennett and colleagues (Jennett 1975, 1982, Jennett et al 1979) have studied the risks of post-traumatic epilepsy in civilian practice (non-missile head injuries). The risks are higher if post-traumatic amnesia extends for 24 h or more, or if the head injury is complicated by intracranial haematoma, depressed fracture or dural tear, and early epilepsy.

After a compound depressed skull fracture, the risk of late epilepsy is 60% if there was also post-traumatic amnesia in excess of 24 h, a dural tear, focal deficit and early seizures. In the event of a compound depressed skull fracture, without a dural tear, neurological deficit or early seizures the risk of late epilepsy is 5% (Jennett 1982). If some of the factors are present the risks are intermediate.

Overall, the risks of late epilepsy in cases with intracranial haematoma (requiring surgical therapy) is 35%, with depressed fracture is 17% and after early epilepsy is 25%. Less than 1% of all those admitted to hospital with head injury without these risk factors will develop late epilepsy, but if more than one of the above factors is present, the risks are accordingly increased. The risk of late epilepsy in the absence of a depressed fracture, intracranial haematoma or early seizures is less than 2%, even if post-traumatic amnesia exceeds 24 h (Jennett 1975).

If early epilepsy has occurred without haematoma or depressed fracture the risk of late epilepsy is 19%. In about one-quarter of cases of early epilepsy, the seizures start within 1 h of the injury and in over half within 24 h of the injury. The seizures are focal in over half, and about 10–15% of cases present in status epilepticus (Jennett 1975).

The risk of late epilepsy after head injury is increased amongst those with early seizures. 25% of patients with early seizures developed late epilepsy, compared to 3% of patients who did not have early seizures. Seizures occurring only at the time of the injury are not associated with an increased risk of late epilepsy.

The risks of developing post-traumatic epilepsy fall with time: 50–60% of cases of late epilepsy have their first late seizure within 12 months of the injury, 85% within 2 years. Most of the remaining cases develop within 5 years (Caveness et al 1979).

*Penetrating (open) head injury*

After a penetrating (open) head injury the risk of epilepsy is much greater. The excess risk is confined to the early years after injury and, if a patient is seizure free after 3 years, there is only a 5% risk of subsequent epilepsy (Caveness et al 1979, Weiss et al 1986). The risk of epilepsy is greatest if the extent of cerebral damage is large, if central, frontal or temporal regions are affected, and if there has been cerebral infection. In penetrating missile injuries during the Vietnam war, epilepsy developed in about 50% of cases. In 75% of cases, seizures were overtly partial (Salazar et al 1985). In this last series, 8% of patients had a single seizure and 53% still had active epilepsy (a seizure within the last 2 years) 15 years after the injury.

## 2.5.2 Epilepsy after neurosurgery

Epilepsy can occur after neurosurgical procedures, albeit at a generally lower frequency than after penetrating head injury. The chance of developing seizures depends on the nature and the site of the surgery, the underlying neurological condition and the presence or absence of focal brain destruction. These risks are an important consideration in deciding upon surgery, and in formulating regulations regarding driving (Ch. 7, 7.2.1). After a burr hole (usually for biopsy or insertion of a ventricular catheter) the reported risk of seizures is between 9 and 13% (Foy et al 1981, Dan & Wade 1986). The site of surgery influences the risk, with frontal shunts associated with a 55% risk of epilepsy while parietal shunts have a 7% risk (Dan & Wade 1986). Shunt operations carry a higher risk in younger patients. In a large series the risk of new epilepsy developing after craniotomy for glioma was 19%, for intracranial haemorrhage 21% and for meningioma removal 22% (Foy et al 1981). All these risks were greatly enhanced if seizures had already occurred preoperatively. Different treatment approaches are associated with differing risks of epilepsy; thus, Cabral et al (1976) found that 20% of patients developed seizures after craniotomy for a posterior communicating aneurysm, compared with 4% treated by carotid ligation. In more recent work by Jennett and colleagues, the risks of epilepsy after surgery for ruptured supratentorial aneurysms have been shown to depend largely on the site of aneurysm and the presence or absence of focal neurological deficits (Jennett et al 1990) (Table 2.21).

**Table 2.21** Risks of late epilepsy after craniotomy for ruptured intracerebral aneurysms followed for at least 12 months after surgery (Epilepsy developed in 14% of patients with single aneurysms and 17% with multiple aneurysms) (Jennett et al 1990)

| | Risk of late epilepsy (%) | | |
|---|---|---|---|
| | All | No fixed deficit | Fixed deficit |
| Posterior communicating aneurysm (*n* = 97) | 10 | 4 | 18 |
| Anterior communicating aneurysm (*n* = 142) | 11 | 4 | 25 |
| Middle cerebral aneurysm (*n* = 98) | 19 | 14 | 23 |

### 2.5.3 Epilepsy in cerebrovascular disease

Epilepsy is common after intracranial haemorrhage; early seizures occurred in 64 (4.6%) and epilepsy in 35 (2.5%) of 1402 patients with intracerebral haemorrhage presenting to a large teaching hospital in Taiwan (Sung & Chu 1989), and 25% of 123 cases in another series from Alabama (Faught et al 1989). In over half of cases, seizures after haemorrhage occur in the first week (usually in the first 24 hours), are often the first sign of the haemorrhage, and status epilepticus occurs in about 10% of cases. Early seizures do not necessarily lead to chronic epilepsy, and in the Taiwanese study, for instance, only 29% of those with seizures in the first week developed long-term epilepsy, compared with 93% of those with late seizures. Chronic epilepsy occurred in 2.5% of the Taiwanese cohort and in 6.5% of survivors in the Alabama series, and 2 years after the haemorrhage the risk of new epilepsy is very small. The incidence of seizures is low in putamenal, thalamic or subtentorial haemorrhage.

In a prospective series of 1000 cases of acute stroke or transient ischaemic attack (TIA), seizures occurred in 4.4%, with the lowest incidence in TIA or in embolic infarction and the highest incidence in haemorrhagic stroke (Kilpatrick et al 1990). In a postmortem study from the Massachusetts General Hospital of 104 brains, with infarction, a history of seizures was obtained in 12.5%, compared with 2.7% in control patients with cerebral arteriosclerosis only (Richardson & Dodge 1954). As with trauma and haemorrhage, in occlusive stroke the seizures typically occur early (the first week or so), do not usually lead to chronic epilepsy and the overall prognosis is good (White et al 1953, Louis & McDowell 1967). In a retrospective review of 104 patients undergoing cerebral arteriography with carotid occlusive disease, a history of epilepsy was found in 17.3% and seizures were the presenting symptom in 6.7% (Cocito et al 1982). The site and size of the infarcted area, not surprisingly, influence the risk of epilepsy, which is higher in large cortical than in small or subcortical infarcts. Cortical venous infarctions, even if small, may be potently epileptogenic and may underlie a significant proportion of apparently spontaneous epileptic seizures complicating other medical conditions. Partial or secondarily generalized seizures can occur in stroke, and EEG changes are often non-specific.

Epilepsy may be the initial or only manifestation of cerebrovascular disease. In a case-control study from the National Hospital, Queen Square (Roberts et al 1988), CT evidence of vascular pathology was found in 15 of 132 patients presenting with epilepsy (and no other neurological features) developing after the age of 40, and in only two age matched control subjects. Similarly, Shinton et al (1987) also found a history of prior epileptic seizures in eight of 176 cases (4.5%) presenting with a first stroke to a general hospital, suggesting that early cerebrovascular disease may result in epilepsy without any other neurological dysfunction. On the basis of these and other figures, it seems likely that overt or occult cerebrovascular disease underlies 10–20% of all cases of adult-onset seizures and 50% of those developing epilepsy after the age of 50 years. Seizures may also result from the cerebrovascular lesions secondary to rheumatic heart disease (Foster 1942), endocarditis (Salgado et al 1989), mitral valve prolapse (Taylor et al 1979), cardiac tumours (Joynt et al 1965), cardiac arrhythmia or after carotid endarterectomy (Kieburtz et al 1990). Improvements in neuroimaging have also demonstrated the importance of haemorrhage and infarction in neonatal seizures. Infarction accounted for seven (14%) of 50 cases of neonatal epilepsy investigated by CT, often with an unremarkable obstetric history and no other neurological signs except lethargy and hypotonia (Levy et al 1985). Conventional antiepileptic drug therapy is usually effective in controlling seizures in adult patients with cerebrovascular disease (Shinton et al 1988, Fish et al 1989).

Large arteriovenous malformations cause seizures in about 40% of cases (Paterson & McKissock 1956, Kelly et al 1969), and were the presenting symptom in 19% in one series (Crawford et al 1986). More common, though, is epilepsy resulting from smaller low flow cavernous arteriovenous malformations (cavernoma), which are often demonstrable only by MRI and in which chronic focal epilepsy is usually the only symptom. Epilepsy occurs occasionally with cerebral aneurysm, with or without subarachnoid haemorrhage, and in about 25% of subdural haematomas. Malignant hypertension, hypertensive encephalopathy and eclampsia of pregnancy can result with seizures (Ch. 6, 6.3.11), as can anoxic encephalopathy after cardiorespiratory arrest or cardiopulmonary surgery.

## 2.5.4 Epilepsy in the primary cerebral degenerative disorders

Epilepsy, although a relatively common symptom of the cerebral degenerative disorders, is seldom the predominant clinical problem, and the seizures are usually well controlled by conventional antiepileptic drug therapy. Seizures develop in up to 33% of cases of Alzheimer's disease, late in the course of the illness, and the seizures are usually infrequent and mild (Radermecker 1974). Pick's disease rarely causes seizures.

Epilepsy occurs in about 5% of cases of Huntington's disease, again usually in the late stages, and is commoner in the juvenile rigid form. Conversely, in dentato–rubro–pallido–luysian atrophy, epilepsy is common and may be the presenting feature.

Epilepsy occurs in about 6% of cases of Wilson's disease (Denning et al 1988). Seizures can occur at any stage of the disease, and may be the presenting feature, but often begin shortly after the initiation of treatment. The seizures may be partial or secondarily generalized, and can be severe, although the response to treatment is usually good and, in 75% of cases, the epilepsy can be controlled. In Creutzfeldt–Jakob disease, epilepsy is common both in the early and established condition; myoclonus occurs in 80% and can be induced by startle or other stimuli, and generalized tonic-clonic or partial seizures occur in about 10% (Will & Matthews 1984). Repetitive periodic discharges are a characteristic EEG pattern in Creutzfeldt–Jakob disease associated clinically with myoclonus, and are seen in almost all cases at some point in the evolution of the condition. In the terminal stages the periodic discharges, the myoclonus and the epilepsy cease.

## 2.5.5 Epilepsy due to alcohol, drugs, and metabolic disturbances

*Alcohol*

Alcoholism can cause epilepsy in a number of ways. Seizures can be due to alcohol withdrawal and also to a direct toxic effect of alcohol. Trauma, subdural haemorrhage, hepatic or renal disease, metabolic disturbances (especially hyponatraemia, hypoglycaemia and hypomagnesaemia), vitamin or nutritional deficiencies and drug abuse can also contribute to the high rate of epilepsy in alcoholic persons. Alcohol withdrawal in chronic alcoholics is particularly associated with seizures (Victor & Brausch 1967, Isbell et al 1967, Brennan and Lyttle 1987), usually taking the form of generalized seizures, within 12–24 h of the cessation of drinking (50% of cases), and with EEG evidence of photosensitivity and sometimes myoclonus and tremulousness. In their large series, Devetag et al (1983) found the incidence of epilepsy in alcoholics to be about 10% and, in about one-third of these cases, the epilepsy occurred unrelated to withdrawal or any other identifiable cause. Alcohol abuse can also complicate established epilepsy. Alcohol was implicated in 41% of patients admitted to hospital in Denver with epilepsy, and the seizures were precipitated by alcohol in 24% (Earnest & Yarnell 1976). The mortality of patients with epilepsy and alcoholism is considerably higher than that of other groups of patients with epilepsy (Pieninkeroinen et al 1992).

*Drugs*

Seizures can result from the ingestion of many drugs (Table 2.22), and drug-induced seizures are probably commoner than is generally appreciated (Boston Collaborative Drug Surveillance Program 1972). Antidepressants, antipsychotics, isoniazid, penicillin, lignocaine and radiographic contrast media are well recognized precipitants of seizures,

**Table 2.22** Drugs which can induce seizures (most centrally acting drugs occasionally cause epileptic attacks: the most important examples are listed here)

| | |
|---|---|
| *Antibiotics* | *Stimulants* |
| Penicillin (especially intravenous or intrathecal) | Aminophylline |
| Isoniazid (especially in slow acetylators) | Doxapram |
| Cycloserine | Theophylline |
| Chloroquine and other antimalarials | Amphetamine |
| *Hypoglycaemic drugs* | *Anaesthetics* |
| Insulin | Methohexitone |
| Phenformin and other oral hypoglycaemic drugs | Ketamine |
| | Halothane |
| *Hormonal/metabolic drugs* | Althesin |
| Prednisone | |
| Oral contraceptives | *Withdrawal seizures* |
| Oxytocin (causing water retention) | Alcohol |
| | Benzodiazepines |
| *Cardiac dysrhythmic agents* | Barbiturates |
| Lignocaine (intravenous) | Other anticonvulsants |
| Procaine (intravenous) | Amphetamine |
| Disopyramide | Opiates |
| *Antidepressant/antipsychotic drugs* | *Radiographic contrast media* |
| Phenothiazines | Meglumine derivatives (Conray, Dimer-X) |
| Tricyclic antidepressants (especially amitriptyline and imipramine) | Metrizamide |
| Anticholinergic drugs | |
| Lithium | |

but many other drugs have also been implicated although in many cases a causal relationship is difficult to prove. Seizures and status epilepticus may also occur in recreational drug abuse (Alldredge et al 1989), especially with newer agents such as crack and ecstasy. Maternal drug abuse can cause withdrawal seizures in the newborn. Drug-induced seizures are more likely after parenteral administration, with high dosages, or in individuals with a pre-existing predisposition to seizures (e.g. those with pre-existing epilepsy or patients with metabolic disorders). Withdrawal of barbiturate, benzodiazepine or other anti-epileptic or psychotropic drugs can also result in seizures (Duncan 1988), especially in those already predisposed to epilepsy. Long-term antiepileptic drug (AED) treatment is usually unnecessary once the offending drug has been withdrawn.

*Metabolic disturbances*

Acute metabolic disorders commonly result in epileptic seizures. In the first weeks of life, hypoglycaemia and hypocalcaemia and pyridoxine deficiency are important causes of seizures. In older children or adults, changes in blood concentrations of sodium, potassium, calcium, magnesium and glucose can all precipitate seizures, as can hyperammonaemia and changes in blood pH, blood oxygenation or bicarbonate levels. Renal, hepatic, pulmonary and cardiac failure cause multiple metabolic or toxic derangements and are commonly associated with seizures. Acute intermittent porphyria can cause epilepsy, often precipitated by injudicious drug administration.

Acute metabolic disorders with rapid changes in metabolite serum concentrations are more likely to induce seizures than conditions inducing slow metabolic changes, and even severe metabolic abnormalities are usually well tolerated if chronic. The hereditary metabolic disorders causing epilepsy include the aminoacidopathies, non-ketotic hyperglycinaemia, galactosaemia, lipid storage diseases and leucodystrophies. Epileptic seizures are not an uncommon sequel to the ingestion of toxins. Encephalopathy due to lead poisoning can present with epileptic seizures, and seizures are a feature of ergotism and of organophosphate intoxication. Heat stroke can present with epileptic seizures, and epileptic seizures are a rare complication of poisoning with many biological venoms.

## 2.5.6 Epilepsy and immunization and infection

*Immunization*

The risk of epilepsy following immunization is very small indeed. An early study, the National Childhood Encephalography Study, suggested that pertussis vaccination resulted in severe brain damage in one in every 310 000 immunizations, but recent evidence from this study and elsewhere suggests that this may be an overestimate and the study has been subject to criticism from various sources (Bowie 1990, Gale et al 1994). More recent work suggests that there is a small excess risk in the first few days after vaccination only. This is an important issue, as the postinfective encephalopathies of childhood are a potent cause of epilepsy and mental retardation.

*Cerebral infection*

Cerebral infection is a potent cause of epilepsy. In a series of 70 patients with bacterial cerebral abscess (Legg et al 1973), 72% of survivors developed epilepsy, and epilepsy was more likely after frontal and temporal abscesses. The epilepsy is likely to develop within 12 months of the acute abscess and is usually severe and often unresponsive to treatment. Epilepsy is also a common presentation of tuberculous abscess, and more rarely is due to fungal infection. Epilepsy is also a frequent sequel to acute viral encephalitis, especially that due to Herpes simplex virus (Meyer et al 1970, Illis & Gostling 1972), and can prove intractable to treatment. 25% of survivors of viral encephalitis who have seizures at the time of the illness develop chronic epilepsy, as do 10% who do not have seizures acutely. The use of advanced techniques for detecting the presence of viral infection may show that viral infection is a more common cause of epilepsy than is currently recognized. Cytomegalovirus, for instance, has been detected in cortical tissue of some cases of Rasmussen's chronic encephalitis (Power et al 1990), and Herpes simplex virus DNA sequences have been found in temporal lobe specimens removed at temporal lobe surgery for epilepsy (Gannicliffe et al 1985).

HIV infection may result in epilepsy, occasionally presenting as seizures (Holtzman et al 1989). Epileptic seizures can occur in 25% of cases of cerebral toxoplasmosis in AIDS, and also in other infective and non-infective syndromes in AIDS (Wong et al 1990). Subacute sclerosing panencephalitis (SSPE) is an important cause of myoclonus and epilepsy in some countries, although where high levels of measles vaccination have been achieved the condition has largely disappeared.

Epilepsy can occur in almost any infective disease with cerebral involvement, for example infection with: protozoans (e.g. *Toxoplasma*), viruses (e.g. Varicella or other viral encephalitides), fungi (e.g. (*Cryptococcus*, *Aspergillus*), bacteria (e.g. bacterial meningitis or encephalitis, including subacute infections with tuberculosis, *Brucella*, *Listeria*) and in conditions of uncertain infectivity (e.g. sarcoidosis, cat scratch fever). Bacterial meningitis carries a 10% risk of subsequent epilepsy if seizures occur acutely and a 3% risk if there are no acute seizures. In some countries, cerebral parasitosis is an important cause of epilepsy. Seizures occur in 2–4% of patients with cerebral involvement (which is common) in schistosomiasis, in 30% of cerebral hydatid, in the great majority of cerebral cysticercosis cases, in 28% of cases of cerebral malaria, and is common in African trypanosomiasis (Bittencourt et al 1988).

Cerebral tuberculosis is potent cause of epilepsy, and in many parts of the world, a tuberculoma is the commonest mass lesion resulting in epilepsy. Transient low-density CT lesions, sometimes mistaken for cerebral tumour, associated with the onset of epilepsy have been reported from India and other developing countries and may be due to tuberculomas or cysticercosis (Shorvon & Bharucha 1992).

## 2.5.7 Cerebral tumour and epilepsy

Cerebral tumours are responsible for about 10% of cases of late-onset epilepsy (McKeran & Thomas 1980). The peak incidence is in middle age and about 40% of adults presenting with newly developing focal epilepsy have an underlying cerebral tumour. The site of the tumour is an important factor in predicting epileptogenicity. Tumours of the cerebral cortex, and especially the frontal or temporal cortex, are most likely to result in seizures. Epilepsy is rare in subtentorial or deep cerebral tumours or in pituitary tumours and, as most childhood tumours are subtentorial, tumour is an uncommon cause of epilepsy in children.

The incidence of epilepsy varies with histological type and rate of tumour growth. It occurs in about 90% of oligodendrogliomas, two-thirds of cases of meningiomas or astrocytomas and about one-third of gliomas. Seizures are the presenting symptom in about 40% of patients with cerebral tumours, and in slow-growing tumours the seizures may be present for decades before other signs become apparent. The EEG is not a useful investigation for the detection of cerebral tumours. The importance of hamartomas, dysembryoplastic neuroepithelial and other benign tumours in epilepsy has been recognized only with the introduction of magnetic resonance imaging, which uncovers lesions in a high percentage of CT negative cases (Ch. 3, 3.3). Most such lesions are potentially treatable by surgery, and high-quality MRI is essential in any patient with chronic, apparently cryptogenic epilepsy in whom surgery could be considered.

### 2.5.8 Other neurological conditions

Epilepsy is a feature of many other conditions affecting the central nervous system. Almost all conditions affecting the cerebral cortex can cause seizures, as can disorders of white matter and of deep cerebral structures, although the exact mechanism is often obscure. The incidence of epilepsy in multiple sclerosis is several times higher than would be expected by chance. Seizures are commoner in patients with large or acute lesions, but can also occur in the chronic condition with plaques in the deep white matter only (Boudouresques et al 1980, Ghezzi et al 1990). Epilepsy is also a not infrequent symptom of acute disseminated encephalomyelitis, other demyelinating disorders and also in the congenital leucodystrophies such as metachromatic leucodystrophy and adrenoleucodystrophy.

Seizures can occur in hydrocephalus of all types, and follow shunt operations for hydrocephalus in up to 10% of cases, and the risk depends upon shunt location. Seizures also occur in some basal ganglia disorders, including Wilson's disease, Hallervorden–Spatz disease, neuro-acanthocytosis, Huntington's chorea and dentato–rubro–pallido–luysian atrophy, but not others such as idiopathic Parkinson's disease, multisystem atrophy, or progressive supranuclear palsy.

### 2.5.9 Congenital and perinatal causes

Epilepsy is commonly congenital in origin, in which case the seizures are commonly associated with mental retardation. In the past, many cases were wrongly attributed to perinatal disorders, but it is now clear that minor perinatal disturbances rarely result in epilepsy. The frequent occurrence of congenital (prenatal) abnormalities is now increasingly recognized due to advances in neuroimaging and genetic investigation. Little is understood about the genesis of many of these conditions. As knowledge advances, undoubtedly some will turn out to be due to genetic defects and others will be found to be caused largely by exogenous factors (e.g. intrauterine exposure to toxins, infections, drugs etc). The exogenously determined conditions are particularly important to identify because of the possibility of prevention.

In a population survey of epilepsy among the mentally retarded (299 cases), in which advanced imaging was not universally applied, identified prenatal factors accounted for 35% of the cases of epilepsy, perinatal factors for 9.5%, postnatal factors for 8.8% and multiple factors for 14.9% (Table 2.23). In 31.5% no cause could be assigned (Forsgren et al 1990). In many of the cryptogenic cases, new imaging or genetic methods would be likely to detect congenital lesions. In a survey of cerebral palsy, epilepsy was found in 52% of those with severe cerebral palsy and 23% of those with mild or moderate cerebral palsy, and the frequency of epilepsy was correlated with the degree of mental and motor disability (Judrjavcev et al 1985).

*Neuronal migrational defect*

Although almost any congenital disturbance of the brain can result in seizures, numerically the most important are those due to abnormalities of neuronal migration. These can produce severe disorders or more subtle changes, of which epilepsy is the only overt clinical sign. Examples

**Table 2.23** Causes of epilepsy in a mentally retarded population (Forsgren et al 1990). A prevalence survey of all those registered as mentally retarded in a northern Swedish country with active epilepsy (299 subjects; 20% of the mentally retarded). Some persons feature in several categories; overall, prenatal factors accounted for 35.5%, perinatal factors for 9.5%, postnatal factors for 8.8%, multiple causes for 14.9% and unknown factors for 31.5%. Cerebral palsy accounted for 33%, Down's syndrome for 4% and fragile X for 2%.

| Cause | % ($n$ = 299) |
|---|---|
| Chromosmal | 8.4 |
| Neurometabolic | 3 |
| Neurocutaneous | 1.7 |
| Other hereditary | 0.6 |
| Multifactorial | 8 |
| Other recognized syndromes (e.g. Rett's) or unknown causes | 11 |
| Phenylketonuria | 0.3 |
| Premature | 1 |
| Low birth weight | 8 |
| Small for dates | 5.7 |
| Other pregnancy-related factors | 12.7 |
| Neonatal asphyxia | 18.7 |
| Neonatal hypoglycaemia | 1 |
| Neonatal haemorrhage/infarct | 2.4 |
| Infection | 11 |
| Trauma | 3 |
| Tumours | 1 |
| Autism | 4 |
| Others | 1.3 |
| Not known | 28 |

of gross lesions caused by disorders of neuronal generation and migration include: agyria, pachygyria, lissencephaly, schizencephaly, heterotopias (diffuse and focal subcortical), polymicrogyria, macrogyria and corpus callosal agenesis. Subependymal heterotopias are an important cause of epilepsy, which may mimic the electroclinical features of idiopathic generalized epilepsy, and sometimes coexist with other abnormalities (Raymond et al 1994a).

The mildest abnormality of neuronal migration is a largely quantitative alteration of neuronal disposition in cortex and subcortical regions known as *microdysgenesis* (Meencke & Janz 1984). The pathological changes comprise unipolar and bipolar cells in the subpial regions, increased cell density in the stratus moleculare, protrusions of nerve cells into the pia, loss of columnar architecture in the cortex and increased numbers of neurones in the white matter. Meencke (1994) demonstrated microdysgenesis in 38% of 591 brains from patients with epilepsy, compared with 8% in 7374 control brains. In 12.3% of the epileptic brains (and 2% of the controls), the changes were severe. Hardiman et al (1988) similarly found severe neuronal microdysgenesis in 21 (42%) of 50 temporal lobectomy specimens (and none of 33 normal controls). Refinements in MRI will increasingly detect small developmental abnormalities and abnormalities of the grey–white interface, indicating subtle cortical organizational disturbances, in a high proportion of patients with apparently cryptogenic partial epilepsy (Barkovich et al 1992, Cook et al 1994).

Congenital disorders can arise at various phases of neural development. During neural tube formation, major defects can result in anencephaly, holoprosencephaly, encephalocele and dysraphism. Disorders of cortical cellular proliferation and differentiation (8–16 weeks) cause microcephaly or megalencephaly. Defects associated with macrocephaly include congenital tumours, tuberous sclerosis, neurofibromatosis type 1, Sturge–Weber, some leucodystrophies and hemimegalencephaly. Epilepsy is common in most of these conditions. The causes of the neuronal migrational and other congenital disturbance are ill understood. Undoubtedly genetic factors are important, and several syndromes have a well defined genetic basis, but most do not. Prenatal environmental and perinatal factors are also involved and numerous possible causes have been identified. Myelination is delayed after complicated pregnancies (e.g. with maternal diabetes, placental insufficiency), or after birth complications (asphyxia), and perinatal and postnatal disorders can also affect the later stages of neuronal migration and maturation. Dysembryoplastic neuroepithelial tumours are a form of tumoural dysplasia which have been differentiated recently and which are a relatively common cause of chronic epilepsy, especially of temporal lobe origin (Raymond et al 1994b). Histologically these tumours are heterogeneous, with dysplastic and proliferative features.

*Sturge–Weber syndrome*

This is an uncommon sporadic developmental disorder of uncertain causation (Alexander 1972, Brett 1991). Genetic factors do not seem important, and the only familial cases that have been described are in identical twins, in whom genetic and exogenous intrauterine influences can not be differentiated.

The condition comprises a facial naevus and related cerebral and ophthalmic lesions. These are probably due to an abnormal persistence of the embryonic primordial vascular plexus, and subsequent growth separates these elements into deep (cerebral) and superficial (skin) parts. The affected cerebral hemisphere is often atrophic with gliosis and neuronal loss. The leptomeningeal angiomatosis is commonly occipital in distribution but can also be in parietal or temporal regions. The cortex is calcified in a gyriform manner, particularly in the middle cortical lamina and around the blood vessels. Neuronal necrosis is common and it has been postulated that the deterioration that occurs with the onset of epilepsy may be due to hypoxia.

The clinical features comprise:

1. *The port wine naevus:* This lesion is situated characteristically on the upper part of the forehead, the cheek, side of the nose and gums and lip. Although largely within the distribution of the trigeminal nerve, it can cross the midline and spread into the dermatomal distribution of the upper cervical nerves. The affected portions of the lip and gum may be enlarged. The naevus is bilateral in up to one-third of cases. It is red and flat and blanches when pressure is applied. Very occasionally more extensive naevi are seen on the trunk and limbs. Sometimes cerebral lesions occur without a cutaneous naevus.

2. *Neurological features:* A triad of neurological features are associated with the skin lesion: seizures, hemiplegia and mental retardation. Epilepsy is usually the earliest symptom, starting most commonly in the first year of life and almost never after the age of 4 years. The seizures can be severe, frequent and are often intractable to treatment. Their form depends largely upon the age of the patient, and can be neonatal convulsions or infantile spasm, although in later childhood and adult life they are usually partial seizures, often evolving to severe secondarily generalized seizures. The partial seizures have motor and sensory features contralateral to the meningeal naevus. Seizures developing in the neonatal period may be very difficult to control and carry a poor prognosis. The onset of seizures in later life may be with abrupt and severe convulsions. Typically, the hemiplegia of Sturge–Weber syndrome develops after a severe burst of seizures and worsens after subsequent bursts. The child's developmental progress can suddenly diminish with the onset of seizures. Mental retardation is nowadays usually not severe in most cases, and this may be due to better control of the epilepsy.

3. *Ophthalmological features:* Intraocular pressure is increased in about 30% of cases, with glaucoma or buphthalmos in some. An homonymous field loss is very common, due to the occipitally placed cerebral lesion. Episcleral haemangioma, choroidal involvement in the naevus and colobomata of the iris occur in some cases.

Variants of Sturge–Weber also occur. There are associations with neurofibromatosis, von Hippel–Lindau syndrome, tuberous sclerosis, Klippel–Trenaunay-Weber syndrome and retinitis pigmentosa.

The diagnosis is made on the basis of the clinical features. Other vascular naevi commonly affect the face, but rarely with the very typical Sturge–Weber distribution and without the intracranial lesions. Diagnostic confusion can occur with the midline linear sebaceous naevus syndrome (Fuerstein's syndrome), which also causes mental retardation and epilepsy. X-ray CT or MRI brain scans will demonstrate the calcified angiomatous meningeal and cerebral lesions.

The epilepsy should be aggressively treated. Surgical resection of the affected cerebral region or hemispherectomy is worthwhile, particularly if carried out early in life. Cosmetic attention to the naevus can be remarkably effective, both with dermatological preparations and with argon laser therapy. Regular ophthalmic monitoring should be carried out to avoid asymptomatic glaucoma developing.

Other uncommon neurocutaneous syndromes without a clear genetic basis, and which also result in epilepsy include neurocutaneous melanosis, incontinentia pigmenti syndrome, Chediak–Higashi syndrome, Klippel–Trenaunay–Weber syndrome and linear sebaceous naevus syndrome.

## 2.5.10 Genetic causes of epilepsy

The idiopathic generalized epilepsies and the epilepsies secondary to other well defined genetic conditions are described below (2.7 and 2.8). It should be emphasized, however, that in many symptomatic cases of epilepsy there is also a genetic contribution. Thus, some studies of head injury have found a family history of epilepsy more commonly in those who develop seizures after trauma than in those who do not; 60% compared with 30% amongst brain-injured soldiers from the Korean War for instance (Caveness et al 1979). Other studies, however, have not found significant differences (Jennett 1975, Salazar et al 1985). Similarly, in patients with infantile hemiplegia, associated convulsions and also EEG changes are much more likely in those with a close family history of epilepsy. It has been argued, indeed, that genetic factors play a significant part in the production of epilepsy in over 50% of patients (Newmark & Penry 1980, Shorvon 1991) (see also Ch. 6, 6.4).

Recently an autosomal dominant form of frontal lobe epilepsy, with a propensity to seizures occurring in sleep, has been described (Scheffer et al 1994) and a full family history should be taken in all patients.

*Tuberous sclerosis*

This is the commonest of the simple mendelian-inherited epileptic conditions causing epilepsy (Gomez 1988, Osborne & Fryer 1991). It is present in about 1 in 10 000 live births and is inherited in an autosomal pattern. Recent linkage studies have suggested loci on chromosome 9q and 16 and the gene on chromosome 16 has recently been cloned (Ch. 6, 6.4.1).

Epilepsy occurs in about 80% of cases and the manifestations are strongly age-related. Seizures may present in the neonatal period, and the condition may also present as the syndrome of *early infantile epileptic encephalopathy*, which is the commonest manifestation of the condition between the ages of 4 and 8 months. Tuberous sclerosis is also the most common identified pathological cause of the Lennox–Gastaut syndrome. Febrile convulsions may be the first manifestation, and later in life tuberous sclerosis can present with partial or generalized seizures. The EEG has no features specific to the condition. Other features of the condition are summarized in Table 2.24.

Mental deficiency is said to occur in about 50% of identified cases. As asymptomatic persons are not detected, the true proportion of cases with learning disability might be less. The incidence of mental handicap is greater in those who develop seizures before the age of 2 years. A wide variety of other neurological deficits can occur, including hemiplegia, ataxia, stroke-like episodes, behavioural disturbance and psychosis. 5% of patients show signs and symptoms of raised intracranial pressure, which

**Table 2.24** The diagnostic features of tuberous sclerosis (from Gomez 1988)

| |
|---|
| *Primary features* |
| (a definite diagnosis can usually be made even if only one of these is present) |
| Classic shagreen patch |
| Periungual fibroma |
| Retinal hamartoma |
| Facial angiofibromata |
| Subependymal glial nodule (on CT or MRI brain scan) |
| Renal angiomyolipomata (bilateral and multiple) |
| *Secondary features* |
| (two or more features are required to make a diagnosis) |
| Atypical shagreen patch |
| Hypomelanotic macule |
| Gingival fibroma |
| Bilateral polycystic kidneys |
| Isolated renal angiomyolipoma |
| Cardiac rhabdomyoma |
| Cortical tuber (histological) |
| 'Honeycomb lungs' |
| Infantile spasms |
| Myoclonic, atonic or tonic seizures |
| First-degree relative with tuberous sclerosis |
| Forehead fibrous plaque |
| Giant cell astrocytoma |

is usually due to obstructive hydrocephalus, caused by a growing hamartoma or astrocytoma close to the ventricular outflow tracts. Malignant change in the cerebral lesions may cause other progressive neurological signs.

Retinal hamartoma or phakomata occur in about 50% of cases and other ophthalmic signs include retinal pigmentary changes, vascular changes in the retina, anomalous discs, megalocornea, pigmentary changes on the iris, cataract, poliosis of the eyebrow, strabismus and oculomotor nerve palsy. Skin lesions are almost invariable. Hypomelanotic patches are found in 90% of cases after ultraviolet light examination (Woods lamp), and other dermatological findings include ash leaf spots, shagreen patches, café au lait spots and depigmented naevi. Facial angiofibroma (adenoma sebaceum) is a characteristic feature of the condition that may be the presenting feature. On the head fibrous scalp patches and poliosis occur. Periungual fibromata of the fingers or toes are found in up to 25% of cases, often with nail changes.

Other organs are affected less prominently, although abnormalities are common. In the renal tract, myolipomas, angiomyolipomas and asymptomatic renal cysts are frequently found, and fibrodysplasia of the renal arteries also occurs; hamatomatous abnormalities occur also in the liver, pancreas, spleen and gastrointestinal tract. Dental changes include gingival fibroma and pit-shaped enamel defects, and angiolipomas of the bones are found on radiographs in over 50% of cases. Cardiac rhabdomyomas occur in perhaps 40% of cases and are often asymptomatic, and pulmonary cysts and fibrosis occur in the lungs. Endocrine abnormalities include sexual precocity, ovarian or testicular defects, and lesions may also occur in the thyroid and adrenals.

In the brain, the condition is characterized by both cortical tubers and subependymal nodules. These are cerebral dysplasias due to abnormal neuronal migration in the prenatal period. The cortical tubers are dysplastic lesions with abnormal cortical lamination, and dysplastic neurones occur in the grey and underlying white matter. The subependymal nodules occur around the ventricles and grey matter nuclei, and are formed of clusters of astrocytic cells, which may undergo malignant transformation into giant cell astrocytic tumours.

Affected individuals show widely varying manifestations and the features within a family may also vary, both across and between generations. Genetic counselling should inform affected individuals that there is a 50% chance of passing the condition to offspring, and unaffected individuals that there is no genetic propensity. In apparently unaffected individuals, screening for the condition should include a thorough clinical examination with scrutiny of the skin under ultraviolet light, an ophthalmic examination, a renal ultrasound and a cerebral CT (or preferably MRI) brain scan. Other tests which can also be considered include echocardiograph and skeletal radiographs. The prognosis is variable. At one extreme are affected individuals with few signs, normal intelligence and only mild epilepsy. At the other are patients with severe epilepsy and mental retardation, who are often dependent in daily activities and whose life span is shortened by the disease. Death is sometimes due to growth or malignant transformation of the cerebral tumours, obstructive hydrocephalus or status epilepticus.

Epilepsy also occurs in other neurocutaneous syndromes in which the genetic pattern has been established. Autosomal dominant conditions include neurofibromatosis, von Hippel–Lindau syndrome and hypomelanosis of Ito. Xeroderma pigmentosa and neuroichthyosis are inherited recessively and incontinentia pigmenti syndrome in an X-linked pattern.

### 2.5.11 Reflex epilepsy

Reflex epilepsy is an unusual form of seizure disorder in which seizures are provoked by a specific external stimulus or event. Usually, seizures occur also at other times, but in rare patients the epileptic attacks only happen when elicited by a specific stimulus, and occasionally every time the stimulus is applied. The term reflex epilepsy is not usually applied to patients whose seizures are precipitated by internal influences, such as menstruation. The definition is therefore rather unsatisfactory, and a variable tendency to reflex seizures is found in many patients with other epileptic syndromes.

The reflex epilepsies are sometimes divided into simple and complex types; in the simple forms, the seizures are precipitated by simple sensory stimuli (e.g. flashes of light, startle) and in the complex forms by more elaborate stimuli (e.g. specific pieces of music). The complex forms are much more heterogeneous and form less well defined syndromes than the simple reflex epilepsies. In hospital practice, about 5% of patients show some features of reflex epilepsy. The stimuli reported to cause seizures include flashing lights and other visual stimuli, startle, eating, bathing in hot water, music, reading, other cognitive activities and movement.

The commonest reflex epilepsies are those induced by visual stimuli. Flashing lights, bright lights, moving patterns, eye closure and viewing specific objects and colours have all been described. The most frequent, known as photosensitive epilepsy, designates those individuals whose seizures are precipitated by flickering lights.

*Photosensitive epilepsy*

Photosensitive epilepsy usually presents between the ages of 7 and 19 years and may account for 10% of all new cases of epilepsy presenting in this age group (Ch. 3, 3.2.5). There is a 3 : 2 female preponderance and greatest expression in adolescence. The commonest seizure types are generalized tonic-clonic, absence and myoclonic seizures. The resting EEG is often normal, or may show generalized spikewave discharges, and photic stimulation will produce the photoconvulsive response in most cases. The most frequent environmental triggers are television, electronic screen games and other computer graphics (Fish et al 1994), and other precipitants include discotheque lighting, sudden emergence into bright light, flickering of sunlight during travelling and sunlight reflected by water or snow. The sensitivity to television is in part frequency-dependent, and most photosensitive persons are most vulnerable at flicker rates of 10–30 Hz. The dangers of electronic screens inducing seizures in people with photosensitivity can be reduced by:

- Using a small screen relative to the viewing distance
- Changing channels using a remote control
- Using a 100 Hz television screen or a non-interlaced computer screen with a high refresh rate or liquid crystal display
- Closing one eye or using polarizing glasses
- Keeping the screen contrast and brightness low
- Avoiding exposure when sleep-deprived (Ch. 4, 4.1.3)
- Avoiding looking at a fixed flickering pattern

Photic-induced seizures and EEG evidence of photosensitivity are also found in patients with idiopathic generalized epilepsy who have spontaneous seizures, and in some patients with progressive myoclonus epilepsy. Some photosensitive individuals are susceptible to moving patterns rather than flickering light, and the EEG activity is dependent upon the spatial frequency, orientation and contrast of the image (Wilkins & Lindsay 1985). Eye-closure will produce spike-wave on the EEG of about 20% of untreated photosensitive persons, but only occasionally seizures. Eyelid myoclonia with typical absences is another unusual epileptic syndrome precipitated by eye-closure in susceptible persons (Appleton et al 1993). Darkened or polarized glasses will reduce the risk of photic-induced seizures, and in mild cases no other therapy is needed. Valproate will abolish photosensitivity and prevent seizures in most cases of photic induced epilepsy (Harding et al 1978), and benzodiazepine drugs and ethosuximide are also effective (Ch. 4, 4.4.2).

*Startle-induced seizures*

Epilepsy with startle-induced seizures is a syndrome characterized by stimuli of various modalities, which cause seizures only if unexpected (Alajouanine & Gastaut 1955, Bancaud et al 1975). The commonest stimulus is loud noise, but touch and movement can also trigger attacks. Startle sensitivity will often occur transiently in the history of an individual with epilepsy. It is most commonly observed in patients with frontal lobe epilepsy, with lesions or seizure foci in the supplementary motor, medial or lateral frontal areas, or in patients with a gross neurological deficit such as a hemiplegia. The commonest seizure type is a focal tonic seizure, and the scalp EEG can show a variety of changes or may be normal. Antiepileptic drug therapy may be disappointing, although carbamazepine and the benzodiazepine drugs are said to be most effective.

Epilepsy with startle-induced seizures should be differentiated from the rare condition hyperekplexia although there may be an overlap in some cases (Andermann & Andermann 1986). The finding of cortical abnormalities on imaging and neurophysiological investigation, the presence of other forms of epileptic seizure and non-startle-induced attacks, an abnormal interictal EEG and a history of slowed motor development are all typical of startle-induced epilepsy but not of hyperekplexia. The latter condition is commonly familial with dominant inheritance, and neurophysiological and imaging abnormalities point to a brainstem origin in many cases.

*Other reflex epilepsies*

Other simple reflex epilepsies include patients whose seizures are induced by movement, touching or tapping. These should be differentiated from startle-induced epilepsy, paroxysmal kinesogenic choreo-athetosis and stimulus-sensitive myoclonus. Hot-water epilepsy is a remarkable syndrome which seems common in parts of India and rare elsewhere (Satischandra et al 1988). The seizures are precipitated by the pouring of hot water over the head or immersion in hot water. The attacks take the form of tonic-clonic or partial seizures.

The complex reflex epilepsies are a heterogeneous group. Primary reading epilepsy is an uncommon form of reflex epilepsy in which attacks are triggered by reading, usually for long periods of time, and in which spontaneous seizures do not occur. Typically, the attacks start with clonic jerking of the jaw, which will progress to a generalized tonic-clonic seizure if the sufferer continues to read. There is a family history in about 25% of cases. The resting EEG is normal, but generalized or focal epileptic paroxysms may occur while reading. Care must be taken to distinguish apparent vertex spikes from movement artefact due to jaw jerks. Comprehensive studies have been undertaken of the aspects of reading which result in epilepsy, with conflicting results in different individuals. The seizures have been related to oro-facial movement, reading difficult or unfamiliar passages, reading foreign languages, reading music, reading emotional material or nonsense, and in others also occur when talking, playing chess or undertaking mathematical calculations. About 60 cases have been recorded and the epilepsy is classified as a specific localization-related syndrome (Wolf 1992a).

Other reflex epilepsies with complex forms include seizures precipitated by eating (Fiol et al 1986), language, sounds, decision-making (e.g. mental arithmetic, chess playing), thinking (Wilkins et al 1982) and music (Reder & Wright 1982, Forster 1977). The latter conditions are heterogeneous in terms of aetiology, EEG and seizure types; the stimulus is only occasionally highly specific (e.g. a particular fragment of music), and non-reflex seizures also occur. The mechanisms underlying these (and other) reflex epilepsies are uncertain and specific 'reflex arcs' have not been identified.

### 2.5.12 Cryptogenic epilepsy

Although epilepsy may result from a variety of different causes, only some of which have been listed above, in many cases no cause is found. In the pre-MRI era, this accounted for about two-thirds of all patients. This proportion is markedly reduced with the advent of high resolution MRI that identifies minor structural developmental abnormalities (Ch. 3, 3.3). Such cases are best designated cryptogenic rather than idiopathic epilepsy, which is a term reserved for the genetically determined idiopathic generalized epilepsies (see below, 2.7).

Some apparently cryptogenic cases that develop in adult life are due to perinatal trauma, although a causal relationship is often difficult to confirm (Nelson & Broman 1977; Bergamasco et al 1984). Others are undoubtedly due to minor head trauma, unsuspected encephalitic illnesses, undetected cerebral malformation or other occult conditions. In many such cases, however, investigation during life and also neuropathological examination after death reveals no obvious cause. Some such cases may have biochemical rather than structural causes, which are presently beyond detection by conventional investigation. The identification and characterization of such biochemical syndromes of epilepsy is a major research goal and the subject of ongoing efforts, both in vivo and in vitro.

## 2.6 CHILDHOOD EPILEPSY SYNDROMES

### 2.6.1 Neonatal seizures

The clinical and EEG features, the cause and the anatomico-pathological basis of neonatal epilepsy differ from those of the epilepsies of later childhood or adult life. Clinical signs are by necessity limited to motor phenomena, and other features, if they occur, are beyond the current limits of detectability. EEG signs, too, are often variable and non-specific and their interpretation difficult. Seizures in the neonatal period are an ominous development, not only because they often indicate cerebral disease, but also because they possibly damage the developing brain. Seizures have been shown to inhibit DNA, RNA, protein and cholesterol synthesis in neonatal rats, and result in diminished brain weight and cell numbers; similar damage is likely to occur in human infants also (Wasterlain & Dwyer 1983, Dwyer & Wasterlain 1983). The seizures are usually repeated or continuous, amounting in many cases to neonatal status epilepticus.

Because of difficulties in detection and definition, the frequency of epileptic seizures in the neonatal period is difficult to assess accurately. Estimates of the incidence vary between 5 and 16/1000 live births (up to 23% in premature infants). The mortality is high (16–60%) and morbidity even higher (35–70%) (Kellaway & Hrachovy 1983, Anonymous 1989, Brett 1991, Aicardi 1992).

Seizures are often polymorphic and poorly organized because of the immaturity of cerebral development. Some seizures resemble isolated fragments of seizures seen in older individuals, and are perhaps due to the poor synaptic connectivity of the immature cortical architecture preventing synchronization of epileptic activity and seizure propagation. While most neonatal seizures are undoubtedly epileptic, especially when accompanied by paroxysmal EEG changes, the nature of some 'seizures' is controversial (especially forms of subtle or tonic seizure). The lack of EEG abnormality in these seizures has prompted the suggestion that subcortical mechanisms (release phenomena), not epilepsy, may be responsible. Stimulus sensitivity, graduated forms and spatial and temporal summation are cited to support this view (Kellaway & Hrachovy 1983, Camfield & Camfield 1987). Indeed, repeated clinical (clonic and subtle) and electrographic seizures have also been observed in an infant with complete atelencephaly (Danner et al 1985). This is not simply a semantic problem, as prognosis differs in non-epileptic and epileptic seizures, and treatment will vary.

Several 'seizure types' are recognized (Volpe 1987, Mizrahi & Kellaway 1987).

*Subtle (minimal) seizures* are sometimes overlooked. Typical motor features are slight jerking or deviation of the eyes, fluttering of the eyelids, orofacial movements, apnoea, autonomic changes, rowing, pedalling, swimming or boxing movements, brief myoclonic movements of the trunk or limbs and tonic spasms. These may continue for hours or days. The EEG can be normal or can show high-voltage slow activity, rhythmic slow activity or burst suppression.

*Tonic seizures* are especially common in the premature infant. Rapid extension of all four limbs occurs, with apnoea, upward or lateral deviation of the eyes, and tremor of the extended limbs. They can be generalized, focal or asymmetric and sometimes stimulus sensitive. The EEG can be normal or show bursts of high voltage slow or burst suppression activity.

*Clonic seizures*: These may be focal or multifocal, and comprise random or organized jerking of the limbs, which may spread or fluctuate. They can resemble fragments of tonic-clonic seizures. Multifocal clonic seizures, unlike tonic seizures, are rare in pre-term infants. The EEG is abnormal, with focal or multifocal paroxysmal activity, sharp waves or spikes.

*Other seizure types*: Unilateral seizures occur in about 10% of cases; due usually to anoxia, cardiac surgery or structural lesions. True myoclonic seizures also occur in term and pre-term infants, especially in those with developmental brain disorders, and may or may not cause measurable electrographic changes. Electrographic seizures, without obvious clinical signs, also occur. With cerebral function monitoring in 87 neonates, seizure activity lasting 1 h or more without clinical signs was found in 14 (16%), two of whom had never had any obvious clinical seizures (Hellstrom-Westas et al 1985). Eyre et al (1983) found seizure discharges in nine of 20 neonates, and Clancy et al (1988) could not detect clinical correlates in 79% of electrographic discharges in neonates with frequent seizures.

It is likely that some at least of subtle or tonic seizures are 'non-epileptic', and other neonatal phenomena which can also be confused with seizures include jitteriness and tremor, toxic or withdrawal 'seizures' from maternal medication, and the abnormal movements in hypoxic–ischaemic encephalopathy, neonatal intracranial haemorrhage or inborn errors of metabolism. In some instances, it is not possible to decide whether or not a clinical manifestation is epileptic.

The EEG in the neonate reflects the immature nature of cerebral development, and both the normal and abnormal patterns differ greatly from those later in life. The ictal and interictal EEG are highly variable, even in the same infant, showing repetitive paroxysmal activity, spikes or sharp waves, usually focal or multifocal and of varying polarity, bursts of alpha, delta or beta activity and periodic lateralized epileptic discharges (PLEDS). Symmetrical synchronous generalized activity is rare. The background activity is usually abnormal. Electrographic activity can be localized to one hemisphere and may spread across the hemi-

**Table 2.25** Causes of neonatal seizures

| | |
|---|---|
| *Hypoxic–ischaemic encephalopathy* | *Metabolic causes* |
| *Acute cerebrovascular event* | Hypocalcaemia |
| Subarachnoid haemorrhage | Hypoglycaemia |
| Intraventricular haemorrhage | Hyponatraemia |
| Intracerebral haemorrhage | Inborn errors of metabolism |
| Subdural haemorrhage | Bilirubin encephalopathy |
| Cerebral infarction | Hypomagnesaemia |
| | Pyridoxine dependency |
| *Intracranial infection* | *Benign and familial syndromes* |
| Meningitis (esp. Group B streptococcus, *E. coli*) | Benign familial neonatal convulsions |
| Encephalitis (esp. Herpes simplex, toxoplasmosis, Coxsackie B, rubella, Cytomegalovirus) | Benign neonatal seizures |
| Abscess | Benign neonatal sleep myoclonus |
| *Cerebral malformations* | *Toxic or withdrawal convulsions* |
| Neuronal migrational and other developmental defects | Toxins (e.g. mercury, hexachlorophene) |
| Neurocutaneous disorders | Drugs (e.g. penicillin, anaesthetics) |
| Chromosomal anomalies | Drug withdrawal (e.g. maternal barbiturate, alcohol, narcotics) |
| | *Specific epileptic encephalopathies* |
| | Ohtahara's syndrome |
| | Neonatal myoclonic encephalopathy |
| | Early infantile epileptic encephalopathy |

sphere only slowly (Plouin et al 1981). Both subtle and tonic seizures can occur without any EEG sign.

Seizures in the newborn are always symptomatic and there are a wide variety of potential causes (Table 2.25) (Rose & Lombroso 1970, Eriksson & Zetterstrom 1979, Lombroso 1983, Kellaway & Hrachovy 1983, Fenichel 1985, Volpe 1987, Mizrahi & Kellaway 1987). Neonatal hypoxic–ischaemic encephalopathy is the commonest cause, and can be prenatal, perinatal or postnatal in origin. The seizures usually take a clonic form and, when perinatal in origin, present in the first 12 h, reach maximum severity at 24–48 h and resolve after 72 h.

Neonatal infection usually presents in the second week of life. Meningitis is usually caused by group B streptococcus, *E. coli*, *Citrobacter* and *Proteus mirabilis*. Cerebral abscess or meningoencephalitis are usually due to Herpes simplex, toxoplasmosis, Coxsackie B, rubella or Cytomegalovirus. Intracranial haemorrhage may be intraventricular, especially in premature infants, subarachnoid, subdural or intracerebral, and may result from coagulation defects. Modern imaging has shown cerebral infarction to be commoner than previously thought (14% of one series of 50 full-term infants with seizures (Levy et al 1985). Many rare congenital cerebral anomalies can present as neonatal seizures, and can be differentiated best by MRI imaging.

Hypoglycaemia presents in the first 3 days of life. Hypocalcaemia and/or hypomagnesaemia is rare as an isolated cause of neonatal seizures and usually occurs in the first 5–10 days of life. Pyridoxine dependency should always be considered, and intravenous pyridoxine administered. Other metabolic causes or inborn errors of metabolism are rare.

*Early infantile epileptic encephalopathy (EIEE)* (Ohtahara et al 1987) is a rare epilepsy syndrome that becomes manifest during the first few months of life. Affected children develop increasingly frequent seizures with characteristic tonic spasms, severe mental regression and cerebral palsy, which is accompanied by burst suppression on the EEG. The clinical picture can evolve into that of the Lennox–Gastaut syndrome. Various underlying pathological causes and brain malformations have been reported. The prognosis is very poor, death in the first year of life occurring in one-third of cases and survivors develop severe epilepsy and profound mental handicap.

*Neonatal myoclonic encephalopathy* is another severe epileptic encephalopathy, in which erratic fragmentary myoclonus is the predominant seizure type. This can be focal or generalized, and associated with partial motor seizures and tonic spasms (Aicardi & Goutieres 1978; Aicardi 1992). Identified causes include non-ketotic hyperglycinaemia, D-glutaric acidaemia, methylmalonic acidaemia, propionic acidaemia and hemimegalencephaly (Aicardi 1992). The EEG is severely abnormal with frequent bursts of epileptic activity, or burst suppression. Antiepileptic drug treatment is ineffective and most affected infants die in early childhood; those surviving do so in a vegetative state.

*Benign familial neonatal seizures*: This is a rare condition, inherited as an autosomal dominant, with an about 85% penetrance (Plouin 1992) (Ch. 6, 6.4.1). The male and female incidence is equal. Convulsions develop in the first week of life in 80% of cases, with peak incidence of onset on the third day. Seizures remit within a few months in about one-third of cases, and in the first year in 70%. Seizures continue beyond the age of 5 years in only about 10% of patients. There are no specific EEG changes.

*Benign neonatal convulsions* are repetitive seizures between days 4 and 6 of life ('fifth day fits'), which continue for a few days and then remit. The aetiology is unclear and the prognosis is good.

## 2.6.2 Infantile spasm (West's syndrome)

Dr W. J. West, a general practitioner in Tonbridge, Kent described this 'peculiar form of infantile convulsion' in his own 4-month-old son (West 1841). The condition is rare, with an annual incidence of about 0.25–0.42/1000 live births, and a prevalence of 0.14–0.19/1000 in children between 0 and 9 years of age. There is a family history of epilepsy in about 7–17% (Lacy & Penry 1976). The spasms rarely develop before the age of 3 months, 90% start in the first year of life, and the peak incidence is at 4–6 months. Neurological deficit is present before the onset of spasms in up to 80% of patients. The spasms take the form of sudden brief contractions of the head, neck or trunk, usually in flexion but sometimes in extension. Some attacks are less dramatic and take the form of simple head-nodding, elevation of the eyeballs or shoulder-shrugging. The attacks last a few seconds and cluster, and hundreds of attacks can occur in a day (Coulter 1986). The spasms are usually generalized, but can be asymmetrical or even unilateral. In about two-thirds of patients the interictal EEG exhibits hypsarrhythmia (Gibbs & Gibbs 1952), which is a disorganized and chaotic pattern of high-voltage slow waves with intermingled multifocal asynchronous spike and sharp waves which is often asymmetric, although modified forms also occur (Table 2.26) (Ch.3, Fig. 3.17).

The physiological basis of the spasms are unknown. They are best considered as an age-specific epileptic response of the developing brain to cerebral pathology, and the epileptic encephalopathy can be caused by

**Table 2.26** Features of infantile spasms (West's syndrome)

- Rare epileptic syndrome
- Commonly develop between 4 and 8 months of age
- Development usually normal prior to onset, but subsequent development retarded
- 'Salaam attacks', short-lived, in clusters
- EEG typically shows hypsarrhythmia
- Good response to corticosteroid drugs
- Seizures usually remit on therapy or spontaneously
- Long-term prognosis poor, with mental retardation and continuing epilepsy common sequelae

**Table 2.27** Causes of infantile spasms

*Disorders of cerebral development*

- Neuronal migrational and other developmental defects
- Neurocutaneous syndromes (e.g. tuberous sclerosis, Sturge–Weber syndrome, neurofibromatosis)

*Metabolic and degenerative disorders*

- Metabolic disorders (e.g. phenylketonuria, non-ketotic hyperglycinaemia, pyridoxine deficiency, Leigh's disease, histidinaemia, hyperammonaemia, leucine-sensitive hypoglycaemia)
- Degenerative disorders of uncertain aetiology (e.g. leucodystrophies, Alper's disease, Tay–Sachs disease)

*Perinatal or postnatal chronic acquired cerebral lesions*

- Hypoxic–ischaemic encephalopathy and cerebral infarction
- Haemorrhage (intracranial, subarachnoid, subdural)
- Infection (meningitis, encephalitis, abscess, intrauterine infection)
- Cerebral trauma
- Cerebral tumour
- Maternal toxaemia
- Metabolic and endocrine disorders
- Infantile spasms evolving from neonatal seizure syndrome

In approximately 40% of cases, no cause is found (of whom 10–15% show some preceding developmental disturbance)

many prenatal, perinatal and postnatal cerebral disorders (Table 2.27). The most frequent causes are tuberous sclerosis, brain dysgenesis and chronic acquired lesions. No specific cause can be found in about 40%, but only about 10–15% of cases are free of pre-existing mental, developmental or neurological abnormalities (cryptogenic cases). A small group of idiopathic cases also exist, with a mild condition and a good prognosis (Dulac et al 1986). About 20–60% are prenatal in origin, 15–40% perinatal and less than 10% postnatal. There is probably no causal relationship between immunization and infantile spasm.

Infantile spasms can develop from pre-existing epileptic or non-epileptic encephalopathies, for instance from Ohtahara's syndrome or neonatal myoclonic encephalopathy. The prognosis is generally poor. The response to ACTH or vigabatrin therapy is good (Ch. 4, 4.4.3), with 60% of cases remitting. Between 5% and 20% of infants die during the active phase (Lacy & Penry 1976). The long-term outlook is generally poor. Although the spasms cease, about 70–90% of infants develop mental retardation, which is usually severe, and 35–60% have chronic epilepsy. Only about 5% make a complete recovery (Dulac et al 1986, Hrachovy & Frost 1990).

### 2.6.3 Febrile convulsions

A febrile convulsion is defined as an epileptic seizure occurring usually between 3 months and 5 years of age, associated with fever but without any evidence of acute intracranial disease or infection. Seizures with fever in children with epilepsy (i.e. a prior history of non-febrile seizures) are excluded. Febrile seizures are usually subdivided into simple and complex forms; a complex seizure is defined as one that lasts more than

**Table 2.28** Features of febrile convulsions

- Common (2–5% of all children)
- Peak age of onset 2–4 years of age
- Seizure is usually at onset of febrile illness, and takes a tonic-clonic form
- Febrile convulsions recur in 30–50% of children
- Complex febrile convulsion: duration greater than 30 min; focal features; recurs within 24 h
- Risk of continuing epilepsy small; prognosis worse if age of onset < 13 months, in the presence of prior neurological abnormalities, complex convulsion

30 min, and/or with focal or lateralizing features, and/or which recurs within 24 h (Table 2.28).

In western populations, 2–5% of children have suffered a febrile convulsion by the age of 5 years (Aicardi & Chevrie 1970, Nelson & Ellenberg 1981, Wallace 1988). 50% of the infants have their first febrile convulsion in the second year of life, and 90% before the age of 3 years (Verity & Golding 1991). In Japan and the developing world the incidence might be higher. The condition is more common in males and in those with a family history of febrile convulsion or epilepsy or a prior history of maternal ill-health, prenatal or perinatal disturbance, or prior cerebral dysfunction. Fever is the commonest precipitating cause of epilepsy in this age group, and it has been estimated that 19–41/1000 infants with fever will convulse. A rapid rate of rise of fever and a high temperature seem important risk factors in the precipitation of febrile convulsions. Viral infection is the underlying cause of the fever in over 80% of cases, and 8% of first febrile convulsions will be due to viral or bacterial meningitis. There is a small excess of febrile convulsions after measles vaccination.

The convulsions have a tonic-clonic form in about 80–85%, a tonic form in 15% and an atonic form in 2–5%, and may be unilateral (a highly characteristic feature, not seen in older children) or focal (Aicardi & Chevrie 1970). Prolonged seizures may be followed by a Todd's paresis, or occasionally by permanent neurological deficit. Most prolonged convulsions (febrile status) occur in children under the age of 18 months, especially before the age of 13 months; about 30% of all febrile convulsions in children under 13 months are prolonged (Lennox-Buchthal 1974). After the age of 2 years, the risk of febrile status epilepticus is very much lower. Prolonged febrile seizures are also more likely in children with pre-existing neurological or developmental problems, and prolonged seizures are more likely to exhibit focal features.

In between 30% and 50% of children, the first febrile convulsion will be followed by a second. Less than 10% of children experiencing a febrile convulsion will have three or more. 50% of recurrences occurred with the first 6 months after the first attack and 75% within 12 months. Only an early age of onset and a positive family history of epilepsy increase the risk of recurrence.

More important than the risk of recurrence of febrile seizures is the risk of subsequent epilepsy later in life. This became a particular concern when neurosurgical series showed mesial temporal sclerosis in over 60% of temporal lobe specimens, and the view arose that this pathology was the result of childhood febrile seizures. Early hospital-based studies then painted a rather gloomy picture of the outcome of febrile convulsions, an over-pessimistic view that has been corrected by a series of large scale epidemiological studies, which have found that only between 2% and 7% of children with febrile seizures subsequently developed epilepsy. The National Cooperative Perinatal Project (NCPP) was the first adequate cohort study of this problem. 39 179 children were followed from infancy, of whom 1706 experienced febrile seizures. Of these 1706 children, only 34 (2%) had developed subsequent epilepsy by the age of 7 years, compared to 0.5% of those without a history of febrile seizures. The presence of prior neurological damage was an important predictor of a worse prognosis, with a risk of subsequent epilepsy of only 1.7% in children without and 9.2% in those with prior neurological disturbance. Similar findings were reported by the National Child Development Study in which only 20 (5.4%) of 366 children with febrile seizures developed epilepsy by the age of 11 years, and among a cohort of 16 004 neonatal survivors (98.5% of all infants born in the UK in 1 week in April 1970), 14 676 of whom were studied at 10 years of life. 2.7% (398 cases) had at least one febrile seizure, and of those who were neurologically normal before the first febrile seizure (382 cases) only 2.4% (nine cases) developed subsequent epilepsy (Verity & Golding 1991). Thus, while there is no reasonable doubt that a prolonged febrile seizure is associated with damage to the mesial temporal structures, in population terms this is rare. No death from febrile status was recorded amongst the 2740 children in three prospective large-scale investigations (Nelson & Ellenberg 1981, Annegers et al 1987, Berg et al 1992) and permanent neurological damage was also rare. In the NCPP, a focal paresis occurred after the febrile seizure in only 0.4%, and no child developed the hemiplegia hemiatrophy epilepsy (HHE) syndrome. 6–18% of those admitted to hospital following a febrile seizure have been subsequently reported to be mentally retarded (Wallace 1988), although it is not clear whether or not febrile seizures cause subsequent cognitive difficulties.

The HHE syndrome occurs almost exclusively in children under the age of 3 years, and three-quarters of cases occur after febrile status (Aicardi & Chevrie 1970, 1983, Maytal et al 1989). Now that febrile status is treated rapidly and effectively, HHE is a rare sequel to febrile status in developed countries, although sadly still common in the developing world. The clinical features of the syndrome are permanent hemiplegia or hemiparesis, mental retardation and chronic epilepsy (in about three-quarters), deficits that follow prolonged asymmetrical or unilateral febrile convulsions. Affected children have often been noted to have neurological signs or epilepsy before the episode of status. The duration of status is a critical factor, with hemiplegia likely to result only after very prolonged episodes, in excess of 1.5–2 h (Roger et al 1972). The pathological findings in the acute phase are severe venous congestion and thrombosis, and massive cerebral oedema which can cause arterial occlusion. An MRI or CT brain scan at the time of the convulsion will show unilateral oedema and brain swelling, which later results in progressive atrophy and hypodensity of the whole hemisphere and unilateral ventricular enlargement.

### 2.6.4 Childhood myoclonic epilepsy syndromes

The nosology of the myoclonic epilepsies of childhood is extremely confused and contentious. In most cases, no cause for the epilepsy is identifiable (best referred to as *cryptogenic myoclonic epilepsy*). Symptomatic myoclonic epilepsy may be caused by various prenatal pathologies and less often perinatal injury (e.g. hypoxic–ischaemic encephalopathy, perinatal haemorrhage). Although causing only a small proportion of cases, myoclonic status is also a frequent symptom of hereditary metabolic diseases, including: neuronal ceroid lipofuscinosis (four variants – early infantile (Santavuori–Hagberg), late infantile (Jansky–Bielschowski), juvenile (Batten's, Spielmeyer–Vogt), late childhood (Kufs)); sialidosis; GM1 and GM2 gangliosidoses; Gaucher's disease type 3; mitochondrial disease; non-ketotic hyperglycinaemia; D-glyceric acidaemia; Lafora body disease.

Other childhood myoclonic syndromes include *benign myoclonic epilepsy of infancy* (Dravet & Bureau 1981), the *syndrome of severe myoclonic epilepsy in infants*, and the *syndrome of myoclonic status in non-progressive encephalopathy* (Dalla Bernadina et al 1992). The first is a benign epilepsy syndrome with excellent prognosis and is probably the first type of idiopathic generalized epilepsy to develop (see below, 2.7.7). In contrast, the latter two are severe encephalopathies, with progressive myoclonus, frequent episodes of non-convulsive and convulsive status epilepticus, and psychomotor regression. The prognosis is poor both in terms of control of the seizures and intellectual functioning. In practice the boundaries between the non-progressive forms and other myoclonic epilepsies and encephalopathies in childhood can be difficult to define, particularly early in the course of the disease.

*Myoclonic–astatic epilepsy* is another childhood myoclonic syndrome characterized by myoclonic and astatic or myoclonic–astatic seizures. It accounts for 1–2% of all childhood epilepsies in some series (Doose 1992). Whether it is a true syndrome separate from other myoclonic syndromes in childhood is contentious. In the 117 cases described by Doose, the onset was between 2–5 years, 74% were male, the EEG showed bilateral synchronous irregular and regular 2–3 Hz spike or polyspike and wave, with a slow background. About 40% of patients exhibit at least one episode of absence status. Differentiation from the Lennox–Gastaut syndrome can be difficult but Doose (1992) lists the following criteria as being useful in the differential diagnosis: genetic predisposition, normal premorbid development, absence of an underlying neurometabolic or degenerative disorder, lack of neurological deficit, lack of atypical absence or daytime tonic seizures, generalized EEG pattern without focal abnormalities.

### 2.6.5 Benign rolandic epilepsy and other benign epilepsy syndromes of childhood

A number of benign epilepsy 'syndromes' have been delineated. The best defined is benign rolandic epilepsy. These benign epilepsies usually occur in children with otherwise normal neurological and psychological functioning, there is often a family history, the seizures respond to simple conventional antiepileptic drug treatment and the ultimate prognosis is generally good (Table 2.29).

**Table 2.29** Features of benign rolandic epilepsy

- Common condition (15% of all childhood epilepsies)
- Usual age of onset 5–10 years
- Partial seizures involving face, oropharynx, and arm, usually with preserved consciousness initially and commonly with secondary generalization
- Typically occur during sleep
- Seizures usually infrequent
- Normal intelligence and no other neurological abnormalities
- Family history in many cases
- EEG typically shows high amplitude focal centrotemporal spiking
- Excellent response to antiepileptic drugs
- Excellent prognosis with remission usual by the mid-teenage years

*Benign rolandic epilepsy*

Benign rolandic epilepsy (also known as benign epilepsy of childhood with rolandic spikes and benign epilepsy with centrotemporal spikes) is a well defined childhood syndrome accounting for up to 15% of all childhood epilepsies, with an annual incidence of about 20/100 000 children. The age of onset is between 3 and 13 years, with a peak incidence between 5 and 10 years. The seizures are typically focal, involving the face and oropharynx, often with secondary generalization, and have a strong tendency to occur during sleep. The focal onset of the attack is typically with clonic jerking of the face or mouth, dysarthria or speech arrest, difficulty moving the mouth, guttural sounds, hypersalivation and drooling. These motor phenomena are usually associated with sensory disturbances and with clonic unilateral jerking of the upper limb. Simple partial seizures occur in about 60% of cases. In about two-thirds of patients, secondarily generalized tonic-clonic seizures also occur, almost always during sleep. The epilepsy is mild in most cases, about 15% of patients having only a single attack and only 20% frequent seizures. There are generally no associated neurological abnormalities, and intellect is usually normal. There is a family history in a substantial proportion of patients (variously estimated as between 10% and 60%) and the condition may have autosomal dominant inheritance. The picture is complicated by the fact that the EEG changes of the condition can occur without a history of seizures (indeed EEG changes without seizures may be 10 times commoner than EEG changes with seizures).

The diagnosis can be made by the typical clinical features and confirmed by the characteristic EEG findings. These consist of remarkably focal high-amplitude midtemporal spike or spike/wave discharges. The focus is unilateral in 40% of cases and can less commonly be situated in occipital or frontal regions. The background activity is normal but the morphology of the sharp waves is characteristic, they are usually exacerbated by sleep and the discharges can occur frequently. There is a striking contrast between the active EEG and the benign clinical picture. Similar EEG features, however, may sometimes occur in symptomatic partial epilepsies.

The prognosis of the condition has been well characterized (Loiseau et al 1988). Of 168 patients, seizures continued for less than 1 month in 31%, for between 1 and 12 months in 21%, for between 1 and 5 years in 39% and for more than 5 years in only 10%. Seizures persisted beyond the age of 14 years in only two cases. On follow up 2% of the group had mild pyramidal signs and 17% mild cognitive deficits. Once the seizures have remitted, long-term antiepileptic medication is not required.

*Benign occipital epilepsy*

The nosological position of this syndrome is much less well defined. Among the patients described there is a male preponderance, the oldest case reported was with onset at 17 years and the peak age of onset is 7 years (Panayiotopoulos 1989). Two-thirds of patients have a family history of epilepsy and about one-sixth of cases have a history of febrile convulsions.

The partial seizures have occipital symptomatology: amaurosis, hemianopia, elementary visual hallucinations and visual illusions. Head deviation and blinking are common motor phenomena, and the seizures may evolve to complex partial seizures with temporal symptomatology, to hemimotor seizures and to secondarily generalized tonic-clonic seizures. Postictal headache, sometimes with vomiting, is characteristic. Prolonged seizures, often lasting several hours are typical of this syndrome (Panayiotopoulos 1989). In one series, non-convulsive (or convulsive) status was reported in nine of 62 children, often as the first epileptic manifestation (Kivity & Lerman 1992). The EEG has a normal background with paroxysmal spike wave bursts in the occipital or posterior temporal regions, involving one or both hemispheres. The EEG changes are attenuated by eye opening and unaffected by hyperventilation or photic stimulation. By definition, no structural cerebral pathology should be present in these cases, but patients with similar clinical and EEG features with overt occipital lobe pathology have been reported. The condition responds well to conventional antiepileptic drug treatment and the prognosis is excellent, with remission from seizures in all cases in late adolescence or early adult life, although 5% of cases develop other seizure types later in life.

*Other syndromes of benign partial epilepsy*

A number of other syndromes have been proposed, with the general characteristics of benign partial epilepsy. These include benign partial epilepsy with affective symptoms, benign epilepsy with extreme somatosensory evoked potentials and benign partial epilepsy with frontal spikes.

## 2.6.6 Electrical status epilepticus during slow wave sleep (ESES)

This syndrome was first described in 1971 (Patry et al 1971) and occurred in 0.5% of children with epilepsy (Morikawa et al 1989), although the condition might be detected more often if routine sleep records were more commonly obtained. ESES is defined by the presence on EEG of generalized spike/wave discharges occupying at least 85% of non-REM sleep. The clinical features of the syndrome include seizures, mental retardation and, infrequently, other neurological features. Overt seizures are almost invariable, usually developing between the ages of 1 and 14 years and can take various forms. The sleep-related EEG abnormalities that define the syndrome, however, are not usually associated with any overt clinical seizure activity. Over half of the recorded cases have normal intellectual function prior to the development of ESES, but mental regression subsequently occurs, which is sometimes marked. Language functioning is particularly affected, mutism can develop and also impairments of memory, spatial orientation, hyperkinetic behaviour and psychosis.

Drug treatment may or may not abolish the ESES, although overt seizures are usually helped (Jayakar & Seshia 1991, Yasuhara et al 1991). The seizures and the ESES tend to remit by the age of 15 years, but adults with similar EEG findings are also encountered. The intellectual deficit that develops during the phase of ESES may improve but seldom returns to premorbid levels; indeed, many patients are left with profound mental deterioration.

There are identifiable causes in about 25% of cases, including previous meningitis, birth asphyxia and CMV infection. 3% of children have a family history of epilepsy and 15% a history of febrile convulsions (Morikawa et al 1989). ESES has similarities with and can occur in cases of the Landau–Kleffner syndrome and the Lennox–Gastaut syndrome, and the differentiation of these syndromes can be difficult. The pathophysiological mechanisms of ESES are obscure and its causes diverse, and it remains possible that the ESES pattern is simply an extreme of a spectrum of sleep-activated EEG changes in severe epilepsy.

### 2.6.7 Acquired epileptic aphasia (Landau–Kleffner syndrome; Worster-Drought syndrome)

A syndrome of persisting acquired aphasia associated with severe focal EEG abnormalities was first described by Landau & Kleffner (1957) and Worster-Drought (1971). Since then over 200 cases have been reported (Beaumanoir 1992, Landau 1992). The exact incidence or prevalence of the condition are unknown, but it is an uncommon condition, usually without a family history and with a male preponderance (about 2 : 1). The pathogenesis and pathophysiology are quite unclear (Landau 1992) and reported underlying pathological abnormalities have included non-specific gliosis, possible encephalitis, tumour and vasculitis.

Development is usually previously normal. The aphasia may evolve in a subacute or gradual fashion, over weeks or even several years. In 70% of cases, this develops before the age of 6 years. The speech disorder is usually a disturbance of verbal comprehension in combination with a motor aphasia. An auditory agnosia (word deafness) is also said to occur. In time, there is an almost total mutism. The aphasia may fluctuate in a striking manner, and transient but complete remission of all symptoms may occur. Other clinical features can occur including hyperkinesis, personality disturbances and intellectual deficits. The EEG shows repetitive high voltage spikes or spike/wave discharges with a generalized focal or multifocal distribution, which is activated in slow wave sleep and may attain the continuous or nearly continuous activity of electrographic status.

Overt epileptic seizures are manifest in only about 70% of patients and are usually mild. The epilepsy, but not the EEG disturbance, can usually be controlled by antiepileptic drug treatment.

The prognosis is variable and, although speech and language usually improve, recovery is often incomplete. In some cases speech functions are permanently severely disrupted (Bishop 1985). The EEG abnormalities usually disappear after the resolution of the speech disturbance. Antiepileptic drug or steroid therapy is usually recommended to try to abolish the electrographic changes in the hope that this will ameliorate language (Lerman et al 1991).

### 2.6.8 Lennox–Gastaut syndrome

The nosology of this condition is confused. The clinical and EEG picture can occur in mild and severe forms, can evolve from other types of epilepsy and can be caused by a great number of different pathological disorders. Whether this condition deserves the title 'syndrome' or whether this clinico-electrographic pattern is simply a relatively non-specific developmental response of damaged brain is uncertain. There is however no doubt that patients with this clinical and EEG pattern have a profound epileptic encephalopathy, and the term has acquired wide clinical usage.

The disorder is characterized by severe epilepsy and mental deterioration (Table 2.30). Seizures are frequent and severe and are atypical absence, tonic, myoclonic and tonic-clonic in form (usually in combination). The patients often fall and sustain injury. Overt status epilepticus is common in the condition, with atypical absence, tonic, tonic-clonic, complex partial or minor motor forms. Subclinical status is also a frequent feature of the condition. The age of onset is generally between 1 and 7 years. In a series of 265 patients, (Ohtahara et al 1988) all cases developed epilepsy between the ages of 4 months and 14 years, with the great majority between 11 months and 6 years. However, apparently adult-onset patients are also encountered, as are adult patients with static clinical features who developed the condition in childhood. The condition can develop in patients with infantile spasm or West's syndrome, or partial epilepsy, and there is overlap both clinically and electrographically

**Table 2.30** Features of the Lennox–Gastaut syndrome

- Onset in childhood
- Severe epileptic disorder with multiple seizure types, including myoclonic, atypical absence, tonic and tonic-clonic seizures
- Seizure precipitated by drowsiness or understimulation, not by hyperventilation or photic stimulation
- Progressive mental retardation
- Status epilepticus common (especially non-convulsive forms)
- EEG shows 1–2.5 Hz spike and wave complexes with various other abnormalities and abnormal background rhythms, without photosensitivity
- Many causes, although about 25% are cryptogenic in origin
- Poor response to antiepileptic drug treatment
- Prognosis for seizure control and mental development poor

with the other forms of myoclonic epilepsies, post-traumatic partial epilepsies, ESES and acquired epileptic aphasia.

The characteristic EEG pattern is the 1–2.5 Hz spike/wave complex, which is spread widely in both hemispheres with varying asymmetry, roughly bilaterally synchronous and with a bifrontal predominance. The EEG record can be dominated by these discharges for hours or days at a time. The complexes are rarely induced by hyperventilation or by photic stimulation, in this respect differing from the 3 Hz spike/wave of petit mal, and are enhanced in non-REM sleep. The background activity is slow during wakefulness, and normal arousal and sleep potentials are diminished or absent. Bursts of generalized rhythmic fast spikes often occur during sleep. The ictal and interictal EEG changes may be very similar.

The syndrome has a multitude of causes. In one large series (Ohtahara et al 1988), 26% were cryptogenic, 12% had an identifiable cerebral lesion causing mental retardation, 28% cerebral palsy, 12% were postencephalitic, 8% developed from West's syndrome and 4% had tuberous sclerosis. Other causes included congenital cerebral malformations, chromosomal and inherited metabolic disorders and neurocutaneous syndromes.

The prognosis is dependent upon the underlying aetiology, but in general outcome is poor. Few children acquire a normal intellect and most continue to have epilepsy. Mortality rates will be high if the aetiology is progressive but even in the static encephalopathies the seizures and mental regression usually persist. The seizure disorder usually improves in adult life, although complete remission from epilepsy is rare. Mental retardation persists without progression. About half of the patients surviving into adult life are totally dependent or institutionalized.

## 2.7 THE IDIOPATHIC GENERALIZED EPILEPSIES

The idiopathic generalized epilepsies (IGEs) are a spectrum of epileptic conditions with a genetic basis and characteristic clinical symptoms (Table 2.31). It has been estimated that IGEs comprise 10% of all epilepsies and 40% of those with tonic-clonic seizures. In an epidemiological study of 814 newly diagnosed patients with epilepsy, 66 (8.1%) had IGE, including 13 (1.6%) with childhood absence epilepsy and 9 (1.1%) with juvenile myoclonic epilepsy (Manford et al 1992a).

The syndromes have highly specific clinical and EEG manifestations, and it is quite wrong to allocate any case of epilepsy without a known aetiology to this category; these cases are best categorized as cryptogenic epilepsy. This diagnostic confusion has bedevilled previous literature.

Within the general compass of these conditions, separate subgroups have been identified. Whether these are best considered simply as part of the overall spectrum of IGE or as a series of separate syndromes is controversial (Berkovic et al 1987, Duncan & Panayiotopoulos 1995). Among the recognized subgroups are included childhood absence epilepsy, juvenile absence epilepsy, juvenile myoclonic epilepsy, epilepsy with generalized tonic-clonic seizures on awakening, and epilepsy with myoclonic absences.

**Table 2.31** Features of the idiopathic generalized epilepsies (typical features of the core syndrome – not all features need to be present in any individual case)

- Seizure disorder comprising: generalized tonic-clonic, myoclonic and/or absence seizures
- Seizures may show a marked diurnal pattern
- Seizure precipitated by sleep deprivation, menstruation, fatigue, stress, alcohol, photic stimulation
- Strong genetic basis, with age-specific expression
- Absence of other neurological abnormalities, and normal intelligence
- Generalized EEG changes, typically with 3 Hz spike/wave, with a normal background, no focal features, and with photosensitivity
- Excellent response to specific antiepileptic drug therapy (especially to valproate and the benzodiazepine drugs)

The genetic contribution both to the clinical and electrographic features of IGE has been intensively studied. There is undoubtedly a strong heritable basis. The exact mode of inheritance has not been established and may differ for the various subtypes. It seems likely that some if not all of the IGEs have an autosomal dominant pattern of inheritance with marked age-specific expression. In the common forms of the condition, the genetic expression of both the clinical and electrographic findings is greatest between the ages of 5 and 15 (Ch. 6, 6.4.2). No other aetiological factors should be present in these idiopathic epilepsies. No gross pathological lesion is found in the brains of patients with IGE, although there have been neuropathological studies in 12 cases in which microscopic developmental abnormalities (microdysgenesis) have been found (Meencke 1994). Microdysgenesis is a neuronal migrational defect in which the normal highly ordered layering of the cerebral cortex is lost and in which ectopic neurones lie in abnormal positions, both in the grey and white matter. The findings, however, are controversial, and the status of these neuropathological changes is unclear. Recently more marked neuronal migration defects, subependymal heterotopia, have been reported in patients with an electroclinical diagnosis of typical absences (Fish 1995). The significance of these pathological abnormalities to the aetiology of IGE is uncertain at present.

The pathophysiology of the IGEs and the 3 Hz spike-wave EEG pattern are controversial. The centroencephalic theory proposed that the bilaterally synchronous cortical discharges were due to a dysfunction at the level of thalamus. More recently, Gloor and co-workers have postulated that the primary defect is diffuse cortical hyperexcitability rather than a primary thalamic abnormality, and that the spike-wave patterns are produced by enhanced synchronization. In man, studies of cerebral blood flow using positron emission tomography indicate that the thalamus has a key role in the production of absence seizures (Prevett et al 1995). The current consensus is that the generation of generalized spike wave discharges and typical absences depends on an abnormal synchronized cycling of cortico-thalamic and thalamo-cortical neurones.

It remains uncertain at what site the abnormal cycling is initiated. This could occur in the cortex, on the basis of diffuse hyperexcitability, or in the thalamus. The thalamus certainly has a major role in the synchronization and continuation of spike wave discharges, mediated by activation of $GABA_B$ receptors and low threshold calcium currents (Crunelli & Leresche 1991, Coulter 1995, Bowery et al 1995).

The exact mix of clinical and EEG features depends on the syndromic subgroup. There is a group of patients with rather non-specific features within the general rubric of the condition, and there are others with characteristic patterns, which may be subcategorized; the commonest of these are outlined below. To what extent syndromic subclassification is justified has been the subject of largely inconclusive debate. In all forms, the tonic-clonic seizures are usually relatively infrequent, but myoclonus and absence attacks often occur on a daily basis. The tonic-clonic seizures may be preceded by increasing absence or myoclonus, which may be a useful premonition. (See above, 2.6.1 for Benign neonatal familial convulsions.)

## 2.7.1 Childhood absence epilepsy

*Incidence*

Absences begin between the ages of 3 and 12 years, most usually between 4 and 8 years. The annual incidence is 6–8/100 000 (Loiseau et al 1990). Patients are more commonly female than male and there is a strong genetic predisposition. Monozygotic twins develop absences in 75% of pairs, as do 5% of dizygotic twins (Gedda & Tateralli 1971); 6–8% of the children of patients with childhood absence epilepsy (CAE) develop epilepsy (Beck-Mannagetta et al 1989).

*Clinical features*

Absences may be noted hundreds of times a day (pyknolepsy), last a few seconds, usually less than 15, and comprise a blank stare and unresponsiveness. Discharges lasting less than 3 s may not be noted clinically but are more likely to be identified if the patient is being closely monitored and involved in a continuous performance task. There is a marked but brief loss of awareness, unresponsiveness and cessation of activity. Eye-opening occurs shortly after onset of spike-wave activity and minor orofacial automatisms are frequently seen (Panayiotopoulos et al 1989). There may also be clonic movements of the eyelids, a transient loss of postural tone resulting in the head, limbs or trunk dropping, and sometimes an increase in tone that leads to retropulsion. The absence ends abruptly, with resumption of the previous activity. Absences are usually reliably precipitated by hyperventilation and also by fatigue, emotional upset, boredom and inactivity.

CAE should be distinguished from other syndromes in which absence seizures are a prominent feature, in particular eyelid myoclonia with typical absences, juvenile absence epilepsy (JAE), juvenile myoclonic epilepsy (JME) and absences occurring in patients with fixed and progressive cerebral pathology, such as frontal lesions (Loiseau 1992, Fish 1995).

40% of patients with CAE develop generalized tonic-clonic seizures, often 5–10 years after the onset of the absences (Gastaut & Broughton 1972). Tonic-clonic seizures are more likely to develop if absences begin at an older age, after 8 years, in boys, if absences do not readily come under control and if the EEG shows photosensitivity and an abnormal background activity (Loiseau 1992). It may of course be argued that such patients should be regarded as having some other IGE syndrome, such as JAE, and not CAE.

A small proportion of patients with CAE (3–8%) have been reported to have myoclonic jerks (Janz 1969, Wolf & Inoue 1984). Some patients develop behaviour and conduct disturbance, which is usually attributable to the attitude of parents and peers, and the adverse effects of medication. Intelligence is generally normal, although frequent absences and high concentrations of medication may adversely affect attention and concentration.

*EEG features*

In CAE the EEG shows generalized, bilaterally synchronous and symmetrical 3 Hz spike and slow wave discharges that are of sudden onset and cessation and occur on normal background activity. The frequency of the spike-wave discharge may slow to 2 Hz towards the end of a discharge, and some patients may have polyspikes. The EEG appearances and ready precipitation by hyperventilation should resolve any difficulties with a differential diagnosis from complex partial seizures. About 20% of children with CAE are photosensitive (Wolf & Goosses 1986).

*Prognosis*

In patients with CAE, absences become less frequent through adolescence and about 80% remit by adulthood. If remission occurs in CAE, it is usually long-lasting and the risk of relapse on tapering AEDs after seizure control for 2–3 years is small (see also Ch. 4, 4.6 and Ch. 8, 8.1.4).

## 2.7.2 Juvenile absence epilepsy

*Incidence*

Juvenile absence epilepsy (JAE) is approximately one-quarter as common as CAE and has an equal gender predominance. One patient in three has a first-degree relative with epilepsy. The age of onset has in many studies been arbitrarily set at 10 years. In contrast, Wolf & Inoue (1984) defined their patient group by the type of seizure, and noted onset of absences at 2–47 years.

*Clinical features*

Absences tend to be less frequent than in CAE, but of longer duration and associated with a less profound impairment of consciousness. About 1 patient in 20 has automatisms as part of the absence (Panayiotopoulos et al 1989).

16% of patients with JAE have myoclonic seizures (Wolf & Inoue 1984). Up to 80% of patients with JAE develop generalized tonic-clonic seizures. In these patients the tonic-clonic seizures most commonly (75%) occur on awakening, with the remainder occurring during sleep (14%) or at any time (11%) (Janz 1969). In some patients, the onset of generalized tonic-clonic seizures precedes the onset of absences, although interpretation must be cautious as the initial absences may have passed unrecognized. In patients with generalized tonic-clonic seizures on awakening and absences it may difficult to decide whether to regard the diagnosis as JAE or generalized tonic-clonic seizures on awakening. This evidence of an overlap would be in keeping with the concept of there being a neurobiological continuum of IGE syndromes.

*EEG appearance*

The background activity is normal. Generalized spike-wave discharges with some frontal predominance occur with a frequency of 3.5–4 Hz, commonly with some slowing of the rate during a discharge. Slow waves may be led by two or three spikes. Discharges of spike-wave are readily precipitated by hyperventilation and by sleep deprivation. Between 10% and 20% of patients with JAE are photosensitive.

*Prognosis*

As with CAE, about 80% of patients with JAE become seizure free with medication. Both absences and generalized tonic-clonic seizures may, however, persist into adulthood. The risk of relapse on subsequent withdrawal of medication is not clearly defined. The clinical and EEG features of JAE place it between CAE and JME, if one accepts the hypothesis of a biological continuum of the various IGE syndromes. In this case, the risk of relapse after 2–3 years freedom from seizures, on medication, is probably between the 10–15% of CAE and the 80–90% of JME, should medication be withdrawn (see also Ch. 4, 4.6 and Ch. 8, 8.1.4).

### 2.7.3 Juvenile myoclonic epilepsy

*Incidence*

Juvenile myoclonic epilepsy comprises 5–10% of cases of epilepsy. The nature of the continuous spectrum of the IGE syndromes, the overlap between them and the likelihood of polygenic inheritance is underlined by the common finding of first-degree relatives each with different subtypes (Greenberg et al 1989, Delgado-Escueta et al 1990) (Ch. 6, 6.4.2).

*Clinical features*

A common presentation is of a teenager who has his first generalized tonic-clonic seizure on awaking, after little sleep, following a late-night party at which he consumed a large amount of alcohol. Enquiry often then reveals a history of early morning myoclonic jerks over the previous months and years.

Three types of seizures occur: myoclonic jerks, generalized tonic-clonic seizures and, in one-third of patients, typical absences. Typical absences usually appear first, at about 10 years of age, followed by myoclonic jerks 1–9 years later and generalized tonic-clonic seizures 1–2 years after that.

The myoclonic seizures may be unilateral or bilateral, predominantly affecting the upper limbs, proximally and distally. The severity of myoclonic seizures is very variable. Severe myoclonic jerks may cause the patient to fall, and mild jerks may be attributed to a tremor. Consciousness is not impaired during the myoclonic seizures of JME, but may be mildly affected if these occur in series, a situation that often results in a generalized tonic-clonic seizure.

Myoclonic and generalized tonic-clonic seizures are precipitated by sleep deprivation and alcohol. Flashing lights and electronic screens may precipitate seizures in the 50% of patients with JME who are photosensitive (Panayiotopoulos et al 1994). There is often a clear diurnal pattern, with myoclonic jerks and generalized tonic-clonic seizures frequently occurring within an hour of awaking. Patients may not regard early morning twitches of the limbs as significant and it is often helpful to imitate myoclonic jerks and to ask specifically whether they are clumsy and jittery on awaking and have difficulty with shaving or carrying a cup of coffee.

Absences in patients with JME may initially resemble those of CAE, but automatisms are very rare and there is incomplete loss of awareness (Panayiotopoulos et al 1989, Janz & Waltz 1995). In older patients, absences appear to become milder and infrequent, often being attributed to brief daydreams and lapses of concentration.

Patients have a normal intellect and no neurological deficit. The picture may be confused, however, by the iatrogenic effects of antiepileptic drugs and by brain injuries, which may result in the development of cognitive and behavioural impairment and ataxia that can produce a superficial similarity to the syndrome of progressive myoclonic epilepsy (see below, 2.8).

*EEG features*

The EEG shows 4–6 Hz polyspike and slow-wave generalized discharges that last up to 20 s with normal background activity. The number and size of the spikes is variable. The frequency of the discharge is fastest at the outset, but unlike JAE there is no gradual slowing (Panayiotopoulos et al 1989). The discharge commonly fragments as it develops. Discharges are provoked by hyperventilation and half of patients show photoconvulsive responses. More than 50% of patients have focal abnormalities on their EEGs, comprising focal slow waves, spikes or sharp waves, or asymmetry of generalized discharges (Panayiotopoulos et al 1994).

Treatment with sodium valproate frequently normalizes the EEG, but abnormalities may often be apparent on recordings undertaken in sleep and on awakening, particularly if the patient has been deprived of sleep.

*Prognosis*

Up to 90% of patients with JME become seizure-free with optimal medication. There is a very high relapse rate if medication is subsequently withdrawn, even if the patient has been seizure-free for several years. The prognosis for a relapse in patients in their forties, however, has not been studied in detail and is uncertain at the present time (Grunewald & Panayiotopoulos 1993).

### 2.7.4 Epilepsy with generalized tonic-clonic seizures on awakening

*Incidence*

Five studies have reported 16–50% of generalized tonic-clonic seizures as occurring on awaking. These reports, however, are difficult to compare because of methodological differences with regard to definitions and patient selection (Janz 1969). There is a slight male predominance and a positive history in 12% of cases (Wolf 1992b).

*Clinical features*

The age of onset is usually between 9 and 25 years, with a peak at the time of puberty. About 50% of patients have absences and 30% have myoclonic seizures. Generalized tonic-clonic seizures occur without an aura, but may be preceded by absences or myoclonic seizures. This may take the form of serial absences resulting in absence status, or serial myoclonic jerks.

The usual definition of seizures on awaking is taken as 'within 2 h of waking from sleep, whatever time of day this occurs. In addition to the association with awaking, seizures may be precipitated by sleep deprivation and by alcohol, and not uncommonly occur in a period of relaxation in the evening. Neurological and psychological examination is unremarkable.

The distinction from JME may be very difficult as generalized tonic-clonic seizures, myoclonic seizures and absences occurring principally on waking are common to both subtypes of IGE. The distinction is often made according to which seizure type developed first. In practical terms, many patients have features that overlap both JME and generalized tonic-clonic seizures on awakening and these probably represent part of the biological continuum of IGE.

*EEG features*

The EEG shows generalized spike-wave activity at 2.5–4 Hz and polyspike and wave activity, particularly on going to sleep and awaking and with enhancement by hyperventilation in some patients. In one study, 13% were photosensitive (Wolf 1992b). Interpretation of these data is difficult without knowing the treatment status of the patients, as valproate will frequently suppress these features.

*Prognosis*

Seizures are controlled with medication in 65% of patients and, similarly to JME, there is a high relapse rate of over 80% if medication is subsequently tapered in patients who have become seizure free (Janz 1969, Janz et al 1983). This fact underlines the need to make a careful syndromic diagnosis when considering patients' antiepileptic drug treatment.

### 2.7.5 Eyelid myoclonia with typical absences

*Clinical features*

Eyelid myoclonia with typical absences (EMA) is an IGE syndrome that is not yet recognized by the ILAE, and underlies the need not to regard typical absences as a single diagnosis (Jeavons 1977, Appleton et al 1993).

EMA is similar to CAE in that typical absences begin in childhood, at a frequency of hundreds per day, with clonic retropulsion of the eyelids and eyes and 3–4 Hz spike and slow-wave discharges. There are, however, clear differences between EMA and CAE. In the former, absences are very short, impairment of consciousness may be mild and eyelid myoclonia is a consistent feature. Eyelid myoclonia consists of rapid clonic eyelid movements with a tonic component of contraction, in contrast to eyelid-blinking-like movements that occur in CAE. Absences are often precipitated by eye closure and patients are usually photosensitive. Most patients with EMA also have generalized tonic-clonic seizures.

*EEG appearance*

The EEG shows polyspike/slow-wave complexes that is often faster than 3 Hz, with discharges being brought on by eye closure.

*Prognosis*

Patients with EMA often continue to have some seizures, even if medication is effective at reducing the frequency of attacks. The condition does not appear to remit in adolescence, but there have not been sufficient long term studies to allow predictions of the prognosis through adulthood.

### 2.7.6 Epilepsy with myoclonic absences

This rare syndrome develops in children (mean age 7 years) with a male preponderance (Tassinari et al 1992). Absences are accompanied by severe bilateral rhythmical myoclonias, causing rhythmic jerking of the shoulders, head or limbs and staggering. Falls occur rarely, but incontinence is common. About 50% of cases show pre-existing mental retardation. The interictal EEG is normal, and the ictal EEG shows 3 Hz spike-wave discharges, similar to those of childhood absence epilepsy. Associated generalized tonic-clonic seizures are common, and in about one-third of cases absence or myoclonic status develops. In some cases, the clinical picture evolves to resemble that of the Lennox–Gastaut syndrome. The nosological position of this syndrome is controversial, and there are features outside the usual spectrum of IGE.

### 2.7.7 Benign myoclonic epilepsy of infancy

This is a rare cause of myoclonus with onset between 16–24 months of life, without other neurological features, and with a normal interictal EEG. The myoclonus may be initially imperceptible but frequent, most attacks lasting 1–3 seconds and being accompanied by spikewave or polyspike discharges on the EEG. Other seizure types do not develop, but there is often a family history of IGE. Treatment is not always required, but the myoclonus will usually be easily controlled by valproate or benzodiazepines. The prognosis is good, most cases remitting spontaneously, but other seizure types may develop later in life.

### 2.7.8 Benign familial myoclonus

This is a rare condition that develops in childhood or early adult life (the average age of onset is 10 years), inherited as an autosomal dominant, at least in some families. The myoclonus is massive and symmetrical and involves the axial and proximal limb muscles initially, becoming more widespread. The myoclonus is often stimulus-sensitive and worsened by stress or fatigue. There are no other neurological abnormalities, the EEG is normal and other seizure types do not develop. If medical therapy is required, valproate or benzodiazepines are the initial choice.

### 2.7.9 Perioral myoclonia with absences

Perioral myoclonia with absences has been recently described (Panayiotopoulos et al 1993) and is not yet recognized by the ILAE. Perioral myoclonus consisting of rhythmic lip protrusion occurs at the time of absences. The small number of patients described with this feature appear to be resistant to antiepileptic drug treatment.

## 2.8 PROGRESSIVE MYOCLONIC EPILEPSY

Progressive myoclonic epilepsy (PME) comprise rare conditions that are characterized by the development of relentlessly progressive myoclonus, dementia, ataxia and other neurological signs. There are a number of well defined aetiologies.

In the initial evaluation of a patient it must be recalled that myoclonus may be a feature of many different forms of epilepsy (Table 2.32), notably IGE, and other cerebral pathologies such as Creutzfeldt–Jakob disease, and may also arise at reticular and spinal level. The term PME should be confined to those cases in which the predominant and initial clinical symptom is myoclonus, and distinguished from other progressive encephalopathies with myoclonus or the progressive myoclonic ataxias (Berkovic & Andermann 1986, Berkovic et al 1989, So et al 1989). Progressive myoclonic epilepsy should be considered when other aetiologies are not apparent and when there is evidence of progression of the clinical condition. It may be difficult to decide early on in a patient's clinical course whether or not deterioration is occurring and re-evaluation after an interval may be very necessary. Conversely, patients with non-progressive conditions such as IGE who are treated with intoxicating doses of AEDs, particularly phenytoin, may appear superficially to have a progressive ataxia, which is iatrogenic and reversible.

The myoclonus is erratic, generalized, multifocal or asymmetrical, and affects limbs and trunk and facial musculature. The myoclonus becomes continuous for long periods of time and is often exacerbated by action or startle. The myoclonus is of cortical origin, often with time-locked EEG potentials. Sometimes a massive increase in the frequency and amplitude of the myoclonus is produced by movement, which may be misinterpreted as a tonic-clonic seizure (the preservation of consciousness should help differentiate these states). Eventually, in some cases, the myoclonus reaches devastating proportions, rendering the patient bed-bound and severely disabled. Focal or restricted myoclonus is much less common. Other seizure types can develop, although these are not generally a serious clinical problem. The occurrence of other neurological features and the severity and rate of progression of the cognitive and neurological deterioration depend on the underlying cause. A causal diagnosis is usually made on the

**Table 2.32** Conditions with myoclonus as a prominent feature

| | |
|---|---|
| *Idiopathic generalized epilepsies* | *Infective* |
| Childhood absence epilepsy | Subacute sclerosing panencephalitis |
| Juvenile absence epilespy | Acute viral encephalitis |
| Juvenile myoclonic epilepsy | Creutzfeldt–Jakob disease |
| Epilepsy with generalized tonic-clonic seizures on awakening | *Other symptomatic or systemic causes* |
| Epilepsy with myoclonic absences | Postanoxic myoclonic epilepsy |
| Benign myoclonus of infancy | Toxic: lead and other poisons, drugs |
| *Childhood myoclonic epilepsies* | Metabolic: renal disease, hepatic disease |
| Infantile spasms | Respiratory disease with hypercapnia |
| Lennox–Gastaut syndrome | *Withdrawal of sedative drugs* |
| Cryptogenic myoclonic epilepsy | Barbiturates, benzodiazepines, alcohol |
| *Progressive myoclonic epilepsies* | |
| Unverricht–Lundborg disease (Baltic myoclonus) | |
| Lafora body disease | |
| Mitochondrial cytopathy (MERRF) | |
| Sialidoses | |
| Ceroid lipofuscinosis | |
| GM1 and GM2 gangliosidoses | |
| Gaucher's disease | |
| Dentato-rubro-pallido-luysian atrophy | |
| Hallervorden–Spatz syndrome | |
| Huntington's disease | |
| Juvenile neuroaxonal dystrophy | |
| Alper's disease | |
| Benign familial myoclonic epilepsy | |
| Menkes disease | |
| Phenylketonuria | |
| Biotin-responsive progressive myoclonus | |

basis of the family history, the age of onset, the rate of progression, the occurrence of associated neurological symptoms and the results of electrodiagnostic tests, imaging and biopsy material (see Ch. 3, 3.7.5 for details of the investigatory strategies to follow in patients with PME).

The EEG in PME usually shows generalized spike or polyspike and slow wave discharges and photosensitivity is often present. There is slowing of the background activity, reflecting the underlying progressive disorder. The EEG patterns do not help to distinguish the different aetiologies.

### 2.8.1 Lafora body disease

The age of onset of Lafora body disease is between 6 and 19 years. Progressive myoclonus is associated with tonic-clonic and partial seizures (the latter often having visual symptomatology) and severe dementia, often with focal cognitive features. Ataxia and dysarthria are common additional features. The clinical course is erratic, with periods of sudden deterioration, but relentless, and death occurs within 10 years of onset. The EEG shows progressive changes, often with focal occipital spike discharges, although these and other EEG findings do not reliably distinguish one form of PME from another. The diagnosis can be confirmed by axillary skin, muscle or liver biopsy. The histopathological marker is the presence of Lafora bodies, which are widespread in brain, skin, muscle and liver. These inclusion bodies are polyglycan deposits, but the underlying enzymic defect has not yet been characterized. The condition is probably inherited by an autosomal recessive mechanism.

### 2.8.2 Unverricht–Lundborg disease

The onset is between the ages of 6 and 15, with an equal sex distribution but marked geographic variation. It is an autosomal recessive condition. Linkage studies have placed the gene on chromosome 21 (Ch. 6, 6.4.1). It presents as myoclonus, initially easy to control but then progressively worsening. Tonic-clonic seizures are infrequent, but ataxia and tremor develop and may become predominant. Slow intellectual decline occurs, but not severe, rapidly developing dementia as is seen in Lafora body disease. The mean duration of the illness is 14 years, death usually occurring in the third decade of life. Investigations fail to reveal a positive cause and the diagnosis is made by exclusion. It is said, on the basis of tenuous evidence, that phenytoin worsens the condition, and this drug should therefore probably not be used in treatment.

### 2.8.3 Mitochondrial disease

Maternally inherited defects in mitochondrial metabolism can produce the myoclonic epilepsy and ragged red fibres (MERRF) syndrome. The clinical form is variable, with onset of symptoms during childhood or adult life. The myoclonus is associated with ataxia in most cases and less consistently with tonic-clonic seizures and dementia. Numerous ass-ociated features have been described in some cases, including short stature, deafness, optic atrophy, endocrine dysfunction, pes cavus and other congenital anomalies, peripheral neuropathy and myopathy. None is consistent, and the diagnosis is made by detecting the leucocyte-mitochondrial DNA mutation and by the characteristic findings of ragged red fibres on muscle biopsy; although occasionally these may not be present. There may be a range of specific mitochondrial defects and genetic mosaicism. The condition is progressive, but the rate of progression varies considerably.

### 2.8.4 Neuronal ceroid lipofuscinosis

Neuronal ceroid lipofuscinosis is an enzyme deficiency, generally inherited autosomal recessively, in which lysosomal inclusions are found in lymphocytes, skin, muscle, liver and brain. The inclusions autofluoresce in ultraviolet light and the storage material comprises excessive amounts of long-chain polyisoprenyl alcohols (dolichols). On electron microscopy there are two types of inclusion: an amorphous osmiophilic granular body and lamellated bodies with a characteristic fingerprint or curvilinear pattern. Electroretinography and evoked potential studies may help define the condition. A definitive diagnosis, however, is made by the examination of lymphocytes and biopsy material (Ch. 3, 3.7.4). The form of the disease differs at different ages of onset.

*The infantile form (Santavuori disease)* has its onset before the age of 2 years, is rapidly progressive and death occurs before the age of 10. It is characterized by myoclonus, developmental regression, ataxia, hypotonia and blindness. Electroretinogram and visual evoked responses (VERs) are helpful diagnostically. Biopsy shows granular body inclusions.

*The late infantile form (Bielschowski–Janski disease)* is the most common form, with onset between the ages of 2 and 4 years. It presents with myoclonus and other seizure types, and then progressive ataxia, spasticity and dementia develop. Death occurs before the age of 10 years. Biopsy usually shows lamellated inclusions with curvilinear and fingerprint inclusions.

*Juvenile neuronal ceroid lipofuscinosis (Batten disease or Spielmeyer–Vogt disease)* is also a common form. The onset is between the ages of 4 and 15 years, and 60% of patients present with visual loss. Progressive massive myoclonus develops with other epileptic manifestations within 1–4 years of the onset of the condition. Dementia is an early sign, but is usually relatively mild, and extrapyramidal and cerebellar signs and then pyramidal motor signs develop as the condition progresses. Dysarthria is common and the patients develop a characteristic stooped gait before becoming wheelchair-bound. Psychotic and other psychiatric symptoms may complicate the progressive course. Death usually occurs by the age of 20 years. The diagnosis can be made by the finding of abnormal storage and vacuolization in lymphocytes and by fingerprint membranous profiles on EM studies of skin or muscle biopsy.

*Adult-onset neuronal ceroid lipofuscinosis (Kufs disease)* presents as progressive myoclonus with prominent dementia, and other signs such as seizures, ataxia, pyramidal and extra-pyramidal signs, including choreoathetosis, are common. Motor signs are prominent but visual loss is not, in contrast to the forms in younger age groups. The progression is rapid and death usually occurs within 10 years. The diagnosis is made by the demonstration of abnormal deposits and osmiophilic granular bodies on liver, muscle or brain biopsy.

### 2.8.5 Dentato-rubro-pallido-luysian atrophy (DRPLA)

This autosomal dominant condition is a comparatively common form of PME in Japan, although also occurring in other parts of the world. The condition can develop in childhood or adult life and is slowly progressive. The presenting symptoms can vary within one affected family. About 50% of cases present as a progressive myoclonic epilepsy. Dementia and cerebellar ataxia are prominent and other pyramidal and extrapyramidal motor signs and psychiatric disturbance also develop. The diagnosis is made by the characteristic pattern of brainstem, basal ganglia and cerebral atrophy on MRI scanning.

### 2.8.6 Other causes of progressive myoclonic epilepsy

There are a number of other causes of the syndrome, each of which is rare. These include other lysosomal storage diseases such as sialidosis (types I and II), Gaucher's disease, $GM_2$ gangliosidosis, juvenile neuroaxonal dystrophy, poliodystrophy, Huntington's disease, biotin-responsive progressive myoclonus, childhood Huntington's disease, action myoclonus/renal failure syndrome, and Hallervorden–Spatz syndrome. In half the patients encountered in our own adult neurological practice, however, no specific cause can be found despite detailed investigation.

## REFERENCES


Aicardi J 1992 Diseases of the nervous system in childhood. Clinics in Developmental Medicine No. 115/118. Blackwell, Oxford

Aicardi J, Chevrie JJ 1970 Convulsive status epilepticus in infants and children. Epilepsia 11: 187–197

Aicardi J, Chevrie JJ 1983 Consequences of status epilepticus in infants and children. In: Delgado-Escueta AV, Wasterlain CG, Treiman DM, Porter RJ (eds) Status epilepticus. Mechanisms of brain damage and treatment. Advances in neurology 34. Raven Press, New York, p 115–128

Aicardi J, Goutieres F 1978 Encephalopathie myoclonique neonatale. Rev d'Electroencephal Neurophysiol Clin 8: 99–101

Alajouanine T, Gastaut H 1955 La syncinésie-sursaut et l'epilepsie-sursaut a declanchement sensoriel ou sensitif inopine. Rev Neurolog 93: 29–40

Alexander GL 1972 Sturge–Weber syndrome. In: Vinken PJ, Bruyn GW (eds) The phakomatoses. Handbook of clinical neurology, vol 14. North-Holland, Amsterdam, p 223–240

Alldredge BK, Lowenstein DH, Simon RP 1989 Seizures associated with recreational drug abuse. Neurology 39: 1037–1039

Andermann F, Andermann E 1986 Excessive startle syndromes: startle disease, jumping and startle epilepsy. In: Fahn S, Marsden CD, von Woert MH (eds) Myclonus. Advances in neurology 43. Raven Press, New York, p 321–338.

Annegers JF, Grabow JD, Groover RV, Laws ER, Elveback LR, Kurland LT 1980 Seizures after head trauma: a population study. Neurology 30: 683–689

Annegers JF, Hauser WA, Shirts SB, Kurland LT 1987 Factors prognostic of unprovoked seizures after febrile convulsions. N Engl J Med 316: 493–498

Anonymous 1989 Neonatal seizures. Lancet 2: 135–137

Appleton R, Panayiotopoulos CP, Acomb AB et al 1993 Eyelid myoclonia with absences: an epilepsy syndrome. J Neurol Neurosurg Psychiat 56: 1312–1316

Asconape J, Penry JK 1984 Some clinical and EEG aspects of benign juvenile myoclonic epilepsy. Epilepsia 25: 108–114

Bancaud J, Talaraich J, Lamarche M, Bonis A, Trottier S 1975 Hypothèses neuro-physiopathologiques sur l'épilepsie-sursaut chez l'homme. Rev Neurolog 117: 441–453

Barkovich AJ, Gressens P, Evrard P 1992 Formation, maturation, and disorders of brain neocortex. Am J Neuroradiol 13: 423–446

Beaumanoir A 1992 The Landau–Kleffner syndrome. In: Roger J, Bureau M, Dravet C, Dreifuss FE, Perret A, Wolf P (eds) Epileptic syndromes in infancy, childhood and adolescence, 2nd edn. John Libbey, London, p 231–244

Beck-Mannagetta G, Janz D, Hoffmeister G, Behl I. Scholz G 1989 Morbidity risk for seizures and epilepsy in offspring of patients with epilepsy. In: Beck-Mannagetta G, Anderson VE, Doose H, Janz D (eds) Genetics of the epilepsies. Springer-Verlag, Berlin, p 119–126

Berg AT, Shinnar S, Hauser WA et al 1992 A prospective study of recurrent febrile seizures. N Engl J Med 327: 1122–1127

Bergamasco B, Benna P, Ferrero P et al 1984 Neonatal hypoxia and epileptic risk. Epilepsia 25: 131–136

Berkovic SF, Andermann F 1986 The progressive myoclonus epilepsies. In: Pedley TA, Meldrum BS (eds) Recent advances in epilepsy 3. Churchill Livingstone, Edinburgh, p 157–187

Berkovic SF, Andermann F, Andermann E, Gloor P. 1987 Concepts of absence epilepsy: discrete syndromes or biological continuum? Neurology 37: 993–1000

Berkovic S, Carpenter S, Evans A et al 1989 Myoclonus epilepsy and ragged red fibres 1. A clinical, pathological, biochemical, magnetic resonance spectrographic and positron emission tomographic study. Brain 112: 1231–1260

Bishop DVM 1985 Age at onset and outcome in 'acquired aphasia with convulsive disorder' (Landau–Kleffner syndrome). Develop Med Child Neurol 27: 705–712

Bittencourt P, Gracia CM, Lorenzana P 1988 Epilepsy and parasitosis of the central nervous system. In: Pedley TA, Meldrum BS, eds. Recent advances in epilepsy 4. Churchill Livingstone, Edinburgh, p 123–160

Blume WT, David RB, Gomez MR. 1973 Generalised sharp and slow wave complexes. Associated clinical features and long term follow up. Brain 96: 289–306

Boudouresques J, Khalil R, Roger J et al 1980 Etat de mal epileptique et sclerose en plaques. Rev Neurolog 136: 777–782

Boston Collaborative Drug Surveillence Program 1972 Drug induced convulsions. Lancet 2: 677–679

Bowery NG, Richards DA, Lemos T, Whitton PS 1995 GABA transmission in absence epilepsy. In: Duncan JS, Panayiotopoulos CP (eds) Typical absences and related epileptic syndromes. Churchill Livingstone, Edinburgh, p 51–58

Bowie C 1990 Lessons from the pertussis vaccine court trial. Lancet 1: 397–399

Brennan FN, Lyttle JA 1987 Alcohol and seizures: a review. J Roy Soc Med 80: 571–573

Brett EM (ed.) 1991 Neurocutaneous syndromes. In: Brett EM (ed) Paediatric neurology. Churchill Livingstone, Edinburgh, p 571-591

Cabral R, King TT, Scott DF 1976 Epilepsy after two different neurosurgical approaches to the treatment of ruptured intracranial aneurysms. J Neurol Neurosurg Psychiat 39: 1052–1060

Camfield PR, Camfield CS 1987 Neonatal seizures: a commentary on selected aspects. J Child Neurol 2: 244–251

Caveness WF, Meirowski AM, Rish BL et al 1979 The nature of post-traumatic epilepsy. J Neurosurg 50: 545–553

Chauvel P, Delgado-Escueta A, Halgren E, Bancaud J 1992a Frontal lobe seizures and epilepsies. Advances in neurology 57. Raven Press, New York

Chauvel P, Trottier S, Vignal JP, Bancaud J 1992b Somatosensory seizures of frontal lobe origin. In: Chauvel P, Delgado-Escueta A, Halgren E, Bancaud J (eds) Frontal lobe seizures and epilepsies. Advances in neurology 57. Raven Press, New York, p 185–232

Chevrie JJ, Aicardi J 1972 Childhood epileptic encephalopathy with slow spike-wave. A statistical study of 80 cases. Epilepsia 13: 259–271

Clancy RR, Legido A, Lewis D 1988 Occult neonatal seizures. Epilepsia 29: 256–261

Cocito L, Favale E, Reni L 1982 Epileptic seizures in cerebral arterial occlusive disease. Stroke 13: 189–195

Commission on Classification and Terminology of the International League Against Epilepsy 1981 Proposal for revised clinical and electroencephalographic classification of epileptic seizures. Epilepsia 22: 489–501

Commission on Classification and Terminology of the International League Against Epilepsy 1989 Proposal for revised classification of epilepsies and epileptic syndromes. Epilepsia 30: 389–399

Cook MJ, Free SL, Fish DR, Shorvon SD, Straughan K, Stevens JM 1994 Analysis of cortical pattern. In: Shorvon SD, Fish DR, Andermann F, Bydder G, Stefan H (eds) Magnetic resonance scanning and epilepsy. Plenum Press, London, p 255–257

Coulter D 1986 Continuous infantile spasms as a form of status epilepticus. J Child Neurol 1: 215–217

Coulter DA 1995 Neurophysiological studies in animal models of absence. In: Duncan JS, Panayiotopoulos CP (eds) Typical absences and related epileptic syndromes. Churchill Livingstone, Edinburgh, p 19–28

Crawford PM, West CR, Shaw MDM, Chadwick DW 1986 Cerebral arteriovenous malformations and epilepsy: factors in the development of epilepsy. Epilepsia 27: 270–275

Crunelli V, Leresche N 1991 A role for GABAB receptors in excitation and inhibition of thalamocortical cells. Trends Neurosci 14: 18–21

Dalla Bernadina B, Fontana E, Sgro V, Colamaria V, Elia M 1992 Myoclonic epilepsy (myoclonic status) in non-progressive encephalopathies. In: Roger J, Bureau M, Dravet C, Dreifuss FE, Perret A, Wolf P (eds) Epileptic syndromes in infancy, childhood and adolescence, 2nd edn. John Libbey, London, p 89–96

Dan NQ, Wade MJ 1986 The incidence of epilepsy after ventricular shunting procedures. J Neurosurg 65: 19–21

Danner R, Shewmon A, Sherman MP 1985 Seizures in an atelencephalic infant: is the cortex essential for neonatal seizures? Arch Neurol 42: 1014–1016

Delgado-Escueta AV, Bascal FE, Treiman DM 1982 Complex partial seizures on closed circuit television and EEG: a study of 691 attacks in 79 patients. Ann Neurol 11: 292–300

Delgado-Escueta AV, Greenberg DA, Weissbecker K et al 1990 Gene mapping in the idiopathic generalized epilepsies: juvenile myoclonic epilepsy, epilepsy with grand mal seizures and early childhood myoclonic epilepsy. Epilepsia 31(suppl 3): S19–S29

Denning TR, Berrios GE, Walshe JM 1988 Wilson's disease and epilepsy. Brain 111: 1139–1155
Devetag F, Mandich G, Zaiotti G, Toffolo GG 1983 Alcoholic epilepsy: a review of cases and proposed classification and etiopathogenesis. Ital J Med Sci 3: 275–284
Doose H 1992 Myoclonic astatic epilepsy of early childhood. In: Roger J, Bureau M, Dravet C, Dreifuss FE, Perret A, Wolf P (eds) Epileptic syndromes in infancy, childhood and adolescence, 2nd edn. John Libbey, London, p 103–114
Dravet C, Bureau M 1981 L'épilepsie myoclonique bénigne du nourisson. Rev d'Electroencephalog Neurophysiol Clin 11: 438–444
Dulac O, Plouin P, Jambaque I, Motte J 1986 Spasmes infantiles epileptiques bénins. Rev d'Electroencephalog Neurophysiol Clin 16: 371–382
Duncan JS 1988 Neuropsychiatric aspects of sedative drug withdrawal. Hum Psychopharmacol 3: 171–180
Duncan JS, Panayiotopoulos CP 1995 Typical absences and related epileptic syndromes. Churchill Livingstone, Edinburgh
Duncan JS, Sagar HJ 1987 Seizure characteristics, pathology and outcome after temporal lobectomy. Neurology 37: 405–409
Dwyer BE, Wasterlain CG 1983 Regulation of brain protein synthesis during status epilepticus. In: Delgado-Escueta AV, Wasterlain CG, Treiman DM, Porter RJ (eds) Status epilepticus. Mechanisms of brain damage and treatment. Advances in neurology 34. Raven Press, New York, p 297–304
Earnest MP, Yarnell PR 1976 Seizure admissions to a city hospital: the role of alcohol. Epilepsia 17: 387–393
Eriksson M, Zetterstrom R 1979 Neonatal convulsions. Acta Paediat Scand 68: 807–811
Eyre JA, Cozeer RC, Wilkinson AR 1983 Diagnosis of neonatal seizure by continuous recording and rapid analysis of the electroencephalogram. Arch Dis Child 58: 785–790
Faught E, Peters D, Bartolucci A, Moore L, Miller PC 1989 Seizures after primary intracerebral haemorrhage. Neurology 39: 1089–1093
Fenichel GM 1985 Neonatal neurology. Churchill Livingstone, New York
Fiol ME, Leppik IE, Pretzel KL 1986 Eating epilepsy: electroencephalographic and clinical study. Epilepsia 27: 441–445
Fish DR 1995 Blank spells that are not typical absences. In: Duncan JS, Panayiotopoulos CP (eds) Typical absences and related epileptic syndromes. Churchill Livingstone, Edinburgh, p 253–262
Fish DR, Miller DH, Roberts RC, Blackie JD, Gilliatt RW 1989 The natural history of late-onset epilepsy secondary to vascular disease. Acta Neurol Scand 80: 524–528
Fish DR, Quirk JA, Smith SJM, Sander JWAS, Shorvon SD 1994 National survey of photosensitivity and seizures induced by electronic screen games (video games, console games, computer games). Department of Trade and Industry, HMSO, London
Forsgren L, Edvinsson S-O, Blomquist HK, Heijbel J, Sidenvall R 1990 Epilepsy in a population of mentally retarded children and adults. Epilepsy Research 6: 234–248
Forster FM 1977 Reflex epilepsy, behavioural therapy and conditional reflexes. Charles C Thomas, Springfield, IL
Foster B 1942 Association between convulsive seizures and rheumatic heart disease. Arch Neurol Psychiat 47: 254–264
Foy PM, Copeland GP, Shaw MDM 1981 The incidence of post-operative seizures. Acta Neurochirurgia 55: 253–264
Furman JRM, Crumrine PK, Reinmuth OM 1990 Epileptic nystagmus. Ann Neurol 27: 686–688
Gale JL, Thapa PB, Wassilak SGF, Bobo JK, Mendelman PM, Foy HM 1994 Risk of serious acute neurological illness after immunisation with diphtheria–tetanus–pertussis vaccine. JAMA 271: 37–41
Gannicliffe A, Saldanha JA, Itzhaki RF, Sutton RNP 1985 Herpes simplex viral DNA in temporal lobe epilepsy. Lancet 1: 214–215
Gastaut H 1970 Clinical and electroencephalographical classification of epileptic seizures. Epilepsia 11: 102–113
Gastaut H, Broughton R 1972 Epileptic seizures: clinical and electroencephalographic features, diagnosis and treatment. Charles C Thomas, Springfield IL, p 64–85
Gastaut H, Tassinari CA 1966 Triggering mechanisms in epilepsy. The electroclinical point of view. Epilepsia 7: 85–138
Gastaut H, Roger J, Soulayrol R et al 1966 Childhood epileptic encephalopathy with diffuse slow spike waves (otherwise known as 'petit mal variant') or Lennox syndrome. Epilepsia 7: 139–179
Gedda L, Tateralli R 1971 Essential isochronic epilepsy in MZ twin pairs. Acta Genet Med 20: 380–383
Ghezzi A, Montanini R, Basso PF et al 1990 Epilepsy in multiple sclerosis. Eur Neurol 30: 218–223

Gibbs FA, Gibbs EL 1952 Atlas of encephalography, vol. 2. Epilepsy, 2nd edn. Addison Wesley, Cambridge, MA

Gloor P 1979 Generalised epilepsy with spike wave discharge: a reinterpretation of its electrographic and clinical manifestations. Epilepsia 20: 271–288

Gloor P 1991 Mesial temporal sclerosis: historical background and an overview from a modern perspective. In: Luders HO (ed) Epilepsy surgery. Raven Press, New York, p689–703

Gomez MR 1988 Tuberous sclerosis, 2nd edn. Raven Press, New York

Gowers WR 1881 Epilepsy and other chronic convulsive disorders. Churchill, London

Greenberg DA, Delgado-Escueta AV, Widelitz H, Abud P, Park MS 1989 Strengthened evidence for linkage of juvenile myoclonic epilepsy to HLA and BF: Human Gene Mapping Workshop 10. Cytogenet Cell Genet 51: 1008

Grunewald RA, Panayiotopoulos CP 1993 Juvenile myoclonic epilepsy. A review. Arch Neurol 50: 594–598

Hardiman O, Burke T, Phillips J, Murphy S, O'Moore B, Staunton H, Farrell MA 1988 Microdysgenesis in resected temporal neocortex: incidence and clinical significance in focal epilepsy. Neurology 38: 1041–1047

Harding GF, Herrick CE, Jeavons PM 1978 A controlled study of the effect of sodium valproate on photosensitive epilepsy and its prognosis. Epilepsia 19: 555–565

Hellstrom-Westas L, Rosen I, Swenningsen NW 1985 Silent seizures in sick infants in early life: Diagnosis by continuous cerebral function monitoring. Acta Paediat Scand 74: 741–748

Holtzman DM, Kaku DA, So YT 1989 New-onset seizures associated with human immunodeficiency virus infection: causation and clinical features in 100 cases. Am J Med, 87, 173–177

Hrachovy RA, Frost JD 1990 Infantile Spasms. In: Dam M, Gram L (eds) Comprehensive epileptology. Raven Press, New York, p 113–121

Illis LS, Gostling JVT 1972 Herpes simplex encephalitis. Baillière Tindall, Bristol

Isbell H, Fraser HF, Wikler A et al 1967 An experimental study of the etiology of 'rum fits' and delerium tremens. Q J Study Alcohol 16: 1–33

Janz D 1969 Die Epilepsien. Georg Thieme, Stuttgart

Janz D, Waltz S 1995 Juvenile myoclonic epilepsy with absences. In: Duncan JS, Panayiotopoulos CP (eds) Typical absences and related epileptic syndromes. Churchill Livingstone, Edinburgh, p 174–183

Janz D, Kern A, Mossinger HJ, Puhlmann HU 1983 Ruckfallprognose während und nach Reduktion der Medikamente bei Epilepsiebehandlung. In: Remschmidt H, Rentz R, Jungmann J (eds) Verlauf und Prognose, neuropsychologische und psychologische Aspekte. Georg Thieme, Stuttgart, p 17–24

Jayakar PB, Seshia SS 1991 Electrical status epilepticus during slow-wave sleep: a review. J Clin Neurophysiol 8: 299–311

Jeavons PM 1977 Nosological problems of myoclonic epilepsies in childhood and adolescence. Dev Med Child Neurol 19: 3–8

Jennett WB 1975 Epilepsy after non-missile head injuries, 2nd edn. Heinemann, London

Jennett WB 1982 Post-traumatic epilepsy. In: Laidlaw J, Richens A (eds) A textbook of epilepsy, 2nd edn. Churchill Livingstone, Edinburgh, p 146–154

Jennett B, Murray A, Carlin J et al 1979 Head injuries in three Scottish neurosurgical units. Brit Med J 2: 955–958

Jennett B, Crandon I, Kay M 1990 Late epilepsy after aneurysm surgery. J Neurol Neurosurg Psychiat 53: 812

Joynt RJ, Zimmerman G, Khalifeh R 1965 Cerebral emboli from cardiac tumors. Arch Neurol 12: 84–91

Judrjavcev T, Schoenberg BS, Kurland KT, Groover RV 1985 Cerebral palsy: survival rates, associated handicaps and distribution by clinical sub-type. Neurology 35: 900–903

Kellaway P, Hrachovy RA 1983 Status epilepticus in newborns: a perspective on neonatal seizures. In: Delgado-Escueta AV, Wasterlain CG, Treiman DM, Porter RJ (eds) Status epilepticus. Mechanisms of brain damage and treatment. Advances in neurology 34. Raven Press, New York, p 93–99

Kelly D, Alexander E, Davis CH et al 1969 Intracranial arteriovenous malformations: a clinical review and evaluation of brain scans. J Neurosurg 31: 422–428

Kieburtz K, Ricotta JJ, Moxley RT 1990 Seizures following carotid endarterectomy. Arch Neurol 47: 568–570

Kilpatrick CJ, Davis SM, Tress BM, Rossiter SC, Hopper JL, Vandendriessen ML 1990 Epileptic seizures in acute stroke. Arch Neurol 47: 157–160

Kivity S, Lerman P 1992 Stormy onset with prolonged loss of consciousness in benign childhood epilepsy with occipital paroxysms. J Neurol Neurosurg Psychiat 55: 45–48

Kotagal P, Luders H, Williams G, Wyllie E, Nichols T, McPherson J 1988 Temporal lobe

complex partial seizures: analysis of symptom clusters and sequences. Epilepsia 29: 661
Lacy JR, Penry JK 1976 Infantile spasms. Raven Press, New York
Landau WM 1992 Landau–Kleffner syndrome: an eponymic badge of ignorance. Arch Neurol 49: 353–359
Landau WM, Kleffner F 1957 Syndrome of acquired aphasia with convulsive disorder in children. Neurology 7: 523–30
Legg NJ, Gupta PC, Scott DF 1973 Epilepsy following cerebral abscess – a clinical and EEG study of 70 patients. Brain 96: 259–268
Lennox WG, Davis JP 1950 Clinical correlates of the fast and slow spike-wave electroencephalogram. Pediatrics 5: 626–641
Lennox-Buchthal MA 1974 Febrile convulsions. In: Magnus O, Lorentz de Haas AM (eds) The Epilepsies. Handbook of clinical neurology, vol 15. Amsterdam, North-Holland, p 246–263
Lerman P, Lerman-Sagie T, Kivity S 1991 Effect of early corticosteroid therapy for Landau–Kleffner syndrome. Devel Med Child Neurol 33: 257–266
Levy SR, Abroms IF, Marshall PC, Rosquete EE 1985 Seizures and cerebral infarction in the full-term newborn. Ann Neurol 17: 366–370
Loiseau P 1992 Childhood absence epilepsy. In: Roger J, Bureau M, Dravet C, Dreifuss FE, Perret A, Wolf P (eds) Epileptic syndromes in infancy, childhood and adolescence, 2nd edn. John Libbey, London, p 135–150
Loiseau P, Duche B, Cordova S, Dartigues JF, Cohadon S 1988 Prognosis of benign childhood epilepsy with centrotemporal spikes: a follow up study of 168 patients. Epilepsia 29: 229–235
Loiseau J, Loiseau P, Guyot M, Duche B, Dartigues AF, Aublet B 1990 Survey of seizure disorders in the French Southwest. I: Incidence of epileptic syndromes. Epilepsia 31: 391–396
Lombroso CT 1983 Prognosis in neonatal seizures. In: Delgado-Escueta AV, Wasterlain CG, Treiman DM, Porter RJ (eds) Status epilepticus. Mechanisms of brain damage and treatment. Advances in neurology 34. Raven Press, New York, p 101–113
Louis S, McDowell F 1967 Epileptic seizures in nonembolic cerebral infarction. Arch Neurol 17: 414–418
Lugaresi E, Pazzaglia P, Frank L et al 1973 Evolution and prognosis of primary generalised epilepsies of the petit mal absence type. In: Lugaresi E, Pazzaglia P, Tassinari CA (eds) Evolution and prognosis of the epilepsies. Aulo Gaggi Editore, Bologna, p 3–22,
McKeran RO, Thomas DGT 1980 The clinical study of gliomas. In: Thomas DGT, Graham DI (eds) Brain tumours. Butterworth, London, p 194–230
Majkowski J 1990 Post-traumatic epilepsy. In: Dam M, Gram L (eds) Comprehensive epileptology. Raven Press, New York, p 281–288
Malonado HM, Delgado-Escueta AV, Walsh GO, Swartz BE, Rand RW 1987 Complex partial seizures of hippocampal and amygdalar origin. Epilepsia 29: 420–33
Manford M, Shorvon SD 1992 Prolonged sensory or visceral symptoms: an underdiagnosed form of focal (simple partial) status epilepticus. J Neurol Neurosurg Psychiat 55: 714–716
Manford M, Hart YM, Sander JWAS, Shorvon SD 1992a National General Practice Study of Epilepsy (NGPSE): the syndromic classification of the ILAE applied to epilepsy in a general population. Arch Neurol 49: 801–809
Manford M, Hart YM, Sander JWAS, Shorvon SD 1992b National General Practice Study of Epilepsy (NGPSE): partial seizure patterns in a general population. Neurology 34: 1911–1917
Margerison JH, Corsellis JAN 1966 Epilepsy and the temporal lobes: a clinical electroencephalographic and neuropathological study of the brain in epilepsy, with particular reference to the temporal lobes. Brain 89: 499–530
Marseilles Consensus Group 1990 Classification of progressive myoclonus epilepsies and related disorders. Ann Neurol 28: 113–116
Mauguiere F, Courjon J 1978 Somatosensory epilepsy. Brain 101: 307–332
Maytal J, Shinnar S, Moshe SL, Alvarez LA 1989 Low morbidity and mortality of status epilepticus in children. Pediatrics 83: 323–331
Meencke HJ 1994 Minimal developmental disturbances in epilepsy and MRI. In: Shorvon SD, Fish DR, Bydder G, Andermann F, Stefan H (eds) Magnetic resonance scanning and epilepsy. Plenum Press, New York, p 127–136
Meencke HJ, Janz D 1984 Neuropathological findings in primary generalised epilepsy: a study of eight cases. Epilepsia 25: 8–21
Meyer JS, Bauer RB, Rivera-Olmos VM et al 1970 Herpesvirus hominis encephalitis. Neurological manifestations and use of Idoxuridine. Arch Neurol 23: 438–450

Mizrahi EM, Kellaway P 1987 Characterisation and classification of neonatal seizures. Neurology 37: 1837–1844

Morikawa T, Seino M, Watanabe Y, Watanabe M, Yagi K 1989 Clinical relevance of continuous spike-waves during slow wave sleep. In: Manelis J, Bental E, Loeber JN, Dreifuss FE (eds) The XVIIth Epilepsy International Symposium. Raven Press, New York, p 359–363

Nelson KB, Broman SH 1977 Perinatal risk factors in children with serious motor and mental handicaps. Ann Neurol 2: 371–377

Nelson KB, Ellenberg JH 1981 Febrile seizures. Raven Press, New York

Newmark ME, Penry JK 1980 Genetics and epilepsy: a review. Raven Press, New York

Niedermeyer E, Fineyre F, Riley T, Biro B 1979 Myoclonus and the electroencephalogram, a review. Clin Electroencephalog 10: 75–95

Ochs R, Gloor P, Quesney F et al 1984 Does headturning during a seizure have lateralizing or localizing significance? Neurology 34: 884–890

Ohtahara S, Ohtsuka Y, Yamatogi Y, Oka E 1987 The early-infantile epileptic encephalopathy with suppression-burst: developmental aspects. Brain and Development 9: 371–376

Ohtahara S, Ohtsuka Y, Yoshinaga H et al 1988 Lennox–Gastaut syndrome: etiological considerations. In: Niedermeyer E, Degen R (eds) The Lennox–Gastaut Syndrome. Neurology and neurobiology, vol 45. Alan R Liss, New York, p 47–64

Osborne JP, Fryer AE 1991 Tuberous sclerosis. In: Swash M, Oxbury J (eds) Clinical neurology, vol 2. Churchill Livingstone, Edinburgh, pp 1526–1532

Panayiotopoulos CP 1989 Benign occipital paroxysms: a 15-year prospective study. Ann Neurol 26: 51–56

Panayiotopoulos CP, Obeid T, Waheed G 1989 Differentiation of typical absences in epileptic syndromes. A video-EEG study of 224 seizures in 20 patients. Brain 112: 1039–1056

Panayiotopoulos CP, Chroni E, Daskopoulos C, Baker A, Rowlinson S, Walsh P 1993 Typical absence seizures in adults: clinical, EEG, video-EEG findings and diagnostic/syndromic considerations. J Neurol Neurosurg Psychiat 55: 1002–1008

Panayiotopoulos CP, Obeid T, Tahan A 1994 Juvenile myoclonic epilepsy: a 5-year prospective study. Epilepsia 35: 285–296

Parsonage M. 1983 The classification of epileptic seizures. In: Clifford Rose F (ed) Research Progress in Epilepsy. Pitman, Bath, p 22–38

Paterson JH, McKissock W 1956 A clinical survey of intracranial angiomas with special reference to their progress and surgical treatment: a report of 110 patients. Brain 79: 233–266

Patry G, Lyagoubi S, Tassinari CA 1971 Subclinical 'electrical status epilepticus' induced by sleep in children. Arch Neurol 24: 242–252

Penry JK, Porter RJ, Dreifuss FE 1975 Simultaneous recording of absence seizures with videotape and electroencephalography. Brain 98: 427–440

Pieninkeroinen IP, Telakivi TM, Hillborn ME 1992 Outcome in subjects with alcohol-provoked seizures. Alcoholism: Clin Exp Res 5: 955–959

Plouin P 1992 Benign idiopathic neonatal convulsions (familial and non-familial). In: Roger J, Bureau M, Dravet C, Dreifuss FE, Perret A, Wolf P (eds) Epileptic syndromes in infancy, childhood and adolescence, 2nd edn. John Libbey, London, p 3–11

Plouin P, Sternberg B, Bour F, Lerique A 1981 Etats de mal neonataux d'etiologie indeterminee. Rev d'Electroencephalog Neurophysiol Clin 11: 385–389

Power C, Poland SD, Blume WT, Girvin JP, Rice GPA 1990 Cytomegalovirus and Rasmussen's encephalitis. Lancet 331: 1282–1284

Prevett MC, Duncan JS, Fish DR, Jones TJ, Brooks DJ 1995 Demonstration of thalamic activation during absence seizures using $H_2{}^{15}O$ and PET. Neurology 45:1396-1402

Radermecker J 1974 Epilepsy in the degenerative diseases. In: Magnus O, Lorentze de Haas AM (eds) The epilepsies. Handbook of clinical neurology, vol 15. North-Holland, Amsterdam, p 325–372

Raymond AA, Fish DR, Stevens JM, Sisodiya SM, Shorvon SD 1994a Subependymal heterotopia: a distinct neuronal migration disorder associated with epilepsy. J Neurol Neurosurg Psychiat 57: 1195–1202

Raymond AA, Halpin SFS, Alsanjari N et al 1994b Dysembryoplastic neuroepithelial tumours: features in 16 patients. Brain 117; 461–475

Reder AT, Wright FS 1982 Epilepsy evoked by eating: the role of peripheral input. Neurology 32: 1065–1069

Richardson EP, Dodge PR 1954 Epilepsy in cerebral vascular disease. A study of the incidence and nature of seizures in 104 consecutive autopsy proven cases of cerebral infarction and haemorrhage. Epilepsia 3: 49–65

Roberts RC, Shorvon SD, Cox TCS, Gilliatt RW 1988 Clinically unsuspected cerebral infarction revealed by computed tomography scanning in late onset epilepsy.

Epilepsia 29: 190–194
Roger J, Bureau M, Dravet C et al 1972 Les hemiplégies cérébrales infantiles. Les données EEG et les manifestations epileptiques en relation avec l'hemiplégie cérébrale infantile. Rev d'Electroencephalog Neurophysiol Clin 2: 5–28
Rose AL, Lombroso CT 1970 Neonatal seizure states: a study of clinical, pathological and electroencephalographic features in 137 full-term babies with a long-term follow-up. Pediatrics 45: 404–405
Salazar AM, Jabbari B, Vance SC et al 1985 Epilepsy after penetrating head injury: 1. Clinical correlates. Neurology 35: 1406–1414
Salgado AV, Furlan AJ, Keys TF, Nichols MS, Beck GJ 1989 Neurologic complications of endocarditis. Neurology 39: 173–178
Sander JWAS, Hart YM, Johnson AL, Shorvon SD 1990 The National General Practice Study of Epilepsy: newly diagnosed epileptic seizures in a general population. Lancet 336: 1267–1271
Satischandra P, Shivaramakrishana A, Kaliaperumal VG, Schoenberg BS 1988 Hot water epilepsy: a variant of reflex epilepsy in Southern India. Epilepsia 29: 52–56
Scheffer IE, Bhatia KP, Lopes-Cendes I et al 1994 Autosomal dominant frontal epilepsy misdiagnosed as sleep disorder. Lancet 343: 515–517
Shinton RA, Gill JS, Zezulka AV Beevers DG 1987 The frequency of epilepsy preceding stroke. Lancet 1: 11–13
Shinton RA, Gill JS, Melnick SC, Gupta AK, Beevers DG 1988 The frequency, characteristics and prognosis of epileptic seizures at the onset of stroke. J Neurol Neurosurg Psychiat 51: 273–276
Shorvon SD 1991 Constitutional epilepsy. In: Swash M, Oxbury J (eds) Clinical neurology, vol 2. Churchill Livingstone, Edinburgh, p 221–232
Shorvon SD, Bharucha NE 1992 Epilepsy in developing countries: epidemiology, aetiology and health care. In: Laidlaw J, Richens AL, Chadwick DW (eds) A textbook of epilepsy, 4th edn. Churchill Livingstone, Edinburgh, p 613–636
So N, Berkovic S, Andermann F, Kuzniecky R, Gendron D, Quesney L 1989 Myoclonus epilepsy and ragged red fibres 2. Electrophysiological studies and comparisons with other progressive myoclonic epilepsies. Brain 112: 1261–1276
Sung C-Y, Chu N-S 1989 Epileptic seizures in intracerebral haemorrhage. J Neurol Neurosurg Psychiat 52: 1273–1276
Sveinbjornsdóttir S, Duncan JS 1993 Parietal and occipital epilepsy: a review. Epilepsia 34: 493–521
Tassinari CA, Bureau M, Thomas P 1992 Epilepsy with myoclonic absences. In: Roger J, Bureau M, Dravet C, Dreifuss FE, Perret A, Wolf P (eds) Epileptic syndromes in infancy, childhood and adolescence, 2nd edn. London, John Libbey, p 151–160
Taylor J (ed) 1931 Selected writings of John Hughlings Jackson, vol. 1. Lectures on the diagnosis of epilepsy. Hodder & Stoughton, London
Taylor D, Horenstein S, Williams G, Weins R 1979 Syncope, seizure and stroke in the mitral-valve prolapse syndrome. Trans Amer Neurolog Assoc 104: 114–116
Theodore WH, Porter RJ, Penry JK 1983 Complex partial seizures: clinical characteristics and differential diagnosis. Neurology 33: 1115–1121
Todd RB 1854 Clinical lectures on paralysis, disease of the brain and other afflictions of the nervous system. Churchill, London
Verity CM, Golding J 1991 Risk of epilepsy after febrile convulsions: a national cohort study. Br Med J 303: 1373–1376
Victor M, Brausch J 1967 The role of abstinence in the genesis of alcoholic epilepsy. Epilepsia 8: 1–20
Volpe JJ 1987 Neurology of the newborn. Major problems in clinical pediatrics, 2nd edn, vol. 22. WB Saunders, Philadelphia
Wallace SJ 1988 The child with febrile seizures. Butterworth, London
Wasterlain CG, Dwyer BE 1983 Brain metabolism during prolonged seizures in neonates. In: Delgado Escueta AV, Westerlain CG, Treiman DM, Porter RJ (eds) Status epilepticus: mechanisms of brain damage and treatment. Advances in neurology 34. Raven Press, New York, p 241–260
Weiss GH, Salazar AM, Vance SC et al 1986 Predicting post-traumatic epilepsy in penetrating head injury. Annals of Neurology 43: 771–773
West WJ 1841 On a peculiar form of infantile convulsions. Lancet 724–725
White PT, Bailey AA, Bickford RG 1953 Epileptic disorders in the elderly. Neurology 3: 674–678
Wieser HG 1983 Electroclinical features of the psychomotor seizure. Fisher/Butterworths, Stuttgart
Wieser HG, Kauser W 1987 Limbic seizures. In: Wieser HG, Elgar CE (eds) Presurgical evaluation of epileptics: basis, techniques, implications. Springer-Verlag, Berlin, p 227–249

Wieser HG, Muller RU 1987 Neocortical temporal seizures. In: Wieser HG, Elgar CE (eds) Presurgical evaluation of epileptics: basis, techniques, implications. Springer-Verlag, Berlin, p 252–266

Wilkins A, Lindsay J 1985 Common forms of reflex epilepsy: physiological mechanisms and techniques for treatment. In: Pedley T, Meldrum BS (eds) Recent advances in epilepsy 2. Churchill Livingstone, Edinburgh, p 239–271

Wilkins AJ, Zifkin B, Andermann F, McGovern E 1982 Seizures induced by thinking. Ann Neurol 11: 608–612

Will RG, Matthews WB 1984 A retrospective study of Creutzfeldt–Jacob disease in England and Wales 1970–1979. J Neurol Neurosurg Psychiat 47: 134–140

Williams LB, Thompson EA, Lewis DV 1987 Intractable complex partial seizures: the initial 'motionless stare' and outcome following temporal lobectomy. Neurology 37: 1255–8

Williamson PD, Spencer DD, Spencer SS, Novelly RA, Mattson RH 1985 Complex partial seizures of frontal lobe origin. Ann Neurol 18: 497–504

Wolf P 1992a Reading epilepsy. In: Roger J, Bureau M, Dravet C, Dreifuss FE, Perret A, Wolf P (eds) Epileptic syndromes in infancy, childhood and adolescence. 2nd edn. John Libbey, London, p 281–298

Wolf P 1992b Epilepsy with grand mal on awakening. In: Roger J, Bureau M, Dravet C, Dreifuss FE, Perret A, Wolf P (eds) Epileptic syndromes in infancy, childhood and adolescence, 2nd edn. John Libbey, London, p 329–341

Wolf P, Goosses R 1986 Relation of photosensitivity to epileptic syndromes. J Neurol Neurosurg Psychiat 49: 1386–1391

Wolf P, Inoue Y 1984 Therapeutic response of absence seizures in patients of an epilepsy clinic for adolescents and adults. J Neurol 231: 225–229

Wong MC, Suite ND, Labar DR 1990 Seizures in human immunodificiency virus infection. Arch Neurol 47: 640–642

Worster-Drought C 1971 An unusual form of acquired aphasia in children. Develop Med Child Neurol 13: 563–571

Yasuhara A, Yoshida H, Hatanaka T, Sugimoto T, Kobayashi Y, Dyken E 1991 Epilepsy with continuous spike-waves during slow sleep and its treatment. Epilepsia 32: 59–62

# 3 The investigation of epilepsy

## 3.1 PRINCIPLES OF INVESTIGATION

There is an increasingly sophisticated range of investigations that can be applied to patients with epilepsy. In order to derive the most benefit and to be cost-effective, it is essential not to order investigations blindly but to answer specific questions. It is important to ensure that results are considered in the clinical context and with regard to each other and not in isolation. Investigations of epilepsy may be grouped into those that are structural (MRI and X-ray CT), functional (EEG, psychological, PET, SPECT) and biochemical or histological (e.g. blood tests, CSF examination, muscle biopsy). The principal of establishing concordance of data from different sources is particularly important in the evaluation of patients for possible surgical treatment (Ch. 10), but also applies to patients with new onset and chronic seizure disorders.

The principal objectives of investigating new and chronic patients referred for evaluation are:

- To clarify the diagnosis of epilepsy or non-epileptic attacks
- To determine the nature of the seizure types and epilepsy syndrome
- In the case of partial seizures, to identify the laterality and localization of seizure onset
- To identify the aetiology of the epilepsy
- To identify concomitant problems, both neurological and general
- To monitor the progression of the condition and the consequences of the epilepsy and its treatment

Answers to these questions allow the formulation of a rational treatment plan and the provision to the patient and his/her family of accurate information regarding diagnosis, treatment and prognosis.

## 3.2 CLINICAL NEUROPHYSIOLOGY

### 3.2.1 Uses and abuses of the electroencephalogram (EEG)

In the assessment of a patient with a seizure disorder the EEG is a useful test to address the following questions:

- Are there functional (epileptiform) changes to support the clinical diagnosis of epilepsy?
- Is the seizure disorder likely to be of partial onset or a primary generalized process?

- Does the patient have photosensitivity?
- Is there evidence of an encephalopathy?

An EEG helps to classify the type of epileptic syndrome, especially in childhood and adolescence. Most patients require an EEG in the evaluation of their epilepsy, although in some adults with clear clinical or neuroimaging findings, EEG data is not necessary to make a confident syndromic and aetiological classification.

In clinical practice it must be remembered that:

- A normal interictal EEG does not exclude epilepsy
- The EEG is not specific or sensitive at diagnosing the presence or absence of underlying structural cerebral lesions
- There are important normal EEG variants that may mimic epileptiform activity
- All EEG changes need to be considered in the clinical context
- With the exception of patients with idiopathic generalized epilepsy and 3 Hz spike-wave activity, the interictal EEG is a poor guide to seizure control or to the likelihood of seizure relapse in a patient who has become seizure free and in whom withdrawal of antiepileptic drugs is being contemplated (Ch. 4, 4.6)

### 3.2.2 EEG recording techniques

*Routine EEG*

This comprises 20–30 min recording during the awake, resting state using a standard array of scalp electrodes (the 10–20 system) (Fig. 3.1). It includes activation by overbreathing for 3 min and photic stimulation. Only 30–40% of patients with epilepsy show epileptiform discharges on a single wake record (Ajmone Marsan & Zivin 1970), although of course the sensitivity will vary according to the population.

*Sleep EEG*

A sleep EEG should be requested when the routine EEG is normal or borderline abnormal and further confirmation of the diagnosis or syndromic classification is required. Sleep can usually be achieved by spontaneous afternoon naps, especially if the patient reduces the previous overnight sleep period by a few hours, or may be induced by medication (e.g. chloral hydrate). Epileptiform changes are seen on a sleep EEG in 70–80% of patients with clinical epilepsy. About 50% of patients with unhelpful wake records show definite interictal epileptiform activity during a sleep record (Gastaut et al 1991). Most of the additional yield occurs during drowsiness or light sleep rather than deep sleep.

Overnight sleep deprivation only marginally improves the yield, and there is the risk that significant sleep deprivation may trigger additional seizures. It may occasionally be helpful in suspected idiopathic generalized epilepsy if EEG confirmation is essential. However, sleep deprivation is sometimes followed by the patient rapidly entering a deep sleep, and not developing drowsiness and light sleep, and it is in these stages that epileptiform activity is most likely to be detected.

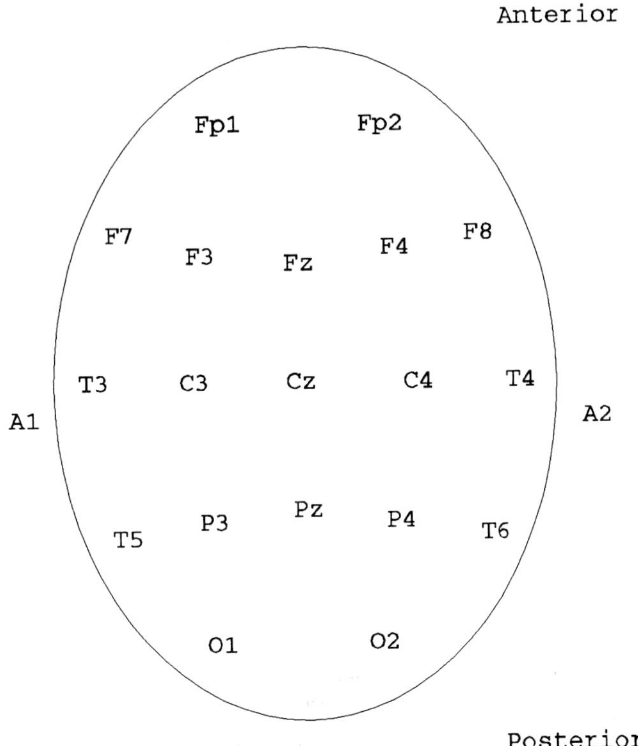


**Fig. 3.1** The standard 10–20 system of scalp electrode placement for EEG recording. Odd numbered electrodes are located on the left side of the head

*Ambulatory EEG*

A portable cassette recorder is used to monitor the EEG continuously over prolonged periods, usually with an internal clock and externally triggered event marker. This allows the detection and quantification of generalized spike and slow wave discharges, the detection of infrequent interictal localized epileptiform discharges and diagnostic screening of ictal events in patients with frequent paroxysmal attacks of unknown nature. Although it is easy to apply, well tolerated and robust the number of channels is usually limited to eight (or sometimes 16), artefact may be difficult to detect without simultaneous documentation of motor behaviour and precise electroclinical correlation is often not possible. The electrodes need to be checked at least once per day, which limits out-patient use. Only definite EEG patterns should be considered to be of diagnostic importance: minor changes or those of questionable origin should be treated with great caution. Digital ambulatory systems may overcome some of these limitations.

*Video-EEG telemetry*

Video-EEG telemetry provides long-term monitoring of the EEG and time-locked video of the patient in a dedicated recording room. It is the most definitive method for the diagnosis of paroxysmal attacks and is feasible if episodes are occurring at a frequency of more than one per week, or can be provoked. Video-EEG telemetry is also used for accurate seizure classification and presurgical evaluation. The patient is usually connected to the recording system by a long, flexible cable, although a few units prefer the greater mobility (but increased potential for extraneous interference) of radio transmitter systems. It is much easier to identify artefact than with ambulatory records, and the technology is more flexible and appropriate for presurgical assessment. Video-EEG telemetry is often used to study patients with suspected non-epileptic attack disorder (NEAD). The act of recording often precipitates an attack in such cases even if they are relatively infrequent in the community. The use of video-EEG telemetry in the evaluation of patients for epilepsy surgery is further discussed in Chapter 10.

*EEG monitoring in intensive care*

Cerebral function monitors identify gross changes in the EEG associated with generalized convulsions or anaesthetic agents such as barbiturates that cause burst suppression or sustained flattening of the EEG. Typically two channels of EEG are recorded and both the ongoing trace and various compressed EEG parameters are displayed, allowing easy review of prolonged periods. Data from these records are complementary to, but not a replacement for a full EEG. Localized abnormalities will often be undetected and poor electrode contact or extraneous artefact (easily occurring in the setting of an ITU) may give rise to spurious results. EEG monitoring is mandatory in patients who have been anaesthetized because of refractory tonic-clonic status epilepticus, as ongoing electrical status epilepticus may no longer have a clinical correlate.

*Sphenoidal electrodes*

None of the standard 10–20 electrodes overlie the anterior or infero-medial temporal lobe. Several alternative additional electrodes have been used to cover this region, applied either to the overlying skin (anterior temporal or zygomatic electrode), inserted subcutaneously (mini-sphenoidal) or inserted through the cheek with the tip resting superficial to the foramen ovale (sphenoidal electrode). Although the latter were much favoured for many years they have a limited role in interictal records (Marks et al 1992a). It is extremely rare for a patient to have epileptiform discharges that are only seen with indwelling sphenoidal electrodes – they are usually evident with the non-invasive alternatives, even though they may be less frequent and of lower amplitude. Sphenoidal electrode recordings do, however, sometimes show slightly earlier changes during ictal recordings (Wilkus et al 1993).

*Brain mapping*

There are various commercially available brain mapping systems to analyse EEG data. These may pictorially display the anatomical distribution of individual waveforms, average the EEG over time or extrapolate to hypothetical point source generators, usually dipoles (Fig. 3.2). Great caution is required in the interpretation of such material, and it is not a substitute for visual inspection of the raw EEG. The EEG recorded on the scalp represents the summation of the excitatory and inhibitory post-synaptic potentials in the apical dendrites of pyramidal neurones occupying several square centimetres of superficial cortex. There is very little con-

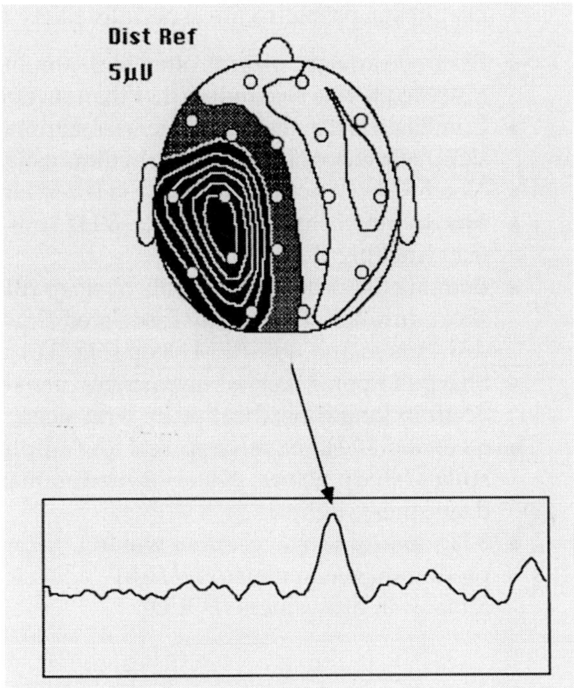


**Fig. 3.2** Brain map (dipole) showing a single localized sharp negative wave maximal in the left parietal region

tribution to the scalp potentials from deep generators and so these cannot be derived from surface measurements.

*Intracranial EEG*

The techniques of intracranial EEG recordings are considered in the context of epilepsy surgery (Ch. 10, 10.2.3).

## 3.2.3 Normal EEG findings

The normal EEG evolves with age and shows considerable variation between subjects. Posterior rhythms are relatively slow in infancy (typically 4 Hz at 6 months of age), increasing to 8 Hz by age 2–4 years and thereafter increasing further to the normal mature pattern of 8–12 Hz (alpha activity). These posterior rhythms are usually symmetrical, and attenuate with eye-opening or alerting (Fig. 3.3). Posterior delta waves (2–4 Hz) may occur intermittently in adolescence or early adulthood (posterior slow waves of youth). Theta activity (5–8 Hz) is often seen in the central regions, particularly with drowsiness. Low-amplitude beta activity (15–22 Hz) is best seen anteriorly.

Important normal EEG variants that can be seen in healthy individuals, may mimic epileptiform discharges (Klass & Westmoreland 1985) and often lead to erroneous support being given to a diagnosis of epilepsy.

Diagnostic problems are especially likely to occur from:

- Electrode artefact: bizarre, often high-amplitude morphology but field restricted to one electrode rather than several adjacent contacts (Fig. 3.4)
- Combined fast and slow frequencies summating to produce an apparent sharp wave: ongoing separate rhythms usually evident, however
- Notched slow activity during overbreathing in children
- Mu rhythm: centro-temporal; 6–8 Hz runs blocked by contralateral fist clenching (Fig. 3.5)
- Benign epileptiform transients of sleep (BETS): low amplitude; very short duration; little if any associated slow wave; restricted to drowsiness and non-REM sleep (Fig. 3.6)
- Sharp temporal theta of drowsiness: usually mid-temporal; may occur in long runs; disappears with sleep.
- 6 Hz and 14 Hz positive spikes: low amplitude bursts of positive spikes/sharp waves; posterior predominance; usually restricted to drowsiness/light sleep
- 6 Hz spike and wave: either waking, high amplitude, anterior predominance in males (WHAM); or occipital, low amplitude, in females in drowsiness (FOLD)

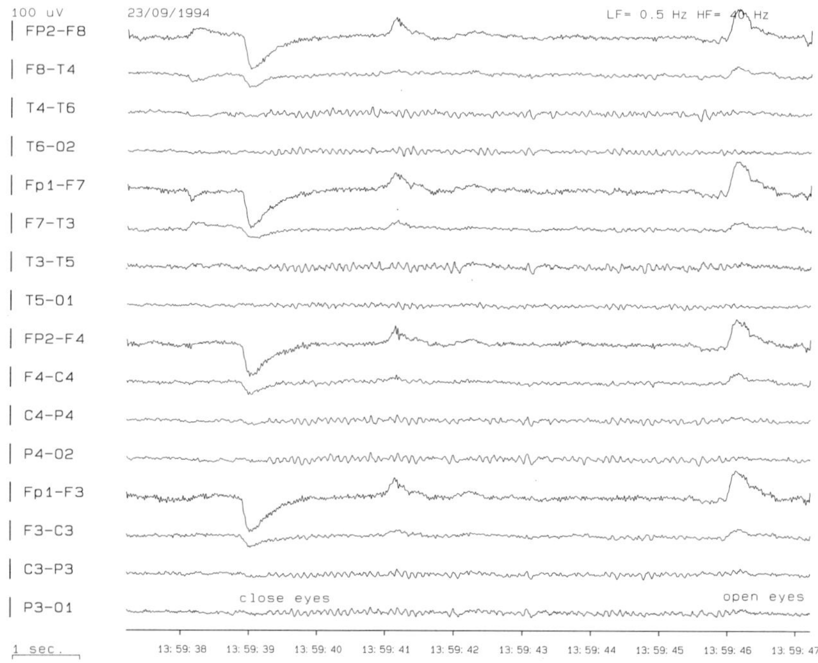


**Fig. 3.3** Normal scalp EEG, showing attenuation of posterior rhythms on eye opening

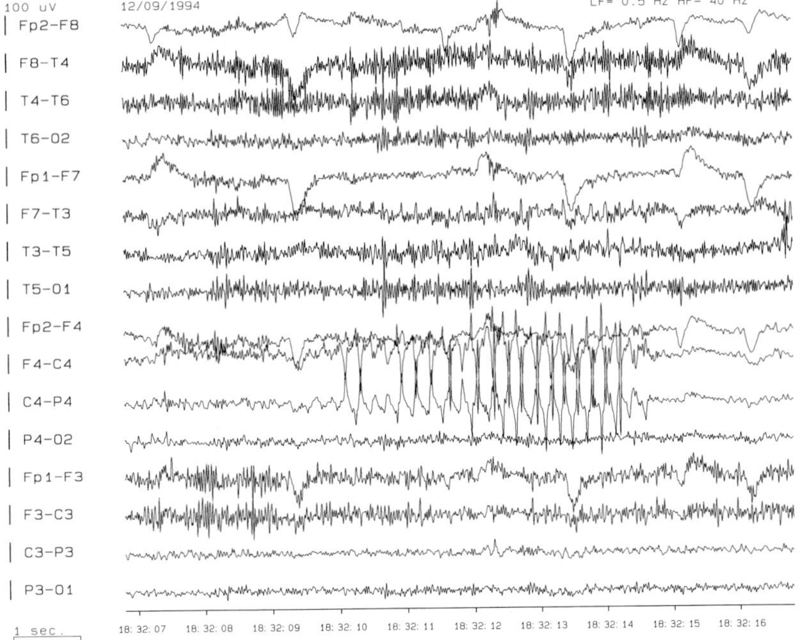


**Fig. 3.4** Electrode artefact. High amplitude waves, restricted to one electrode (C4) rather than several adjacent contacts. Significant muscle artefact is present on most other channels

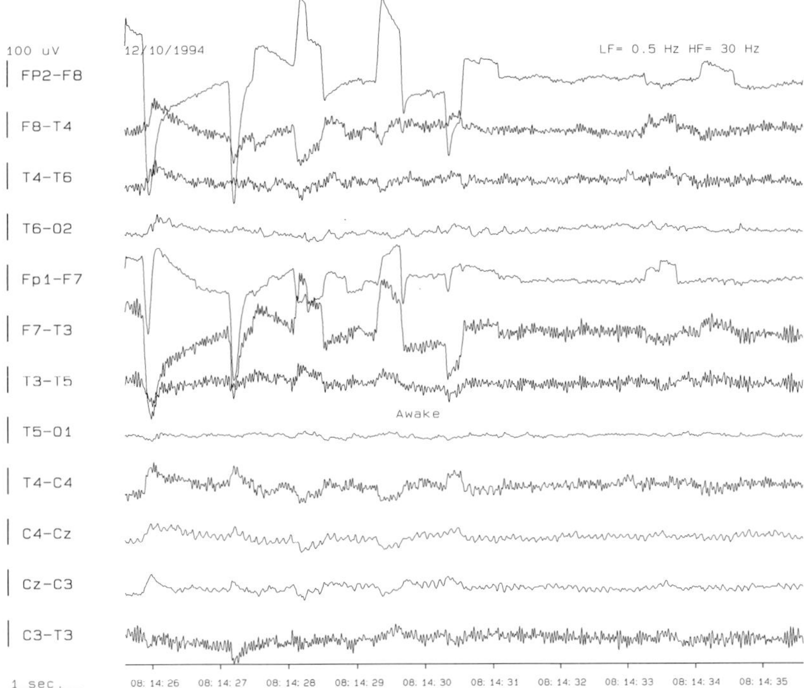


**Fig. 3.5** Mu rhythm. Approximately 8 Hz activity best seen in C4–Cz and Cz–C3. Note the absence of alpha rhythm posteriorly, when the eyes are open

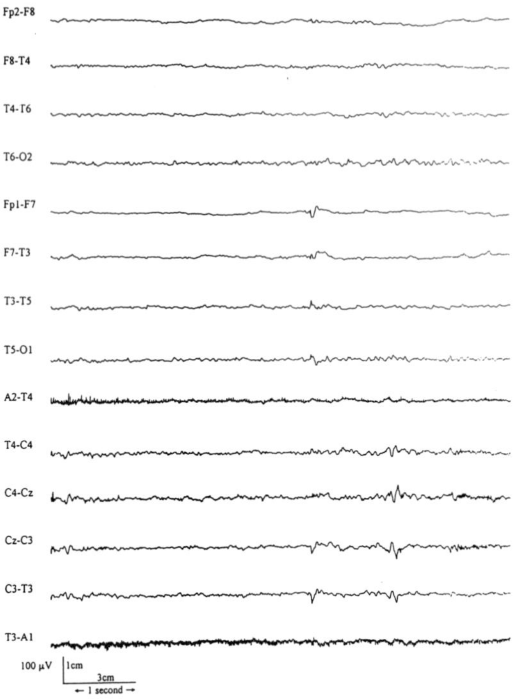


**Fig. 3.6** Benign epileptiform transients of sleep (BETS): low amplitude (note amplitude scale), very short duration, little if any associated slow wave, restricted to drowsiness and non-REM sleep

## 3.2.4 Abnormal EEG findings

These are of three types:

- Interictal epileptiform discharges
- Ictal electrographic activity (i.e. the EEG during seizures)
- Non-epileptiform changes

*Interictal epileptiform discharges*

Interictal epileptiform discharges consist of spikes (duration 20–70 ms) or sharp waves (duration 70–200 ms), with or without associated slow waves. These may be localized (Fig. 3.7), multifocal (Fig. 3.8) or generalized. Provided that normal variants and non-specific disturbances are excluded the false positive rate is very low. Most studies on apparently healthy subjects derive from military screening programs: epileptiform abnormalities are seen in less than 1% of cases without a history of epilepsy (Gregory et al 1993). The false positive rate is higher in patients with other neurological abnormalities: some structural lesions such as cerebral palsy, strokes and tumours may be associated with sharp waves or spikes without any clinical seizures. Previous skull defects may cause 'breach rhythms' (Cobb et al 1979) of variable amplitude and frequencies, sometimes producing apparent spikes, or runs of rhythmic sharp activity mimicking a seizure, but are of no clinical significance (Fig. 3.9). Careful consideration is needed if these changes are seen in patients with known structural abnormalities or previous surgery. Such patients are often referred for EEGs because of odd symptoms that might or might not be

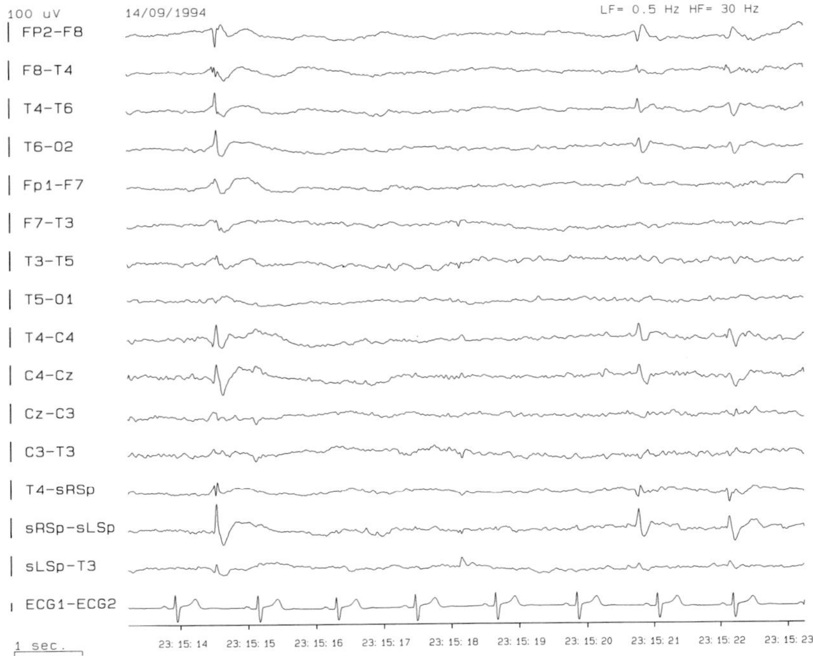


**Fig. 3.7** Interictal epileptiform activity localized to right mid to anterior temporal lobe. This shows phase reversal at the right sphenoidal electrode and is equipotential at F8–T4

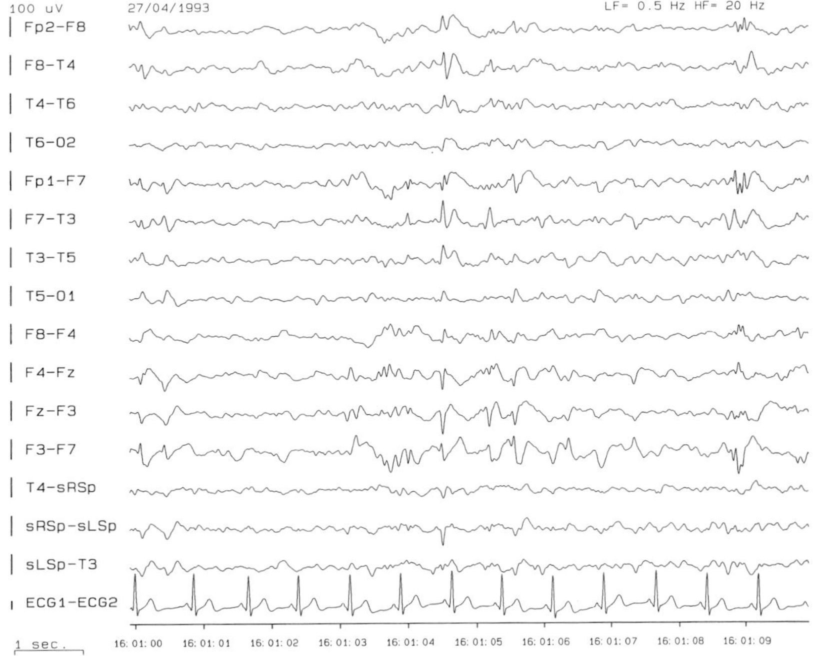


**Fig. 3.8** Multifocal interictal epileptiform activity, predominantly left frontal

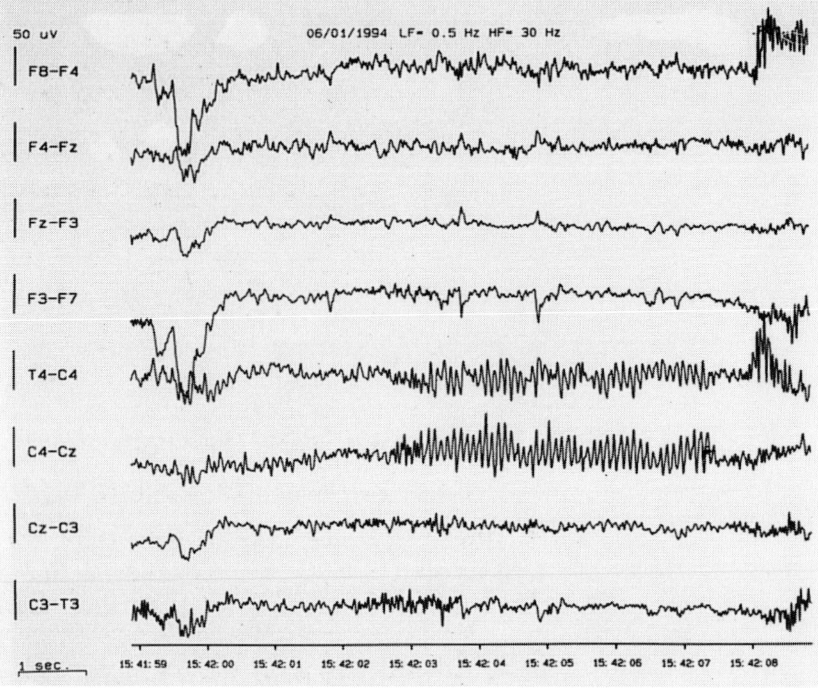


**Fig. 3.9** Breach rhythms caused by a previous skull defect, producing rhythmic spikes mimicking ictal electrographic activity, but of no clinical significance

epileptic. Great caution must be exercised in assessing the importance of interictal EEGs in these situations, and ictal recordings are often needed.

*Ictal electrographic patterns*

An EEG recording taken during an epileptic seizure (an ictal recording) can take a variety of forms, depending upon the seizure type and pathways of spread. They are usually sustained, rhythmic, clearly different from the interictal record and, at least in partial epilepsies, evolve in frequency and/or amplitude (Fig. 3.10), sometimes being followed by flattening of the trace and/or slow activity. Simple partial seizures are often not associated with any discernible change in the scalp EEG. Frontal lobe attacks often have prominent motor components that obscure the EEG, but even when it is readily visible there may be few if any changes.

*Non-epileptiform EEG abnormalities*

These include:

- Asymmetry of amplitude or frequency
- Localized slow waves
- Generalized slow waves

Asymmetries of the background EEG activity may reflect areas of localized damage that cannot produce normal rhythms (Fig. 3.11). Localized irregular slow activity that is persistent may be seen with underlying structural or vascular lesions (Fig. 3.12). Widespread or generalized slow activity suggests an encephalopathic process (Fig. 3.13), including anti-epileptic drug toxicity, and may also be seen postictally (see also 3.2.8).

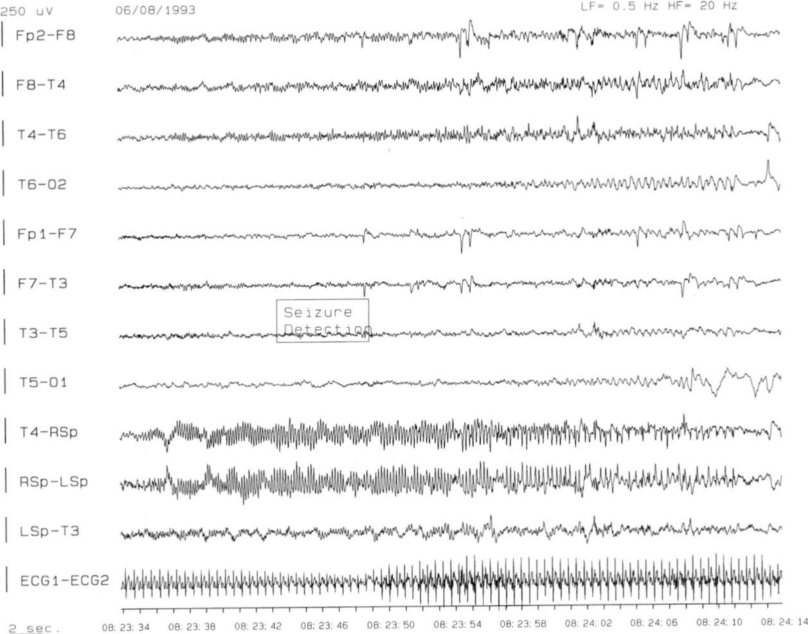


**Fig. 3.10** Ictal EEG recording. Seizure activity is first apparent over the right anterior temporal lobe (T4 – R sphenoidal) and evolves in frequency, slowing towards the end of the event. 'Seizure detection' denotes recognition of this event by an automatic computer

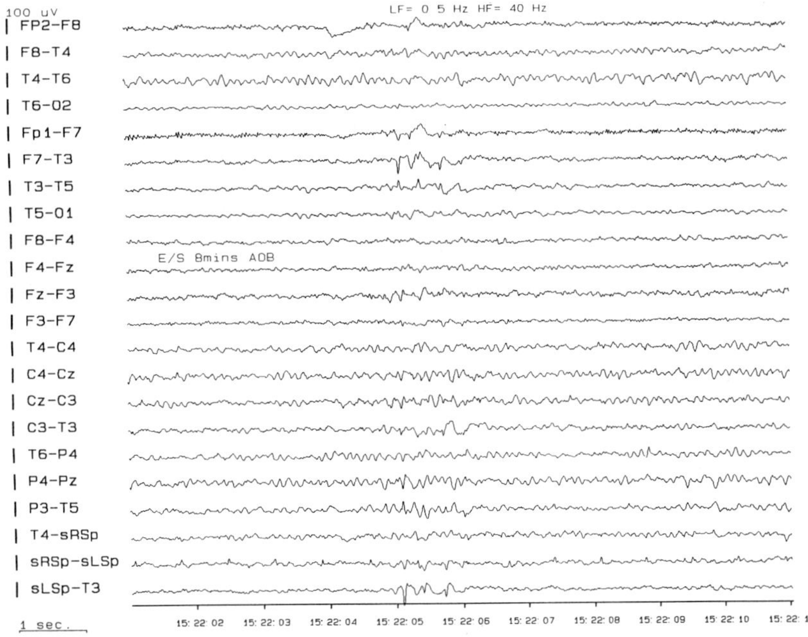


**Fig. 3.11** Asymmetry of the background EEG activity. There is relative paucity of normal rhythms over the left hemisphere (compare T4–T6 with T3–T5) and a burst of slow activity is seen over the left mid-temporal region

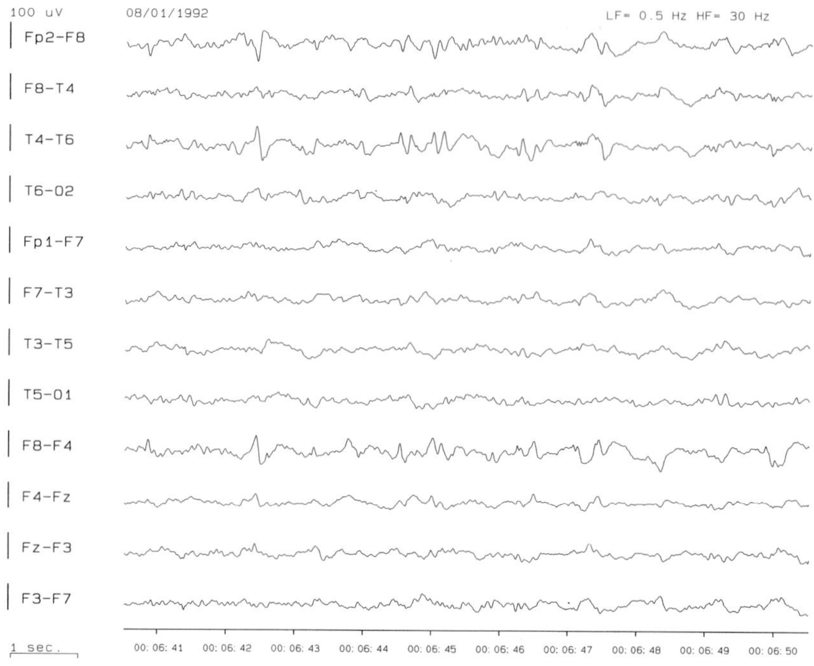


**Fig. 3.12** Localized, persistent, irregular slow activity mixed with sharp waves that overlies a structural lesion in the right temporal lobe

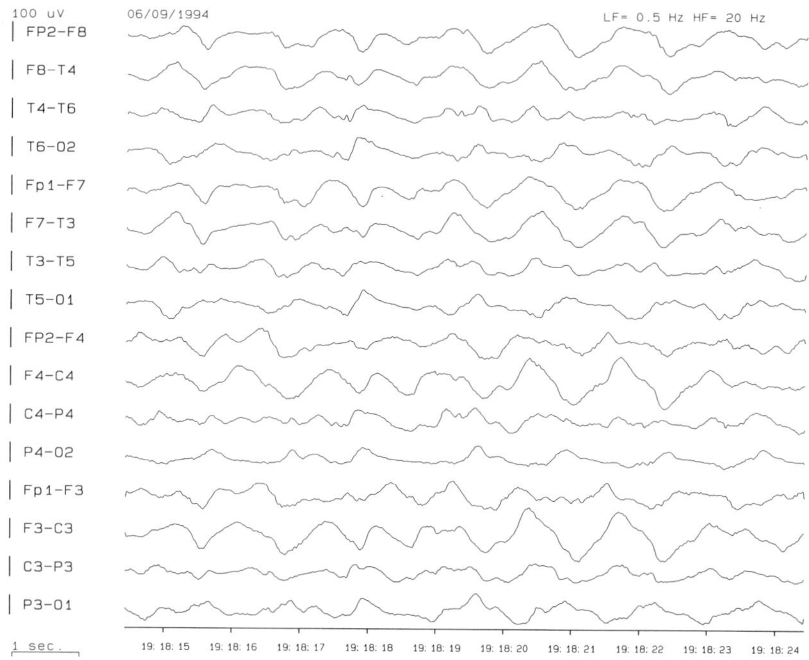


**Fig. 3.13** Generalized irregular delta activity (approximately 1 Hz), suggesting an encephalopathic process

## 3.2.5 EEG findings that are characteristic of epilepsy syndromes

The EEG features of different types of seizures and epilepsies are described in their clinical context in Chapter 2. Syndromes in which the routine EEG is likely to be of diagnostic importance are discussed below, with illustrative EEGs.

### *Idiopathic generalized epilepsy*

The key EEG features of idiopathic generalized epilepsy (Ch. 2, 2.7) are:

- Generalized epileptiform discharges, often at 3 Hz, usually maximum in the anterior parasagittal regions (Fig. 3.14)
- Normal background
- Often photosensitive

They must be distinguished from those of partial epilepsy, which are:

- Focal or multifocal epileptiform discharges
- Background EEG often abnormal
- Rarely photosensitive

Confusion can occur. Focal spikes may propagate to produce bilaterally synchronous discharges mimicking generalized epilepsy. This is most likely to occur with extratemporal epilepsy, especially if due to parasagittal lesions or cortical dysgenesis (Fig. 3.15). EEGs in patients with idiopathic generalized epilepsy may contain quite frequent additional focal discharges or show asymmetries, especially when recorded using temporal rather than parasagittal montages (Grunewald & Panayiotopoulos 1993). Further, occasional patients have both idiopathic generalized and partial epilepsy.

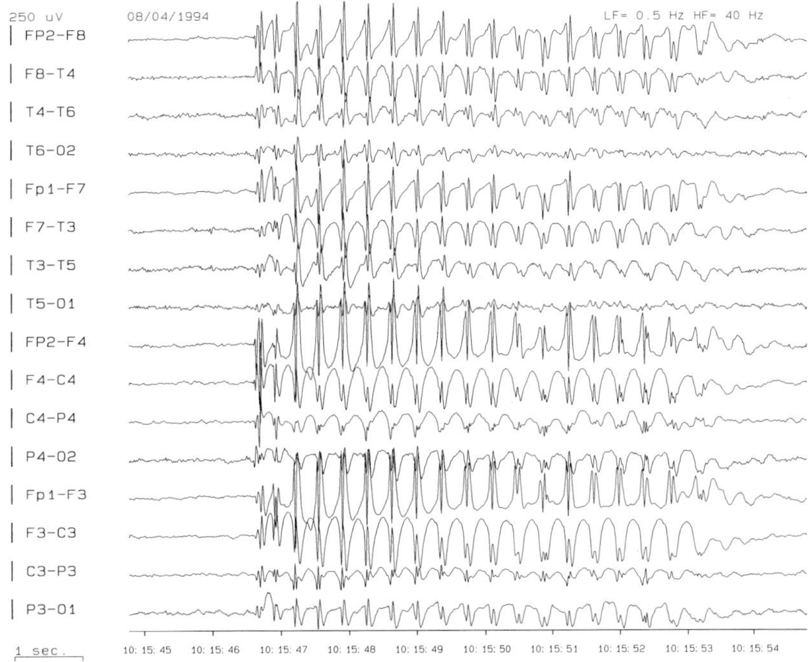


**Fig. 3.14** Generalized 3 Hz spike-wave activity. Onset is abrupt. The frequency of the discharge slows towards the end and becomes less regular

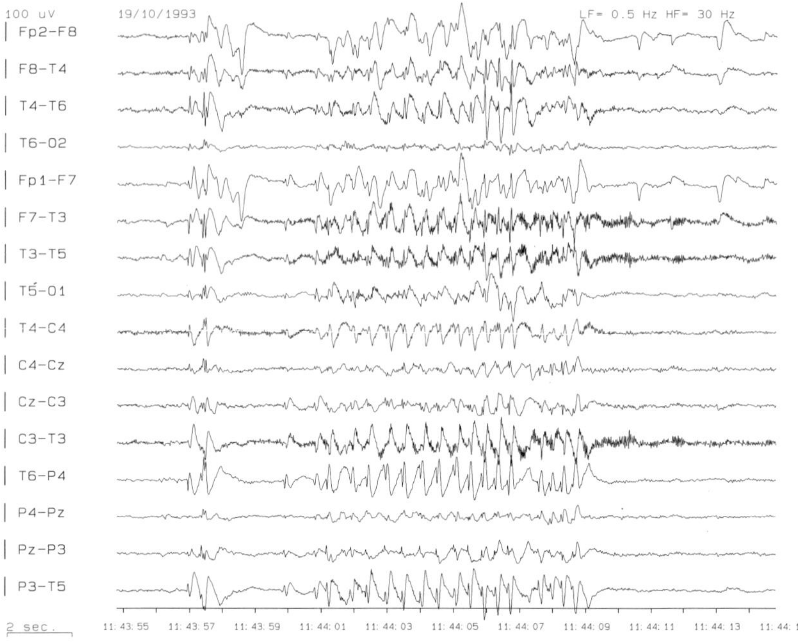


**Fig. 3.15** Secondary bilaterally synchronous discharges mimicking generalized epilepsy, in a patient with a small medial parietal oligodendroglioma

*Photosensitivity* is age-dependent. In the peak age group of 7–19 years, 10% of patients with newly presenting seizures show unequivocal photosensitivity on the EEG, with a female : male ratio of 3 : 2, while it rarely presents at other ages (Ch. 2, 2.5.11) (Fish et al 1993).

Photosensitive EEG responses have been classified by Waltz et al (1992) into four categories:

1. Occipital spikes
2. Occipital spike and slow waves with spread to the parieto-occipital regions
3. Occipital spike and slow waves with frontal spread
4. Generalized spike and slow wave discharges (Fig. 3.16)

Type 4 responses are the most common (Fig. 3.16) and show the strongest association with clinical epilepsy. Previously, greater importance has been placed on discharges that outlast the stimulus (Reilly & Peters 1973), but this is probably of less significance, being in part dependent upon how quickly the stimulus is turned off. Photosensitivity is usually seen in patients with idiopathic generalized epilepsy, but may occur in progressive myoclonic epilepsies (Berkovic et al 1991a), in metabolic disorders and occasionally in occipital partial epilepsies.

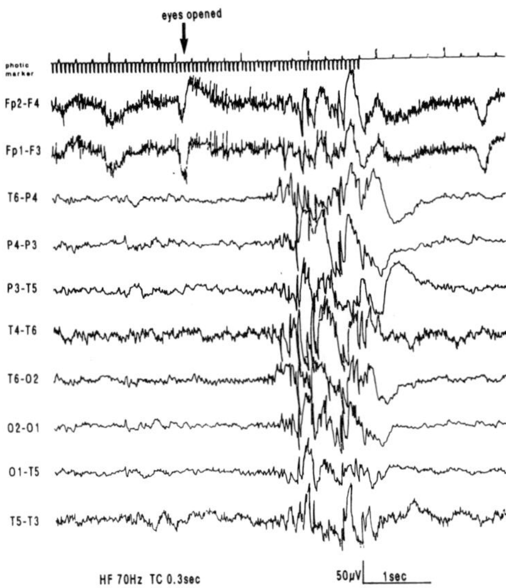


**Fig. 3.16** Grade 4 photosensitivity. There is a generalized spike-wave discharge continuing, in this case, after the end of the stimulus

*EEG findings in partial epilepsies*

The EEG findings in partial seizure disorders reflect both the site of onset and the aetiology of the epilepsy. Foreign tissue lesions are likely to be associated with localized slow activity, while neocortical atrophic processes may be associated with a relative paucity of normal rhythms.

*Temporal lobe epilepsy*: Interictal spikes are usually maximum over the temporal or fronto-temporal regions. Even in patients with unilateral temporal lobe lesions or hippocampal sclerosis who are good surgical candidates the interictal spikes are often bilateral and independent, especially during sleep. The ictal scalp EEG often shows rhythmic theta at the onset that may be localized to the affected temporal lobe or be bilateral.

*Frontal lobe epilepsy*: The scalp EEG is very variable, reflecting the heterogeneity of syndromes and the difficulties in recording from the frontal cortex. The interictal EEG often shows no epileptiform activity, bilaterally synchronous spikes or widespread spiking. Localized unifocal spikes are relatively uncommon. The ictal scalp EEG is often obscured by muscle and movement artefact and, because of rapid seizure propagation, localized changes are rare. Even when movement artefact does not obscure the trace, the scalp EEG may remain unchanged or only show poorly formed postictal slowing.

*Parieto-occipital lobe epilepsy*: Interictal spikes may be localized posteriorly, but there are often more anterior discharges, either over the temporal regions or bilateral, synchronous widespread discharges. The latter may be the most apparent feature, presumably due to rapid propagation. Similarly, ictal scalp recordings may show more anterior changes than would have been expected.

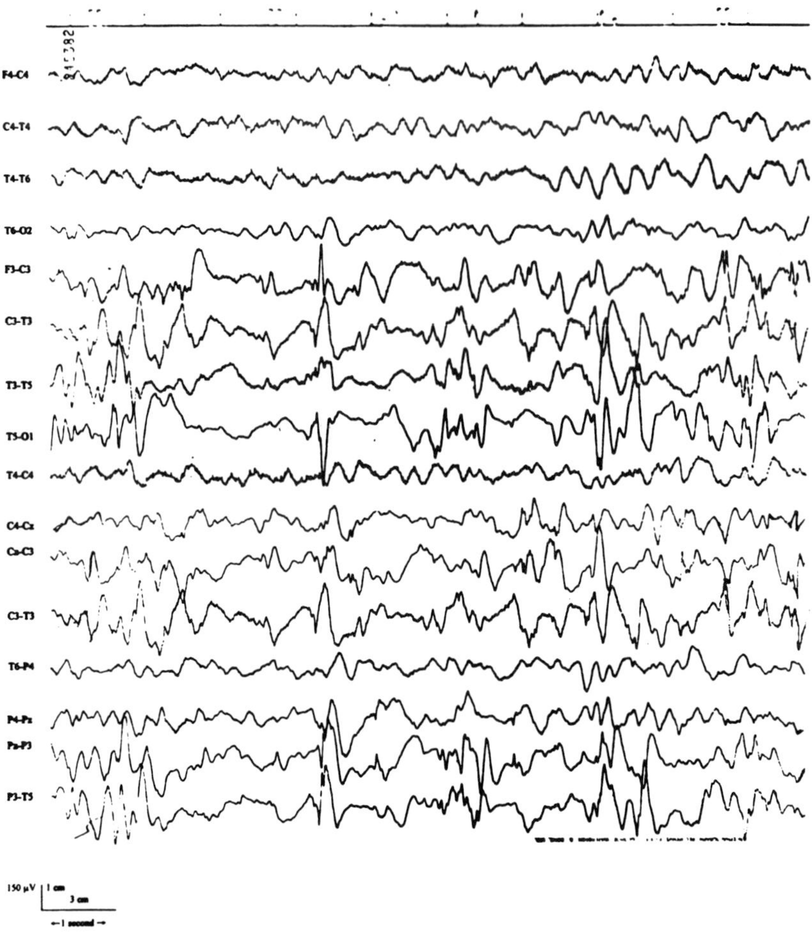

Fig. 3.17 Hemi-hypsarrythmia, with a high amplitude disorganized pattern seen over the left hemisphere, in a 6-month-old child with a right hemiparesis and gross developmental delay (reproduced by courtesy of the Department of Clinical Neurophysiology, St Mary's Hospital, London)

*Infantile spasms*

The resting EEG shows a characteristic disorganized high-voltage pattern, with generalized attenuation during the spasms. Hypsarrythmia may be seen bilaterally or, in some cases, unilaterally (Fig. 3.17) (Hrachovy et al 1984)

*Benign rolandic epilepsy*

This condition is characterized by unilateral or bilateral, triphasic, large-amplitude spikes that are maximum in the central or centro-temporal, without background abnormalities (Fig. 3.18) (Loiseau & Beaussart 1973).

*Benign occipital epilepsy*

Posterior 1.5–3 Hz spike and slow wave discharges may occur singly or in long runs, may be lateralized and usually attenuate with eye-opening. Spread of activity may occur to produce a picture of generalized epileptiform discharges (Newton & Aicardi 1983).

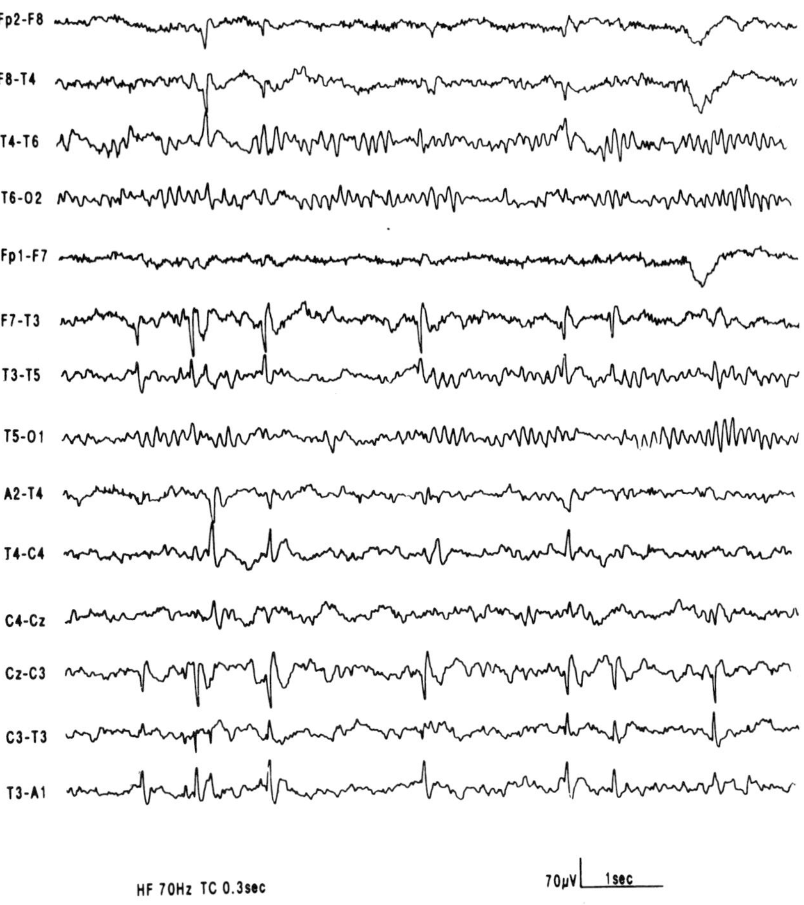


**Fig. 3.18** Benign rolandic epilepsy. There are bilateral, triphasic, large amplitude spikes, maximal in the centro-temporal areas, with normal background activity

*Lennox–Gastaut syndrome*

The background EEG is usually slow and disorganized, with superadded 1–2.5 Hz generalized, anteriorly predominant spike and slow wave discharges. During sleep there are often bursts of fast generalized spikes (Fig. 3.19) (Yaqub 1993).

*Electrical status epilepticus in slow wave sleep*

More than 85% of slow wave sleep shows spike and wave activity, which is usually generalized (Jayakar & Seshia 1991).

## 3.2.6 Non-epileptic seizures

In non-epileptic seizures, rhythmic head movements can produce EEG artefacts that may mimic cerebral ictal activity, and this may lead to erroneous conclusions. In non-epileptic attack disorder (pseudo-

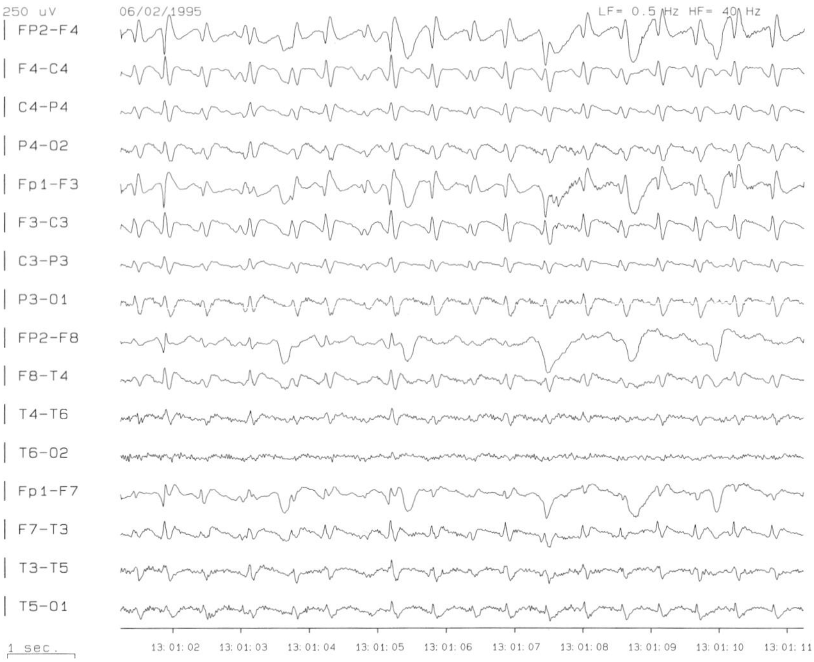


**Fig. 3.19** Generalized, irregular slow spike-wave activity, characteristic of the Lennox–Gastaut syndrome

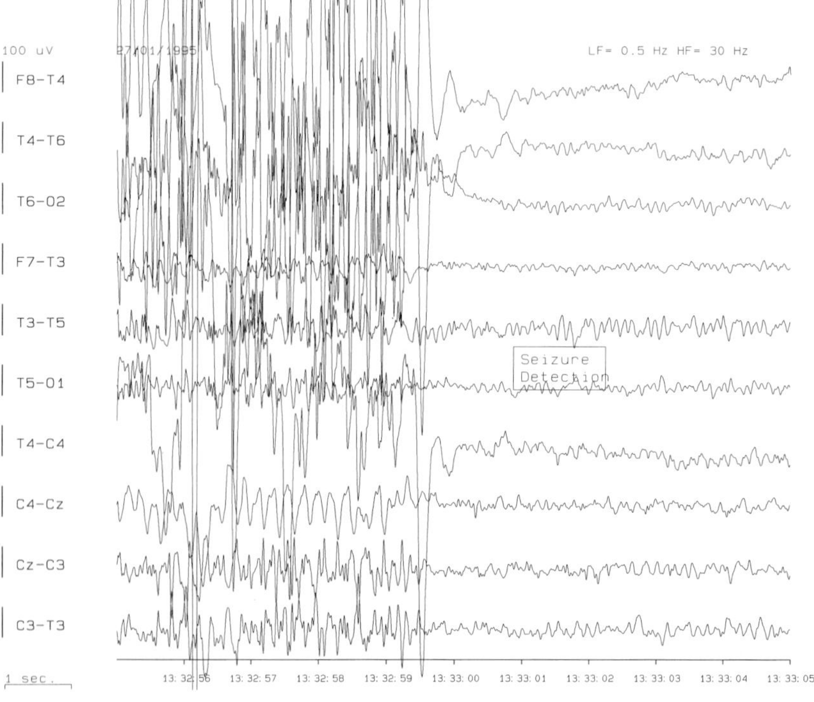


**Fig. 3.20** Non-epileptic attack (pseudoseizure). Intense muscle activity, followed immediately by alpha rhythm, while the patient appears to be unresponsive

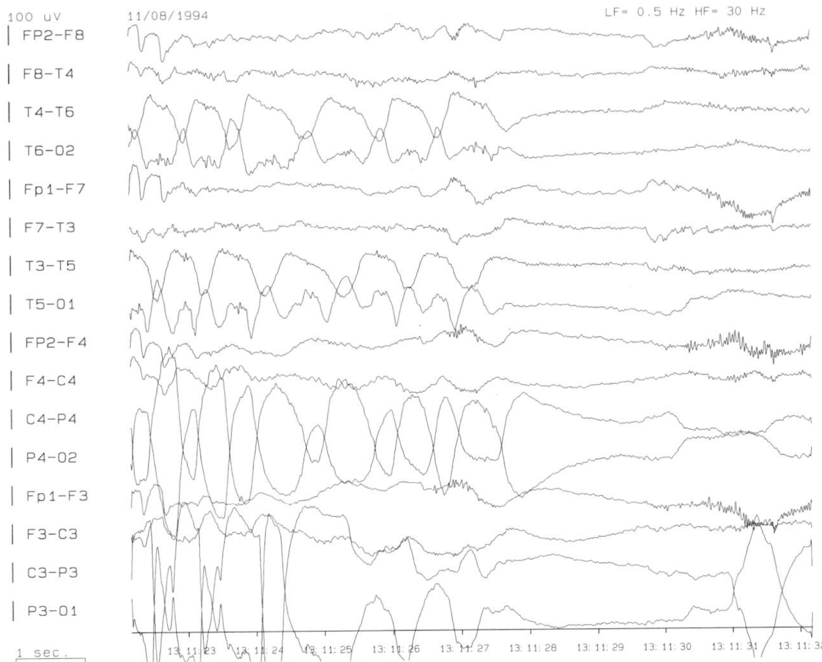


**Fig. 3.21** Non-epileptic attack (pseudoseizure). Rhythmic head movements producing EEG artefacts that resemble cerebral slow waves

seizures), however, the record abruptly returns to normal in between the movements (Figs 3.20, 3.21) and alpha activity may then be seen, which attenuates with alerting stimuli such as calling the patient's name or forced eye-opening (Meierkord et al 1991).

## 3.2.7 EEG in status epilepticus

See Chapter 5 for clinical and treatment aspects of status epilepticus.

*Generalized convulsive status*

The EEG is often obscured during clonic movements, but some changes are always apparent. These include generalized spikes/polyspikes and waves, intermittent attenuation, periodic lateralized epileptiform discharges or slowing between convulsive episodes (Treiman et al 1990).

Patients with generalized convulsive status may need to be anaesthetized and ventilated. EEG monitoring is then essential to confirm cessation of ictal electrographic activity and may also help to monitor anaesthetic effects (e.g. barbiturate-induced burst suppression).

*Non-convulsive status*

This can occur in patients with idiopathic generalized epilepsy ('absence status') or in partial epilepsies. Often there is diagnostic uncertainty on clinical grounds and the prolonged duration of events may raise the possibility of psychiatric, metabolic, infectious or structural cerebral lesions. Urgent EEG studies are crucial and may provide important diagnostic information (Cascino 1993). In idiopathic generalized epilepsies the record usually shows generalized spike and slow wave activity that terminates abruptly with response to treatment (Andermann & Robb 1972). Partial epilepsies show more variable patterns, which fluctuate during individual episodes (Grand'Maison et al 1991). Semi-rhythmic slow activity is common but non-specific and does not differentiate between ictal, postictal or encephalopathic disorders. Ongoing seizure activity is suggested by:

- Continuous rhythmic activity unresponsive to alerting stimuli
- Episodic generalized attenuation
- Intermittent periodic lateralized epileptiform discharges (Fig. 3.22)
- Abrupt cessation of the rhythmic activity with intravenous diazepam

Unfortunately, however, intravenous diazepam often produces non-specific changes due to sleep, and may exacerbate respiratory depression.

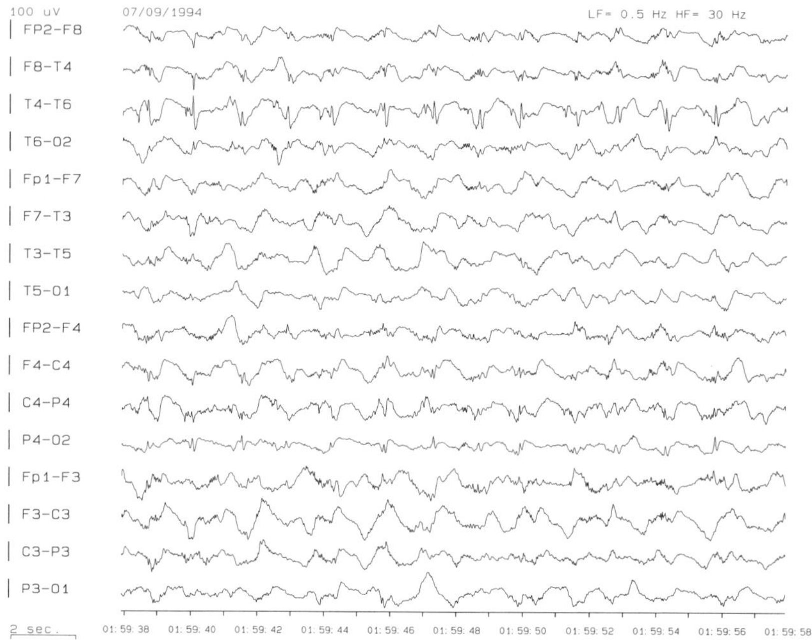


**Fig. 3.22** Intermittent periodic lateralized epileptiform discharges in patient with complex partial status epilepticus

*Epilepsia partialis continua*

Epilepsia partialis continua involves repetitive focal jerking. The EEG only infrequently shows contralateral rhythmic spikes time-locked to the jerks. Often there is only focal slow or poorly associated epileptiform discharges, and sometimes the EEG is remarkably unhelpful (Schomer 1993).

### 3.2.8 Evaluation of possible encephalopathy

In the emergency evaluation of a patient with an acute encephalopathy and seizures, the EEG may give useful evidence of an encephalitis. Herpes simplex encephalitis has a characteristic appearance, with disorganized and slow background rhythms with periodic lateralized epileptiform complexes at 2–4 s intervals that are often particularly evident over the fronto-temporal areas. These features may, however, be lacking or only evolve over several days.

In an encephalopathy caused by a metabolic disturbance, as for example in liver failure, or intoxication by a drug, including anti-epileptic drugs, the background rhythms are slowed and there is widespread excessive theta and delta activity. These appearances, however, are non-specific and the EEG appearances are not a good guide to the cause of an encephalopathy (Fig. 3.13).

In some chronic conditions in which seizures occur, such as subacute sclerosing panencephalitis (SSPE) and Creutzfeldt–Jakob disease (CJD), there may be characteristic EEG features that can help to make a diagnosis. In SSPE there are periodic complexes at intervals of 10 s or more and in CJD the EEG often shows generalized pseudoperiodic sharp wave complexes at regular intervals of less than 1 s.

## 3.3 STRUCTURAL IMAGING OF THE BRAIN

### 3.3.1 Indications for structural imaging

The skull radiograph has no place in the investigation of patients with epilepsy other than in the emergency assessment of patients with significant head injuries in whom there is concern about a skull fracture (Fig. 3.23). The identification of acute traumatic intracranial damage and haematomas is best carried out with X-ray CT scans (Fig. 3.24, 3.25).

The indications for structural imaging of the brain were initially defined in the X-ray CT era, when the prime goal was to identify gross structural lesions such as cerebral tumours. The situation has changed radically with the development of MRI, which can reveal subtle structural abnormalities that underlie epilepsy in a much higher proportion of patients, without ionizing radiation, and also with the development of effective surgical treatment strategies for patients with medically refractory partial seizures (Ch. 10).

The major difficulties with MRI are the lack of ready availability of the instruments in some countries, suboptimal MRI techniques and a paucity of skilled radiographers and neuroradiologists to employ optimal sequences and to interpret the data. If structural imaging of the brain is necessary, optimal MRI rather than X-ray CT is undoubtedly the investigation of choice as the initial technique, depending on the availability of resources. At present, in optimal circumstances, structural imaging of the brain is regarded as being indicated in any of the following circumstances:

- Partial seizures, on history and/or EEG
- Fixed or progressive neurological or psychological deficit
- Onset of generalized seizures before the age of 1 year and after 20 years
- Difficulty obtaining seizure control with AEDs
- Loss of seizure control or status epilepticus, if this does not have a clear explanation such as omission of medication
- Acutely, after significant cerebral trauma

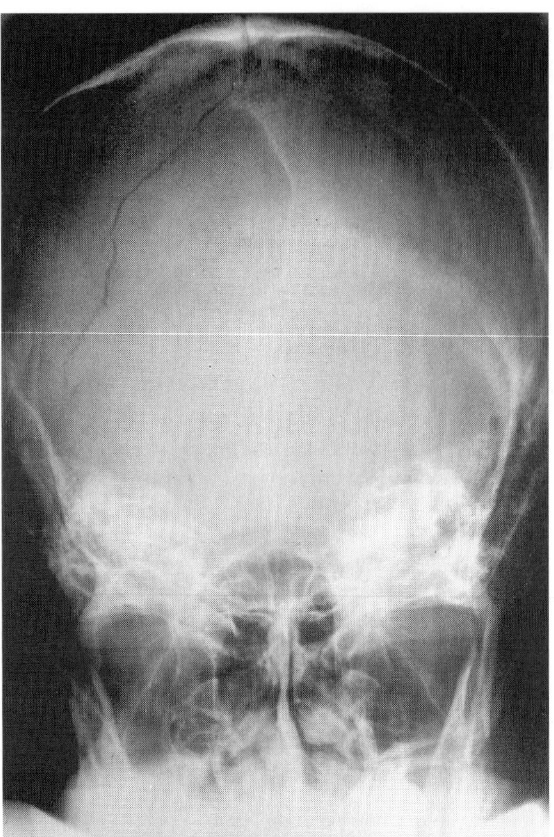

Fig. 3.23 Skull radiograph (PA projection) showing right parietal fracture, sustained during a tonic-clonic seizure

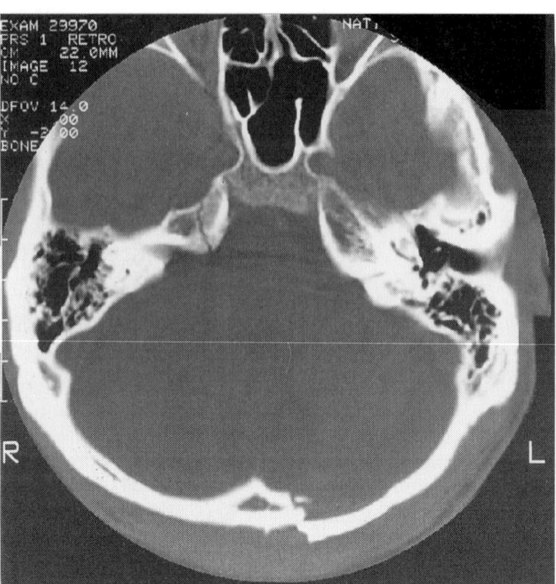


**Fig. 3.24** Axial X-ray CT scan. There is a fracture of the left occiput near the midline and a fracture between the middle and inner thirds of the right petrous bone. These injuries were sustained during a tonic seizure

In practical terms, these indications have the result that patients with onset of generalized seizures between the ages of 1 and 20 years who have no fixed deficit and whose seizures respond quickly to AED therapy will not be scanned. It is also probably reasonable to defer structural neuroimaging in a patient, of whatever age, who has an isolated generalized seizure that has been clearly provoked, such as by alcohol withdrawal, although some authorities feel that all patients who have an epileptic seizure should have neuroimaging. It is also reasonable to defer imaging in a child with a typical clinical and EEG picture of benign rolandic epilepsy. In pregnancy, the same general principles of indications for imaging apply, although if the situation is not acute and there is no other cause for concern it is often reasonable to defer imaging until after the delivery (Ch. 6, 6.3.11).

MRI is indicated in most patients with refractory partial seizures in whom an X-ray CT scan is unremarkable or unclear, and in all patients in whom surgical treatment is under consideration. The superiority of MRI over CT in terms of both sensitivity and specificity for detecting lesions that underlie epilepsy has been demonstrated by numerous studies (Jabbari et al 1986, Lesser et al 1986, Ormson et al 1986, Sperling et al 1986, Theodore et al 1986, Kuzniecky et al 1987, Bergen et al 1989, Franceschi et al 1989, Brooks et al 1990).

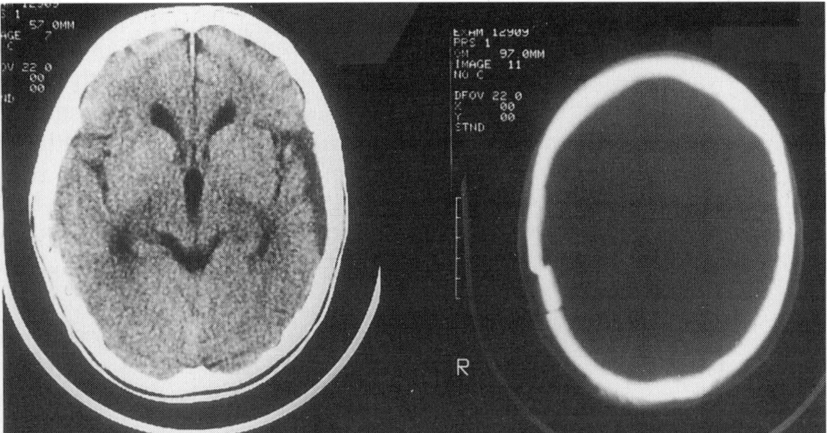


**Fig. 3.25** Axial X-ray CT scan. There is a depressed fracture of the right parietal bone (bone window image: on right) and a contrecoup subdural collection (soft tissue image: on left). Injury sustained during a seizure 10 days previously

X-ray CT may be preferred to MRI if a patient is disturbed or acutely unwell, as the patient is more accessible during an X-ray CT scan, and is also valuable for the investigation of possible acute intracranial haematomas and skull fractures (Figs 3.24, 3.25), and as a supplement to MRI for clarification of possible intracranial calcification, which is not shown easily by the latter technique.

*Problems with MRI*

In addition to problems of limited availability of facilities and the need for highly trained radiographers and interpreting radiologists, together with the operator-dependent nature of optimal MRI, there are some practical difficulties associated with MRI. Some patients cannot tolerate the procedure because of claustrophobia and MRI is contraindicated if the patient has a cardiac pacemaker or ferromagnetic metal clips on cerebral blood vessels. Metal fragments within the eye may move during an MRI because of the magnetic field and cause intraocular damage. Metal objects in the head may also cause severe artefact that renders the images difficult to interpret. Patients who are restless, severely claustrophobic, and young children may require a general anaesthetic to be scanned.

## 3.3.2 Recent developments in MRI

MRI techniques are evolving rapidly in terms of improved spatial and temporal resolution and the development of functional MR measures. Developments in MRI that have led to improved brain imaging include:

- Magnet design and strength
- Use of optimal sequences and scanning planes for demonstrating cerebral structure and abnormalities
- Processing of data post-acquisition, including reformatting, surface-rendering, quantitation of size and morphology of cerebral structures and of signal intensity

It is currently widely held that imaging is optimal using a 1.5 Tesla magnet. Optimal scanning planes are those that demonstrate the length and cross-section of a structure with minimization of partial volume effects. These are best obtained by orienting the plane in which the data is acquired or, less well, by reformatting images for viewing in the preferred plane. Reformatting of a set of MR images is possible if a volume of data is originally acquired in contiguous 1 mm thick slices. An advantage of acquiring data in this way is that the process of reformatting may be used to correct any undesired yaw, roll or tilt that the patient's head has with respect to the instrument. If data is acquired in thick, non-contiguous slices, e.g. using an inversion recovery sequence with a slice thickness of 5 mm and an interslice interval of 2.5 mm, reformatting is not possible and malpositioning of the patient in the scanner cannot be corrected.

As a result of these rapid and continuing developments it is important to recognize that not all MRI scans are of comparable quality and that optimal imaging may reveal abnormalities that were not apparent on a suboptimal sequence obtained on an older instrument.

The basic epilepsy MRI protocol that we currently employ is:

1. A volume acquisition T1-weighted coronal data set that covers the whole brain in 1.5 mm-thick slices. This sequence produces approximately cubic voxels, allowing for reformatting in any orientation, subsequent measurement of hippocampal morphology and volumes, and 3D reconstruction and surface-rendering. The sequences used are IRPF SPGR (GE) or MPRAGE (Siemens).

2. An oblique coronal inversion recovery sequence that is heavily T1-weighted and orientated perpendicular to the long axis of the hippocampus, to best demonstrate the internal structure and T1-weighted signal intensity of the hippocampus.

3. An oblique coronal spin echo (VEMP) (GE) or double-echo STIR (Siemens) sequence that is heavily T2-weighted and orientated perpendicular to the long axis of the hippocampus, to demonstrate any increase in T2-weighted signal intensity. Quantitation of hippocampal T2 relaxation times may also be obtained using various techniques, for example a Carr–Purcell–Meiboom–Gill multiecho sequence, with 16 echo times ranging from 22 to 262 ms.

### 3.3.3 Current MRI developments

It is likely that the spatial resolution of MR images will improve so that the substructures of the hippocampus will be readily identifiable and subtle pathological changes in the neocortex reliably identified in vivo. In part this will be achieved by improvements in instrument hardware, including design of coils, such as surface coils that provide better definition of the cortical ribbon. Software advances include the development of new imaging sequences that may identify abnormalities that are not visible using standard methodologies, such as FLAIR, which gives images that are heavily T2-weighted but in which the signal from cerebrospinal fluid is suppressed and so appears black (Bergin et al 1995). The use of echoplanar imaging techniques allows images to be obtained in less than 100 ms, so that movement artefact may be averted and dynamic changes in diffusion and blood flow followed. Diffusion-weighted imaging, obtained with echoplanar techniques, and magnetization transfer imaging show promise as very sensitive methods for identification of neuronal injury.

Magnetic resonance angiography is likely to replace conventional cerebral angiography in the next 5 years. Functional MRI, which is sensitive to the oxygenation status of haemoglobin, provides images that are sensitive to changes in regional cerebral blood volume and flow, producing data analogous to that obtained with blood flow tracers and positron emission tomography, but with an improved temporal resolution, to the order of 3-5 s. It has already been demonstrated that this technique can detect ictal changes in cerebral blood flow and shows considerable potential for the investigation of seizure disorders in vivo (Jackson et al 1994). A further important use of this technique is to delineate areas of brain that are responsible for specific functions, such as the primary sensory and motor cortex, and to identify their anatomical relation to areas of planned neurosurgical resection (Turner 1994, Pritchard & Rosen 1994).

There are also important advances being made in the post-acquisition of data. Reformatting, three-dimensional reconstruction and segmentation of images will allow easier delineation of areas of abnormal cortical morphology and their relation to normal structures. Co-registration of data from different imaging modalities, such as MRI and PET, is now becoming commonplace and allows precise structure–function correlations to be made, greatly enhancing the interpretation of both sets of data. A surgical application of post-acquisition data processing is the real-time co-registration of previously acquired MRI stereotactic information with that obtained from a pointer used by a surgeon during an operation, so that the surgeon has precise feedback about the extent and location of the surgical field with relation to the brain as a whole.

### 3.3.4 MRI of hippocampal sclerosis

Hippocampal sclerosis (HS) is found in 50–70% of temporal lobes removed for the treatment of epilepsy and is associated with a greater than 60% chance of the patient becoming seizure-free (Babb & Brown 1987, Bruton 1988). Hippocampal sclerosis, then, is the single most important cause of intractable partial seizures, and a reliable means of diagnosing HS in vivo, non-invasively, is a major advance. The ability of MRI to diagnose HS reliably is the result of several factors: appreciation of hippocampal anatomy, awareness of relevant imaging abnormalities, use of optimal orientation of scanning planes, optimal scanning sequences and advances in instrumentation (Duvernoy 1988, Jackson et al 1990, Berkovic et al 1991b). The hippocampus is a curved structure, with its concave surface adjacent to the brainstem and its longitudinal axis at approximately 35° to the orbito-meatal line, that was traditionally used for the axial imaging plane with both X-ray CT and MRI. To minimize partial volume effects the hippocampus is best visualized in two planes: along the long axis and perpendicular to the structure. These imaging planes are readily determined on a sagittal scout image, the axial plane being in the line joining the base of the splenium of the corpus callosum to the inferior posterior border of the frontal lobe (Fig. 3.26) and the coronal plane being perpendicular to this, parallel to the anterior border of the brainstem. If contiguous 1mm thick slices are acquired these may be satisfactorily reformatted into the optical planer to demonstrate hippocampal morphology.

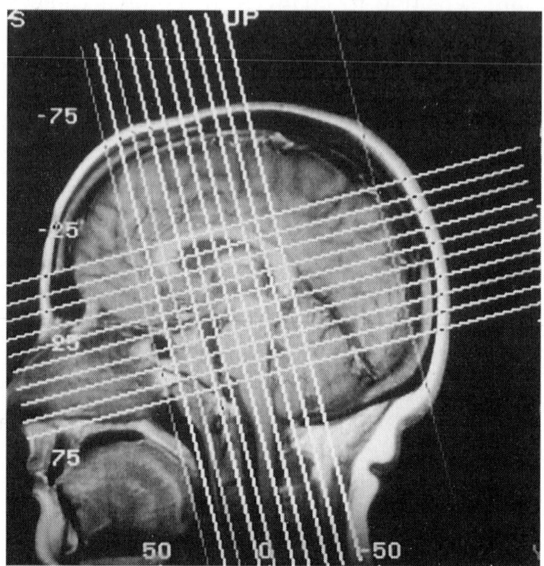


**Fig. 3.26** Sagittal scout image showing imaging planes to demonstrate the hippocampus, along the long axis and perpendicular to the body of the hippocampus

The initially identified MRI features of HS were hippocampal atrophy, demonstrated with coronal T1-weighted images (Fig. 3.27), and increased signal intensity within the hippocampus on T2-weighted spin echo images (Fig. 3.28) (Jackson et al 1990). Increased T2-weighted signal per se is a non-specific finding, and may result from foreign tissue lesions and pixels containing partial volumes of CSF. In order to avoid such errors it is necessary that the finding of T2-weighted signal increase is interpreted in the light of high-quality anatomical imaging. Further MRI features of HS, in addition to atrophy and increased T2-weighted signal and well demonstrated on coronal inversion recovery images, include decreased T1-weighted signal intensity and disruption of the internal structure of the hippocampus (Jackson et al 1993a) (Fig. 3.27). Misalignment of the patient in the magnet may cause difficulties with the assessment of hippocampal atrophy and a potential advantage of volume acquisitions is the facility to reformat the images in any orientation. In addition, atrophy of temporal lobe white matter and cortex and dilatation of the temporal horn are variably accompanying features to the changes of HS but are not reliable in their own right.

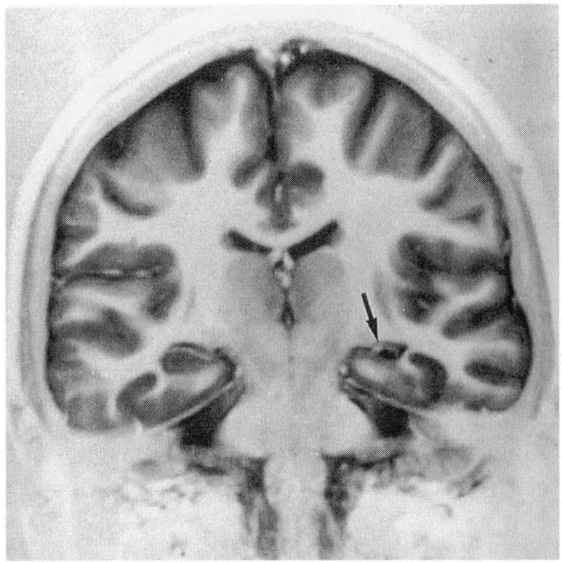

**Fig. 3.27** Coronal T1-weighted inversion recovery image through the body of the hippocampi showing the features of left hippocampal sclerosis: marked atrophy, T1 signal hypointensity and disruption of the internal structure of the hippocampus (arrowed)

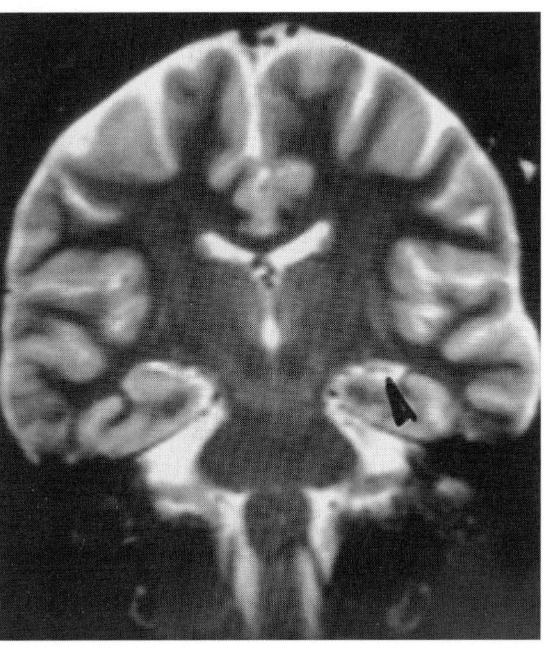

**Fig. 3.28** Coronal T2-weighted image showing increased T2 signal intensity in the body of the left hippocampus (arrowed)

*Measurements of hippocampal volumes*

The identification of hippocampal atrophy can be improved by measurement of the volumes of hippocampi (Jack et al 1990) In this initial study, hippocampal volume measurements gave correct lateralization in 76% with no false lateralizations and were superior to qualitative inspection of hippocampal asymmetry, measurements and visual assessment of anterior temporal lobe and mesial parenchymal T2-weighted signal intensity. The same group subsequently showed hippocampal atrophy on MRI in 14 of 15 patients with mesial temporal sclerosis and in three of nine patients with lesser degrees of neuronal loss or no abnormality (Cascino et al 1991). Further, asymmetric atrophy of the resected hippocampus on MRI was associated with a good prognosis for seizure control; atrophy of the contralateral non-resected hippo-campus was associated with a worse outcome and two patients with bilateral atrophy and no side-to-side difference did poorly (Jack et al 1992).

Cook et al (1992) used approximately 30 contiguous 1.5 mm slices through the hippocampus and amygdala, with a spoiled gradient echo technique, thresholding and a manually driven cursor, to outline the hippocampus and amygdala in individual slices (Fig. 3.29). Automated counting of pixels then generated cross-sectional contour maps that did not find an asymmetry of hippocampi in 10 normal right-handed subjects and demonstrated focal and diffuse hippocampal atrophy in patients with well defined temporal lobe epilepsy (Fig. 3.30). With technological and software developments, quantitative volumetric techniques have advanced considerably in recent years. The use of contiguous thin slices enhances the accuracy and reliability of measurements and permits localization of

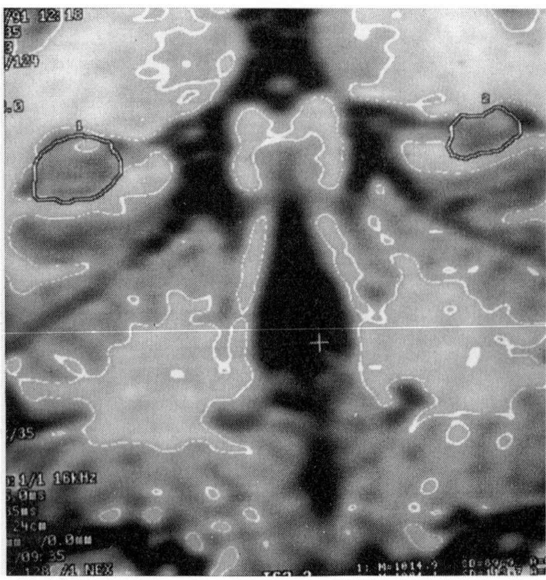

**Fig. 3.29** 1.5 mm thick coronal section demonstrating thresholding of the grey–white interface and outlining of the hippocampi (reproduced with permission from Cook et al 1992)

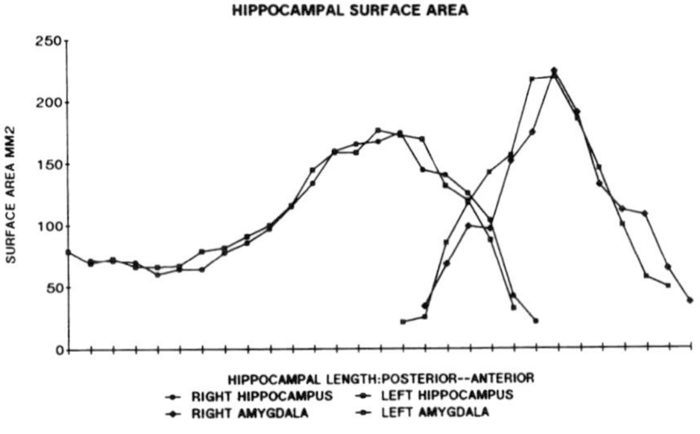


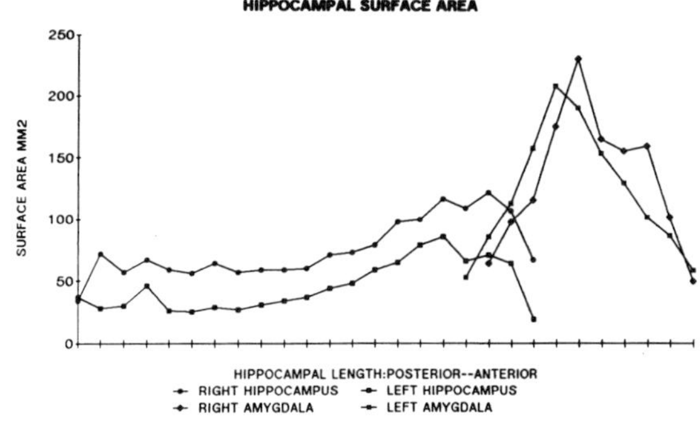


**Fig. 3.30** Cross-sectional area contour maps of hippocampus and amygdala derived from contiguous 1.5 mm slices (above) in a normal subject and (below) demonstrating diffuse left hippocampal atrophy (reproduced with permission from Cook et al 1992)

atrophy along the length of the hippocampus. Images obtained with increased T1 contrast and orientation of images perpendicular to the hippocampus may increase precision further. Attempts are being made to automate the assessment but at present, however, the methodology of hippocampal volumetry is demanding and time-consuming, requiring a post-processing computer and a skilled operator.

*Quantitative relaxometry*

A visually evident increase in hippocampal T2-weighted signal intensity generally has been reported in 0–60% of cases of HS (McLachlan et al 1985, Sperling et al 1986, Kuzniecky et al 1987, Triulzi et al 1988, Brooks et al 1990, Jack et al 1990, Jackson et al 1990, Bronen et al 1991, Ashtari et al 1991). In an analogous way to the quantification of hippocampal atrophy by volumetric analysis, T2-weighted signal intensity may be quantified reproducibly by measurement of T2 relaxation time (Fig. 3.31).

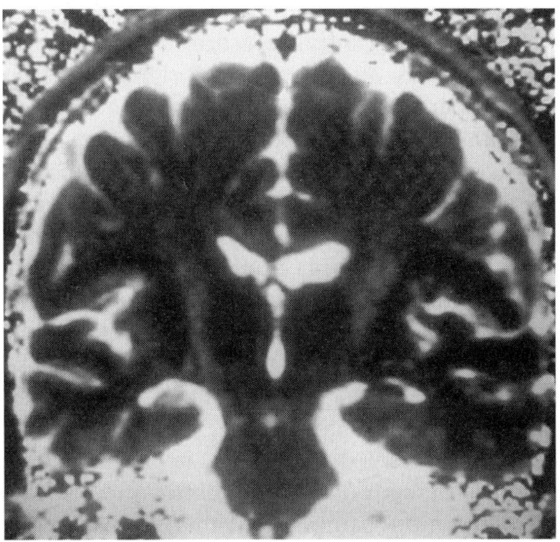

**Fig. 3.31** Calculated coronal T2 map in patient with right hippocampal sclerosis. Right hippocampal T2 relaxation time 124 ms; left hippocampal T2 relaxation time 106 ms

Hippocampal T2 relaxation times may be reproducibly constructed from 16 images, with echo times from 22 to 262 ms (Jackson et al 1993b, Duncan et al 1994, Grunewald et al 1994). The range of hippocampal T2 relaxation times in control subjects was 99–106 ms. These studies concluded that T2 relaxation time measurements are a useful identifier of hippocampal pathology, with T2 times in excess of 116 ms being associated with HS and intermediate values of 106–116 ms being seen in patients without qualitative MRI evidence of HS, contralateral to HS and in some patients with extratemporal seizure onset. T2 times in the hippocampus contralateral to HS were outside the normal range in 32% of patients, possibly reflecting bilateral hippocampal sclerosis. Subsequent studies on the same system have shown HS in patients with a hippocampal T2 of 107 ms and an inverse correlation between hippocampal T2 and neuronal density in the hippocampus (van Paesschen et al 1994). The data from healthy subjects indicate that there is a narrow range of normal hippocampal T2 relaxation times, resulting in the parameter being a potentially useful absolute measure. This is in contrast to hippocampal volume measurements, for which the wide normal range of absolute values at present largely limits assessment to identification of asymmetry and may preclude identification of bilateral HS and lesser degrees of contralateral hippocampal damage. The development of methods of correcting the hippocampal volume for the total intracranial volume may, however, obviate this limitation (Free et al 1995). The technique of T2 mapping can be readily implemented on most modern MRI systems and may be of clinical utility in the assessment of subtle degrees of T2 signal change in the hippocampus, in the identification of bilateral disease and in longitudinal studies of the progression of hippocampal damage.

*Conclusion*

In routine clinical practice, visual assessment of hippocampal size asymmetry and T2-weighted signal intensity provide useful data for the preoperative evaluation of possible hippocampal sclerosis. The further features of disruption of hippocampal internal structure and decreased signal intensity on heavily T1-weighted oblique coronal scans may also aid interpretation. Quantitation of hippocampal volumes provide objective data for assessment of difficult cases and may localize areas of atrophy within a hippocampus, with potentially important consequences for surgical planning, but the techniques are demanding, time-consuming and operator-dependent. T2-mapping software is available on many modern MRI systems, does not require sophisticated post-processing and may be of utility in routine clinical practice in the assessment of equivocal hippocampal T2 changes.

It is likely that research in the next decade will define the role of measurement of tissue volumes and relaxation times in the assessment of the hippocampus and that improvements in spatial resolution will reveal details of hippocampal substructure in vivo. Other MR methodologies will also be developed and evaluated. Proton MR spectroscopy of the temporal lobe shows promise as a technique for investigating biochemical and metabolic abnormalities associated with temporal lobe epilepsy (Connelly et al 1994, Connelly & Duncan 1995).

### 3.3.5 Other structural abnormalities revealed by MRI

Modern MRI frequently reveals the structural basis of epilepsy, which has not been revealed by X-ray CT or by previous MRI scans. Common examples include indolent gliomas, dysembryoplastic neuroepitheliomas, cavernous haemangiomas and disorders of neuronal migration. The finding of a discrete structural abnormality is of great importance when surgical treatment is being considered. Similarly, the finding of a diffuse abnormality, such as widespread cortical dysplasia, argues against surgical therapy being likely to effect seizure control (Ch. 10).

Indolent gliomas are clearly identified using MRI (Figs 3.32, 3.33).

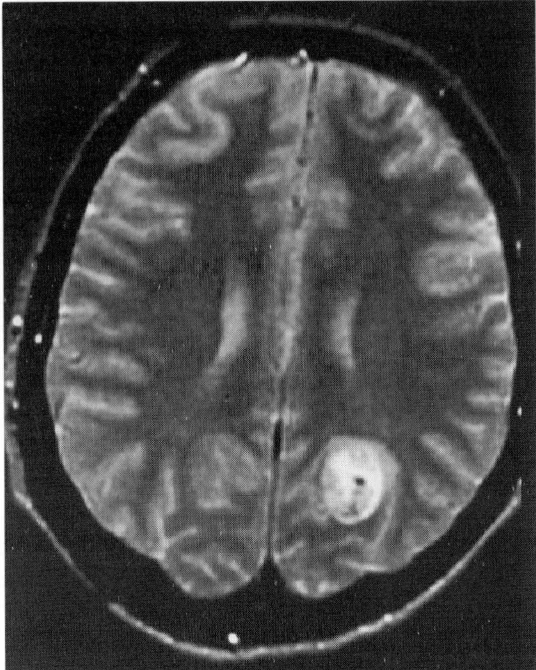

**Fig. 3.32** Indolent occipital lobe glioma. T2-weighted axial MRI scan showing a mass of mixed signal intensity in the left occipital lobe. Previous X-ray CT had shown an area of calcification that had been attributed to a prior head injury. The patient was a 15-year-old girl who had a 7-year history of complex partial seizures that began with the perception of blobs of colour and nausea. The surgical resection specimen showed a grade II glioma and she has been seizure-free for the 3 years following surgery

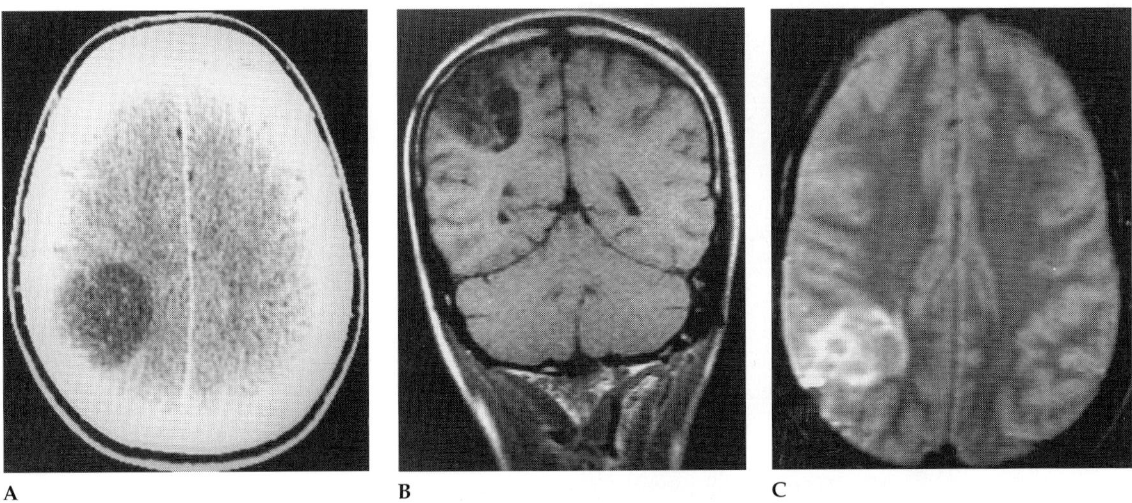

A B C

**Fig. 3.33 (A, B, C)** Indolent glioma in right parietal lobe. The patient was 22 years old and had had refractory complex partial seizures from the age of 14. Pathological examination of the surgical specimen showed a grade II glioma. **A.** Axial X-ray CT scan. **B.** Coronal T1-weighted MRI scan. **C.** Axial T2-weighted MRI scan

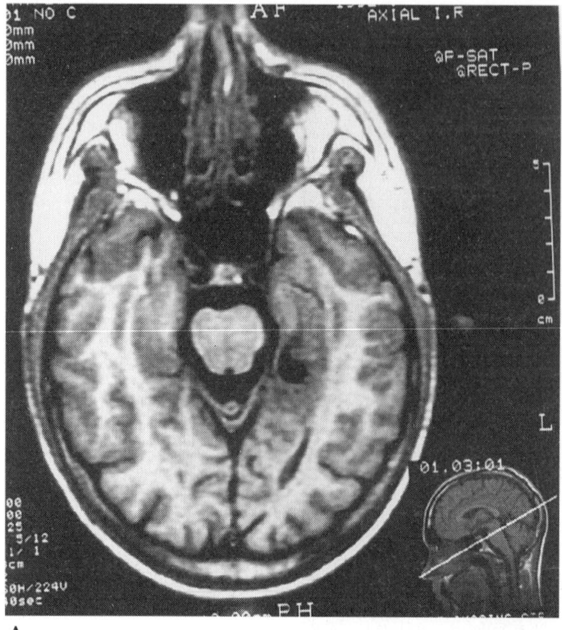

A

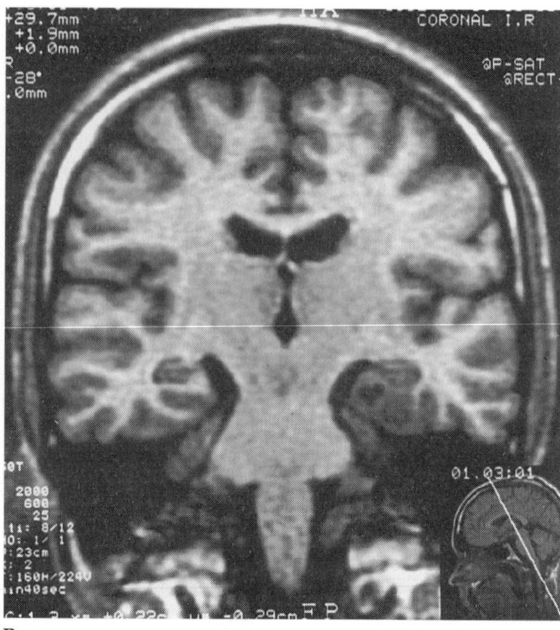

B

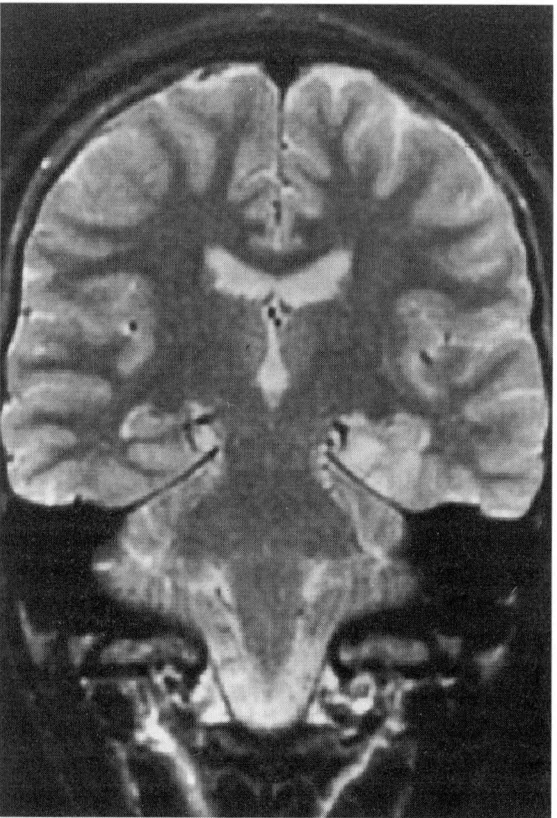
C

**Fig. 3.34 (A, B, C)** Dysembryoplastic neuroepithelioma in medial left temporal lobe. The patient was a 21-year-old secretary with a 6-year history of complex partial seizures that commenced with an epigastric rising sensation, followed by automatisms, that were uncontrolled by AEDs. A previous X-ray CT scan was normal. She is seizure-free 3 years following a left temporal lobectomy. **A.** Axial T1-weighted MRI scan showing a mass with low signal intensity in medial left temporal lobe, involving hippocampus at the level of the posterior brainstem. **B.** Coronal T1-weighted MRI scan showing a mass with low signal intensity in medial left temporal lobe, involving hippocampus. **C.** Coronal T2-weighted MRI scan showing the mass with high signal intensity

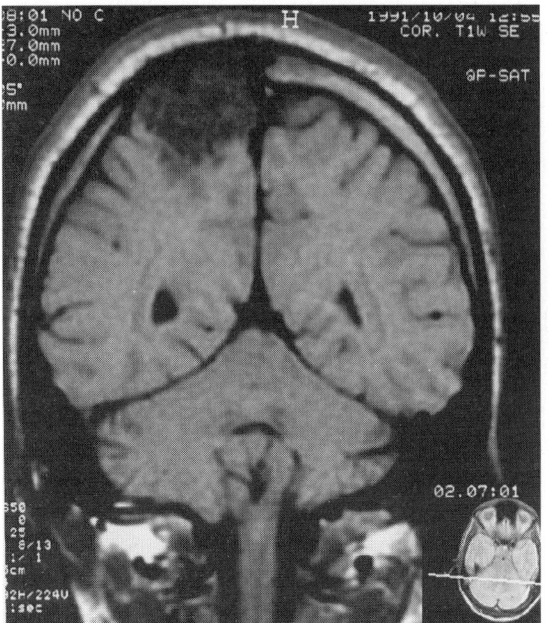


**Fig. 3.35** Coronal T1-weighted MRI scan showing a septated epidermoid cyst with low signal intensity in the superior right parietal lobe, causing erosion of the inner table of the skull

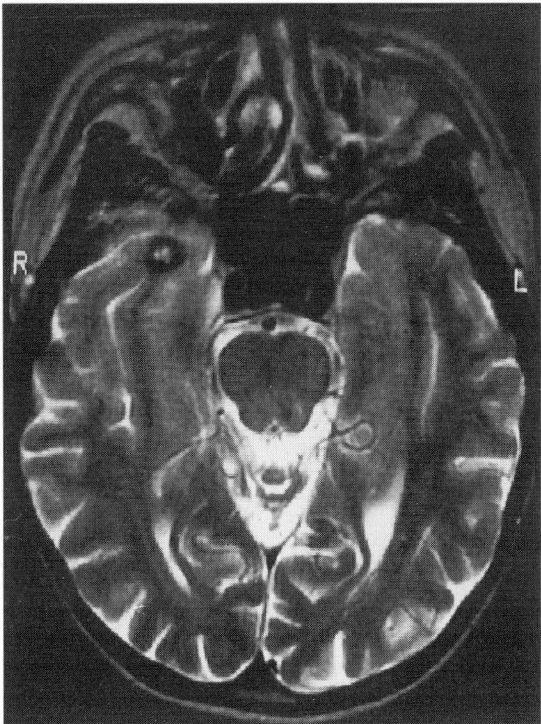


**Fig. 3.36** Axial T2-weighted MRI scan showing cavernous haemangioma in pole of right temporal lobe. There is a high signal centre surrounded by a ring of low signal intensity. The patient was a 56-year-old man who had had complex partial and secondarily generalized seizures from age 25 years, occurring once or twice per month, that were uncontrolled by AEDs.

These lesions are most commonly ill defined and non-cystic, do not enhance with contrast media and appear to arise from white matter.

Dysembryoplastic neuroepitheliomas (Fig. 3.34) are most commonly found in the temporal lobe, may be cystic and calcified and are usually circumscribed and arise in the cortex. If the lesions are in superficial cortex, focal erosion of the cranial vault may occur. One-third enhance and there is no associated cerebral oedema. Associated cortical dysplasia is evident in 20%. Intracranial epidermoid cysts may give rise to refractory partial seizures and a fixed neurological deficit that is stable over many years (Fig. 3.35).

Cavernous haemangiomas (Fig. 3.36) are circumscribed and have the characteristic appearance of a range of blood products. The central part contains areas of high signal on T1- and T2-weighted images, reflecting oxidized haemoglobin, with darker areas on T1-weighted images due to deoxyhaemoglobin. The ring of surrounding haemosiderin appears dark on a T2-weighted image. There may be calcification, which usually appears dark on T1- and T2-weighted images. There is no evidence of arteriovenous shunting. Arteriovenous malformations with high blood flow have a different and distinctive appearance (Fig. 3.37).

The clarity with which neuronal migration defects may be demon-

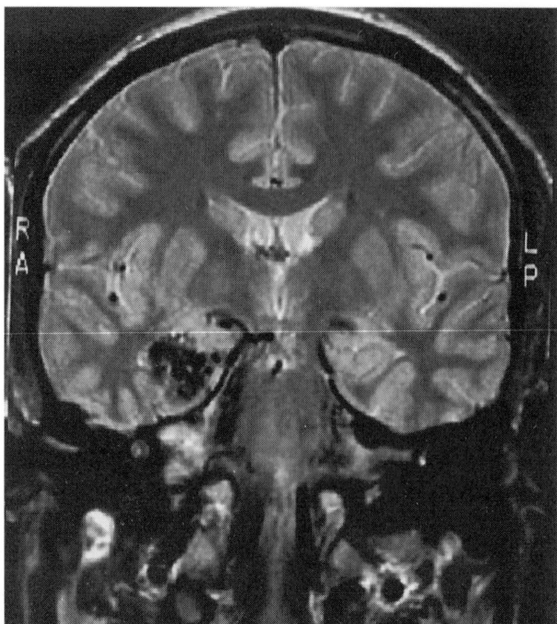


**Fig. 3.37** Coronal T2-weighted MRI scan showing a high blood flow arteriovenous malformation in the right uncus and amygdala, with signal change in the right hippocampus

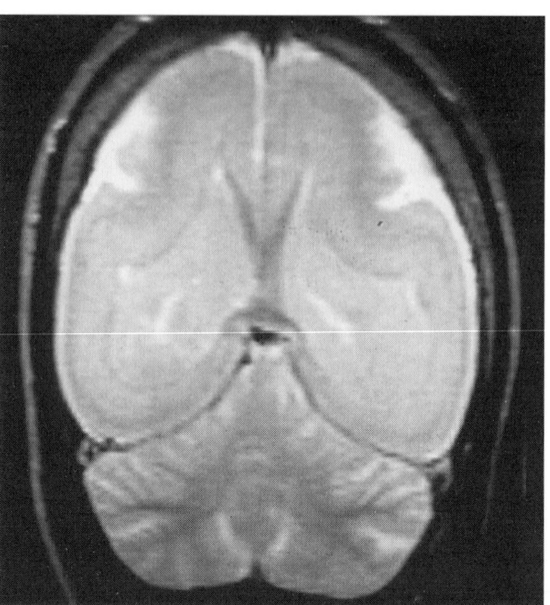

**Fig. 3.38** Coronal T2-weighted MRI scan showing a gross neuronal migration defect, lissencephaly, that on an X-ray CT scan was apparent as a blurring of the grey–white boundary. There is minimal formation of sulci and gyri. The patient was a 21-year-old woman with severe mental retardation and secondary generalized tonic-clonic seizures occurring several times per week

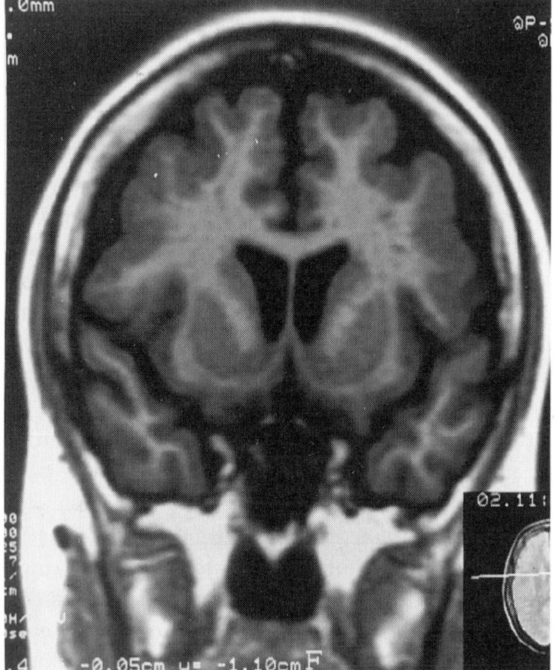


**Fig. 3.39** Coronal T1-weighted MRI scan showing extensive bilateral frontal neuronal migration defects, with only rudimentary gyrus formation. An X-ray CT scan was unremarkable

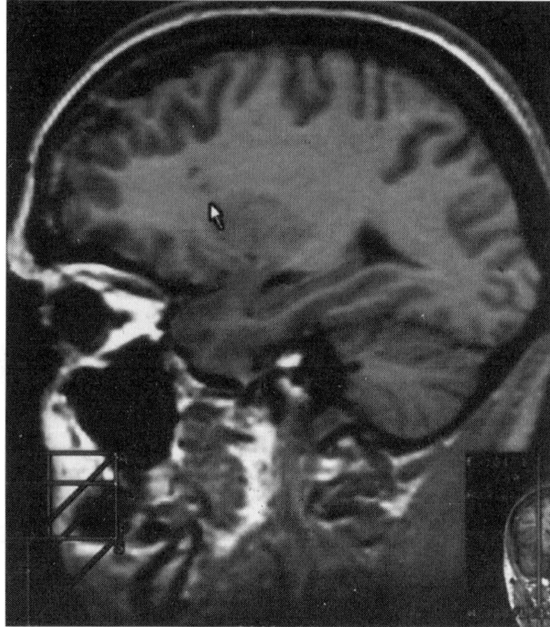

**Fig. 3.40** Sagittal T1-weighted MRI scan showing focal cortical dysplasia in right frontal lobe. The patient was a 23-year-old female with normal intellect and daily tonic and occasional tonic-clonic seizures, who had a single seizure in the 2 years following a right frontal lobectomy

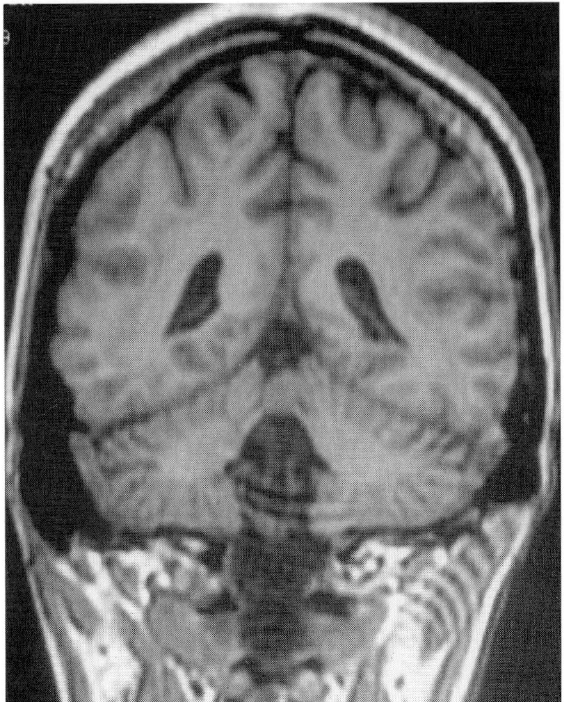

Fig. 3.41 Coronal T1-weighted MRI scan showing band heterotopia. There is a bilateral band of ectopic neurones giving the appearance of a 'double cortex'. The patient was a 29-year-old female with a 12-year history of refractory complex partial and secondary generalized tonic-clonic seizures

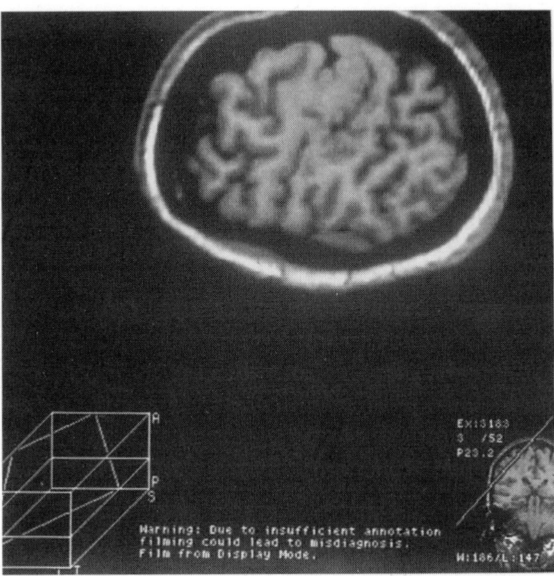


Fig. 3.42 Reformatted tangential slice from a coronally acquired T1-weighted MRI scan, which shows a focal area of polymicrogyria

strated by MRI, compared with X-ray CT, is striking. Gross abnormalities such as lissencephaly or schizencephaly may be identified on CT but are seen much more clearly using MRI (Fig. 3.38). Less pronounced, but extensive, neuronal migration defects may not be identified at all with X-ray CT (Fig. 3.39). More subtle abnormalities such as focal nodular heterotopia (Fig. 3.40) and band heterotopia (Fig. 3.41) may only be apparent if optimal MRI techniques are used.

Minor anomalies of the morphology and arrangement of cortical gyri may only be visualized if the data is processed after acquisition and reformatted to display the abnormalities. At present such detailed analysis is operator-dependent, requires experienced personnel and is very time-consuming. A focal area of polymicrogyria, for example, may not be evident on conventional sagittal, coronal or axial scans, only on a reformatted tangential slice that cuts across the affected area (Fig. 3.42) or a three-dimensional reconstruction of the surface of the brain.

Cerebral infarcts and haemorrhages and areas of post-traumatic cerebral damage are readily and more clearly identified with MRI than with X-ray CT. MRI commonly shows the abnormality to be more widespread than was initially thought, resulting in surgical treatment being inappropriate (Fig. 3.43). Areas of focal atrophy (Fig. 3.44) and

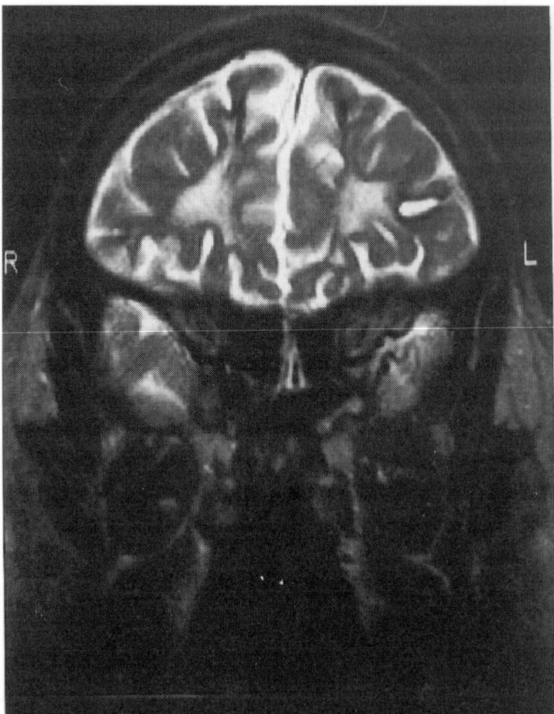


**Fig. 3.43** Coronal T2-weighted MRI scan showing bifrontal atrophy and extensive signal change and haemosiderin in the site of two haematomas in the left frontal lobe, following closed head injury

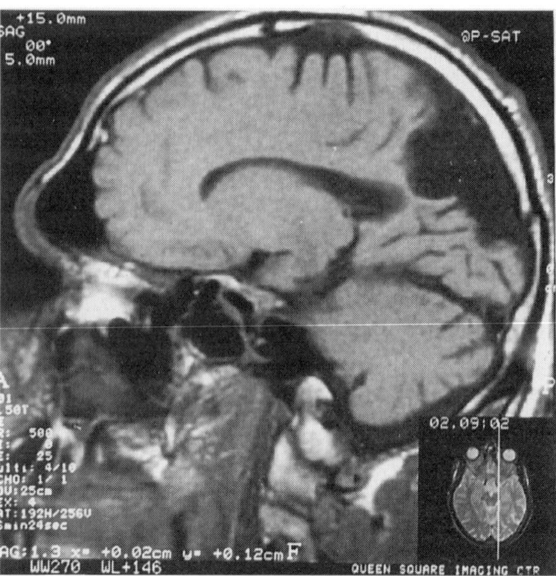


**Fig. 3.44** Sagittal T1-weighted MRI scan demonstrating focal atrophy of the left occipital lobe

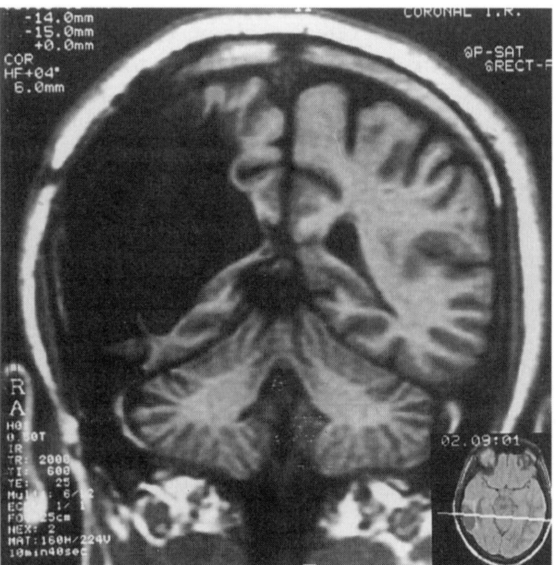


**Fig. 3.45** Coronal T1-weighted MRI scan showing a large right parietal and posterior temporal porencephalic cyst

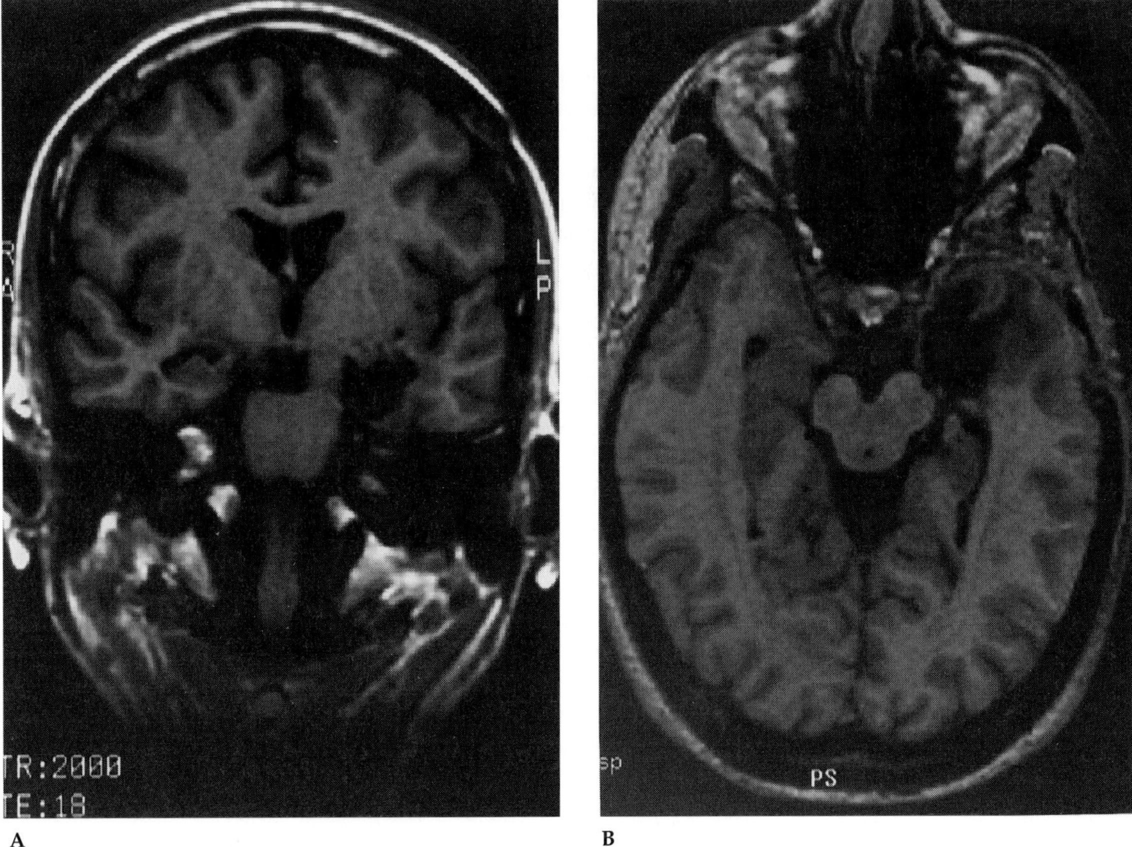


A B

**Fig. 3.46** Coronal **(A)** and axial **(B)** T1-weighted MRI scans 3 months after a selective left amygdalo-hippocampectomy, showing the extent of the resection

porencephalic cysts (Fig. 3.45) are also readily identified using MRI.

In the postoperative assessment of patients who have had epilepsy surgery, MRI is invaluable in determining the extent of the surgical resection and whether pathological tissue remains. It is our practice to obtain postoperative imaging 3 months after surgery, by which time any acute changes have resolved (Fig. 3.46). Not infrequently the actual excision is shown to differ from the surgeon's impressions at the time of operation and, if seizures are continuing several months following surgery and pathological tissue remains, a repeat operation may be recommended (Ch. 10).

## 3.4 FUNCTIONAL IMAGING

### 3.4.1 Single photon emission computerized tomography

Single photon emission computerized tomography (SPECT) may be used to image the distribution of cerebral blood flow and specific receptors in the brain.

The most commonly used SPECT tracer for imaging cerebral blood flow is $^{99m}$Tc-HMPAO (Ceretec, Amersham). This is convenient to use, being given by vein and having 70% brain uptake in 1 min. The subsequent image is stable for 6 h, as after crossing the blood–brain barrier HMPAO reacts with intracellular glutathione, becoming hydrophilic and so much less able to retraverse the blood–brain barrier. A limitation of the tracer is instability after preparation. This is less of a problem for interictal than ictal studies. Derivatives with a longer shelf-life have recently been developed (Neurolite, DuPont; cobalt chloride stabilized Ceretec, Amersham).

Dedicated multiheaded SPECT cameras have more sensitivity than rotating cameras and with technological advances spatial resolution has improved to 7–8 mm. Unlike positron emission tomography (PET) the data remains, at best, semiquantitative, with the use of a reference region as an internal standard. As with MRI, the correct orientation of imaging planes is important to visualize the temporal lobe optimally. The commonly used orbito-meatal line is about 40° off the long axis of the temporal lobe. It follows that partial volume effects between inferior frontal and superior temporal lobe will be maximized, with loss of potentially useful localizing information. If thin slices are acquired this deficit can to some extent be corrected for by reformatting. This is of limited utility, however, if slices are 8 mm thick and it is much more satisfactory to acquire data in the optimum plane.

It is now possible to realign and co-register different imaging modalities in single patients. If an optimal MR image with high resolution of anatomical features and high-resolution SPECT images are available, it is possible to obtain a meaningful co-registration and the ability to co-register MRI with PET and SPECT data allows for a structure–function correlation that greatly enhances the interpretation of both individual data sets and the consensus diagnosis.

*Clinical interictal studies of HMPAO*

The hallmark of an epileptic focus studied interictally is a region of reduced cerebral blood flow. In HMPAO SPECT studies of patients with temporal lobe epilepsy a significant asymmetry of cerebral blood flow has been noted in about 50% of cases; the range in different studies is 11–80% (Fig. 3.47). Concordance with interictal EEG lateralization has been noted in 65%. Localization (e.g. frontal vs temporal) has been shown to be more difficult with, in one large representative series, correct localization in 38% in interictal studies of patients with a unilateral temporal lobe EEG focus (Rowe et al 1991). Localization with a interictal SPECT is more difficult in patients with extratemporal epilepsy, widespread hypoperfusion being seen in two of 12 cases in a recent investigation (Marks et al 1992b). In consequence of this poor sensitivity and specificity, interictal SPECT studies have little place in the routine investigation of patients with epilepsy.

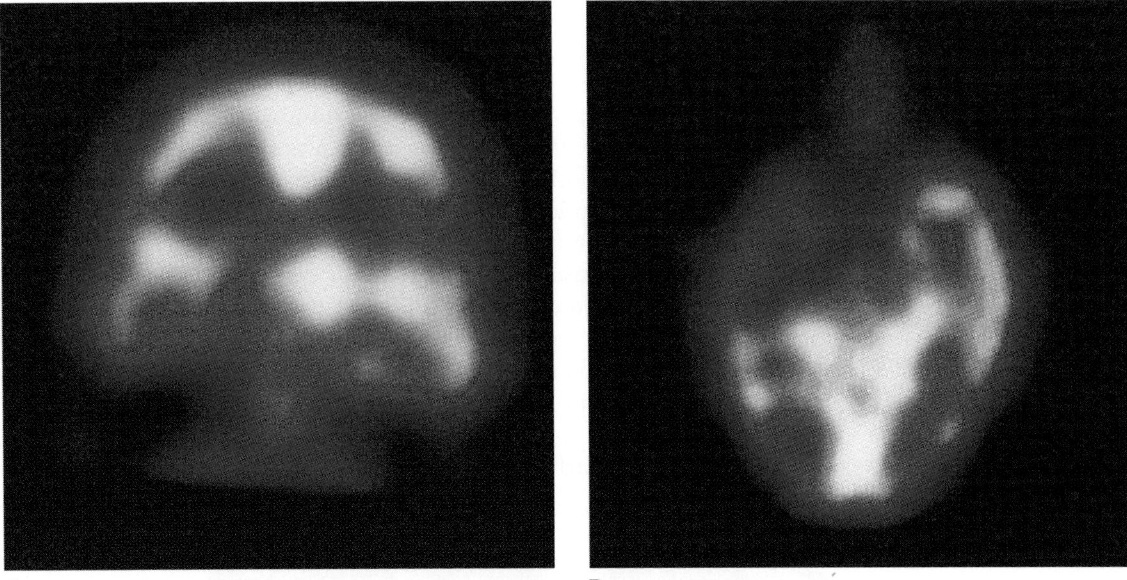

A B

**Fig. 3.47** Interictal HMPAO SPECT scan of a patient with right hippocampal sclerosis, showing reduced cerebral blood flow to the right temporal lobe in the coronal **(A)** and axial **(B)** planes

*Ictal studies using HMPAO*

The increase in cerebral blood flow associated with a seizure and postictal suppression may be detected using SPECT. This may provide useful localizing information in patients with partial seizures. An injection of HMPAO at the time of a seizure results in an image of the distribution of cerebral blood flow 1–2 min after tracer administration, which is then stable for several hours so that the patient may be imaged

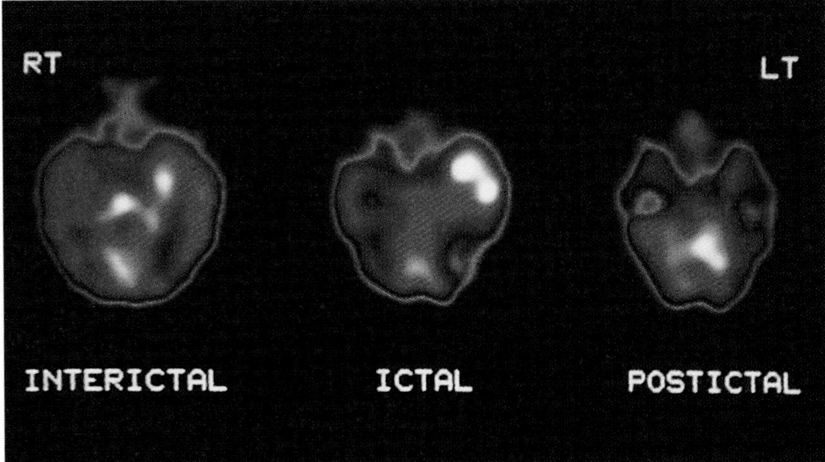


**Fig. 3.48** Interictal, ictal and postictal HMPAO SPECT scans in the axial plane demonstrating ictal hyperperfusion and post ictal suppression of cerebral blood flow (Illustration kindly provided by Dr S. Berkovic)

when the seizure is over. The general pattern is of localized ictal hyperperfusion, with surrounding hypoperfusion, followed by accentuated hypoperfusion in the region of the focus, which gradually returns to the interictal state (Fig. 3.48). Combined data from interictal and ictal SPECT scans give a lot more data than interictal scans alone and may be useful in the evaluation of both temporal and extratemporal epilepsy. In adults with temporal lobe epilepsy correct localization could be made in 69% of cases (Rowe et al 1991) and in 93% of children (Harvey et al 1993a). A characteristic feature of temporal lobe seizures is an initial hyperperfusion of the temporal lobe, followed by medial temporal hyperperfusion and lateral temporal hypoperfusion (Newton et al 1992).

Ictal HMPAO scans may be useful in the evaluation of patients with extratemporal seizures who do not have an identifiable abnormality on MRI. This technique localized the seizure focus in 10 of 12 patients in one recent series, (Marks et al 1992b) and in 20 of 22 in another (Harvey et al 1993b) (Fig. 3.49).

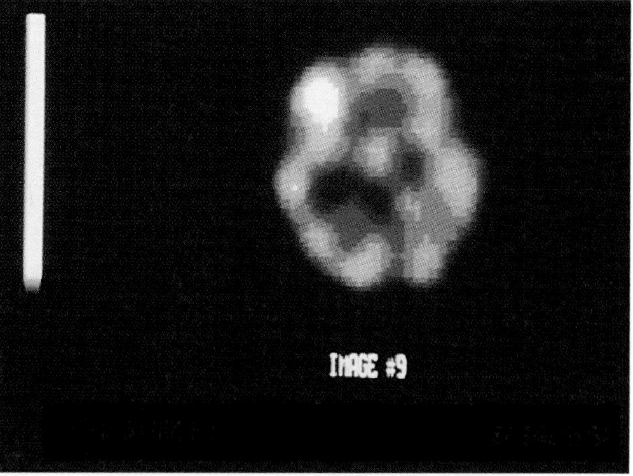


**Fig. 3.49** Ictal HMPAO SPECT scan showing a focal increase in cerebral blood flow in the right frontal lobe (Illustration kindly provided by Dr P. Bartenstein)

Ictal HMPAO scans, however, must be interpreted with caution. Simultaneous video-EEG is essential to determine the relationship between the onset of a seizure and tracer delivery: without this precaution there is risk of confusing ictal and postictal data. A further problem is that spread to other areas of the brain, such as the contralateral temporal lobe, may occur within seconds of seizure onset and so an image of cerebral blood flow distribution 1–2 min after the onset of a seizure may not indicate the site of onset.

Until recently, HMPAO had to be made up immediately prior to injection, resulting in a delay of up to 1 min. A new preparation of Ceretec has now been developed which is stabilized with cobalt chloride. An alternative is Neurolite (DuPont). This allows the labelled tracer to be prepared in advance, and may be injected into a patient at any time over the subsequent 6 hours without the need for further preparatory work. The advantage of this development is that the interval between seizure onset and tracer delivery to the brain can be significantly reduced.

It should also be pointed out that an ictal HMPAO study does not reliably differentiate between epileptic and non-epileptic attacks. Cases of non-epileptic attacks that were not associated with a focal increase in cerebral blood flow have been reported, but a focal increase in cerebral blood flow may occur, particularly if there is prominent motor activity.

*Other SPECT tracers*

$^{123}$I-iomazenil is a derivative of the central benzodiazepine receptor antagonist flumazenil. Early studies with $^{123}$I-iomazenil showed a reduction in binding in region of the epileptic focus (Van Isselt et al 1990, Bartenstein et al 1991). In the latter investigation, 10 of the 12 patients had reduced blood flow demonstrable with HMPAO and it was suggested that $^{123}$I-iomazenil did not confer additional benefits. More recent studies, however, with higher resolution cameras and optimal scan orientation have suggested that the area of reduced specific binding of $^{123}$I-iomazenil is more restricted than the defect of blood flow and possible of greater utility for localization of an epileptogenic focus (Johnson et al 1992). Another tracer that may prove to be of clinical utility is $^{123}$I-iododexetimide, which labels muscarinic acetylcholine receptors (Muller-Gartner et al 1993).

*The utility of interictal SPECT in presurgical evaluation*

The utility of SPECT needs to be re-evaluated in the light of advances in structural imaging with MRI. It could be argued that, if MRI demonstrates a relevant focal lesion that is concordant with clinical, psychological and non-invasive EEG data, SPECT is superfluous. If, on the other hand, EEG or other data is discordant, SPECT might obviate the need for an in-depth EEG investigation.

If there is no lesion seen on optimal MRI, or if dual or diffuse pathology is evident and if clinical, non-invasive EEG and psychological data agree, the utility of a SPECT study is unproven and this has not been the subject of a rigorous investigation. Congruence of SPECT findings with other data may provide sufficient confidence to proceed to surgery, whereas discordance is likely to result in invasive EEG studies. Similarly, if there is no lesion seen on optimal MRI and if clinical, non-invasive EEG and psychological data do not agree, the utility of a SPECT study is unproven. It might be hypothesized that SPECT data would help define the target for intracranial EEG investigations.

## 3.4.2 Positron emission tomography

Positron emission tomography (PET) is much more expensive, and less widely available, than SPECT. The principal differences are that positron-emitting isotopes are generally short-lived and have to be produced by a nearby cyclotron, whereas SPECT tracers are commercially available. The advantage of PET is that spatial resolution is superior (currently 5–7 mm) and, because of the ability to accurately correct for scatter and attenuation of radiation, the data is quantitative. PET may be used to map cerebral blood flow, using $^{15}$O-labelled water, and regional cerebral glucose metabolism, using $^{18}$F-deoxyglucose. PET may also be used to demonstrate the binding of specific ligands, e.g. $^{11}$C-flumazenil to the central benzodiazepine–$GABA_A$ receptor complex and $^{11}$C-diprenorphine and $^{11}$C-carfentanil to opiate receptors. $^{15}$O-labelled water and $^{18}$F-deoxyglucose (FDG) may be produced by commercially available equipment, but $^{11}$C-labelled compounds require the additional expense and complexity of a radiopharmaceutical laboratory.

*Glucose metabolism and blood flow*

The hallmark of an epileptogenic focus, studied interictally, is an area of reduced glucose metabolism, and reduced blood flow, that is usually considerably larger than the anatomical abnormality (Fig. 3.50) (Engel et al 1982, Franck et al 1986, Sackellares et al 1986). The reason for this is not clear; possibilities include inhibition or deafferentation of neurones around an epileptogenic focus or loss of neurones as a result of the epileptic activity. In patients with medial temporal lobe foci the hypometabolism frequently appears more pronounced in lateral neocortex (Sackellares et al 1990). In consequence $^{18}$FDG PET studies are less reliable for answering the question of precise localization of seizure onset, e.g. inferior frontal vs medial or lateral temporal lobe, than for answering the question of lateralization, e.g. left or right temporal lobe.

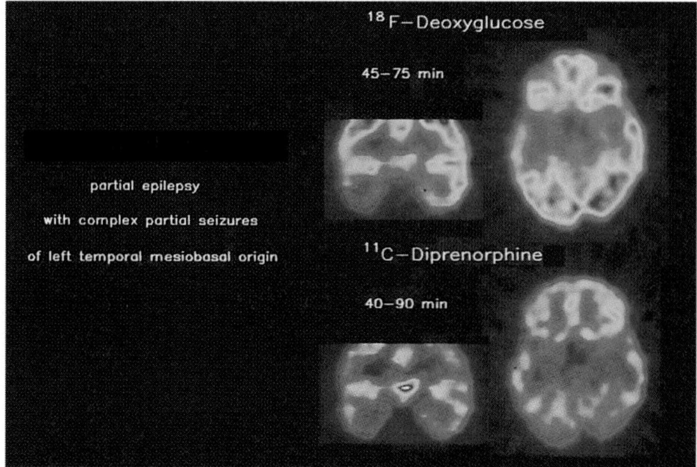


**Fig. 3.50** PET scans of a patient with left temporal lobe epilepsy, on the basis of hippocampal sclerosis. The upper image shows reduced glucose metabolism in the medial and lateral parts of the affected temporal lobe (in this illustration on the left-hand side of the images). The lower images show that there is no significant asymmetry of $^{11}$C-diprenorphine binding to opioid receptors

$^{18}$FDG PET scans provide superior resolution and greater reliability for identifying a focal deficit than do PET scans using $^{15}$O-water or HMPAO SPECT scans (Ryvlin et al 1992). Partial seizures are associated with an increase in regional cerebral glucose metabolism and blood flow in the region of the epileptogenic focus, and often a suppression elsewhere (Engel et al 1983). In general ictal PET scans can only be obtained fortuitously, because of the 2 min half-life of $^{15}O$ and the fact that cerebral uptake of $^{18}$FDG occurs over 40 min after injection, so that cerebral glucose utilization data will reflect an amalgam of the ictal and postictal conditions. Overall the concordance between $^{18}$FDG PET and surface ictal EEG recordings is about 70%. In a further 20%, only one of the PET or the EEG data is localizing, and in the remaining 10% the data are contradictory (Franck et al 1986, Engel et al 1990).

Over the last decade, some epilepsy surgery programmes have relied extensively on $^{18}$FDG PET as a localizing tool. The current place of this technique needs to be re-evaluated in the light of developments in MRI, as the finding a definite focal abnormality such as hippocampal sclerosis may render an $^{18}$FDG scan superfluous (see above, 3.2, and Ch. 10). It is our current practice to carry out $^{18}$FDG PET scans, for clinical purposes, in patients who are candidates for surgical treatment in whom high-quality MRI has not shown a relevant structural abnormality. $^{18}$FDG PET scans may have a greater role to play in the evaluation of children, in whom EEG telemetry can pose particular difficulties.

*Central benzodiazepine and opioid receptors*

The binding of $^{11}$C-flumazenil, analogous to the SPECT tracer $^{123}$I-iomazenil, to central benzodiazepine receptors in epileptogenic foci is reduced by an average of 30%, with no change in the affinity of the ligand for the receptor (Fig. 3.51) (Savic et al 1988, Frey et al 1991, Henry et al 1993, Duncan 1993). These data are of considerable research interest in investigations of the pathophysiology and consequences of epilepsy, and can also be of direct clinical relevance in the evaluation of presurgical patients. In patients with partial seizures, the area of reduced $^{11}$C-flumazenil binding is more restricted than is the area of reduced glucose metabolism, and the technique appears to be superior for

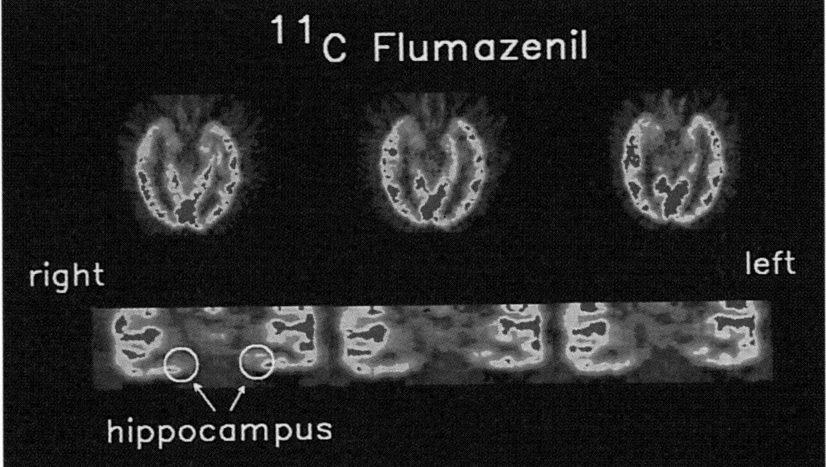


**Fig. 3.51** $^{11}$C-flumazenil PET scan showing reduced binding to the medial right temporal lobe in a patient with right hippocampal sclerosis

the localization of the source of the seizure. At present, however, $^{11}$C-flumazenil PET scans have only very limited availability.

Investigations of opioid receptors have shown an increase of $^{11}$C-carfentanil binding to mu-receptors in lateral temporal neocortex, without a reduction in the amygdala, and no significant side to side asymmetry of $^{11}$C-diprenorphine binding (see Fig. 3.50). The areas of increased binding in the neocortex corresponded to areas of reduced glucose metabolism (Frost et al 1988, Mayberg et al 1991). Diprenorphine binds to all subtypes of opioid receptor with similar affinity and these data suggest a differential alteration of mu and non-mu opioid receptors in patients with partial seizures. Studies of this type advance our understanding of the neurobiology of epilepsy: for example, it has been suggested that these findings may reflect an adaptive tonic upregulation of an endogenous antiepileptic mechanism that functions to contain epileptic activity. The facilities for these investigations, however, are very limited and they are not available to routine clinical practice.

## 3.5 NEUROPSYCHOLOGY

### 3.5.1 Indications for neuropsychological assessment

A minority of patients with epilepsy, particularly those with poorly controlled seizures, are at risk of disorders of cognitive function and require detailed neuropsychological assessment and treatment.

Risk factors that may indicate that a neuropsychological assessment is appropriate include known or suspected underlying brain damage, early age of seizure onset, frequent severe seizures, episodes of convulsive status, the prescription of a combination of AEDs and high serum drug concentrations.

*Assessment of newly diagnosed and chronic patients*

Neuropsychological evaluation has a role in the assessment of both patients with recent onset of seizures and those with chronic epilepsy, if there is a suspicion of focal cerebral disturbance. In such cases testing may confirm the existence of a specific cognitive deficit, e.g. memory impairment, and the measurement of other related functions assists in interpreting the significance of the assessed memory problems. Subsequent assessments may then be used to determine whether there is evidence of progressive impairment of focal or widespread cerebral dysfunction. If there is evidence of a progressive deterioration further investigation is necessary to evaluate the cause of this. Serial neuropsychological assessment is also warranted in such cases to identify the gradient of the deterioration. Parallel versions are available for many neuropsychological tests for use in such circumstances. Practice effects, however, may still give a false picture if tests are repeated more frequently than every 6–12 months.

If patients are being assessed for the first time their reading level gives a reasonable indication of their optimal intelligence as this function is relatively robust and is likely to be preserved even in the presence of significant cognitive decline. Comparison of current scores on measures of intelligence with figures derived from the reading assessment gives a reasonable indication as to whether the patient has declined cognitively.

*Monitoring of the effects of AEDs*

All AEDs, at high doses, have the propensity to cause some impairment of higher cognitive function (Ch. 9, 9.5.1). Barbiturates and phenytoin appear to have more deleterious effects than do more modern agents. The predominant effects of AEDs are slowing on tasks with a motor component and impairment of mental speed, attention and concentration. Neuropsychological assessment can be most useful to identify deficits in these areas and repeat testing after changes in AED therapy may be used as an indicator as to whether function has improved or not. Computerized psychological tests have been developed in recent years and these can add precision to assessments, particularly in recording the speed of processing (Thompson 1991). In practice, however, it may be difficult to ascertain the relative effects of continued seizures, AEDs and fixed cerebral deficit on motor and mental speed, attention and concentration. Further, it should not be taken that detailed repeated, neuropsychological assessments are either feasible or appropriate for every patient with epilepsy who is receiving antiepileptic medication, but should rather be used in patients who are presenting with an impairment.

*Assessment of individual potential*

Neuropsychological assessment can have a valuable role in identifying an individual's potential. People with intractable epilepsy frequently have their abilities either under- or overestimated because a global IQ figure may mask an uneven cognitive profile. Identifying an individual's strengths and weaknesses helps realistic goals to be set regarding independent living and employment and helps identify whether or not they have untapped potential that may respond usefully to a period of rehabilitation. Knowledge of strengths and weaknesses can be conveyed to relatives, teachers and employers as well as to professional carers and this can avoid misunderstandings, particularly when there are hidden deficits such as language problems. Assessment may also determine whether there is evidence of a progressive decline of cognitive functions. Identification of any such deterioration clearly has important implications for investigations of the cause and for the making of care plans.

### 3.5.2 Neuropsychological test schedules

There is no one cognitive deficit characteristic of patients with epilepsy and a broad range of functions needs to be assessed. A neuropsychological battery for epilepsy has been proposed which includes the administration of the WAIS-R and many of the subtests of the Halstead–Reitan Battery and is popular in the United States (Dodrill 1978). The entire assessment, however, takes 6–8 h to complete.

At the National Hospital for Neurology and Neurosurgery the basic neuropsychological schedule for patients with epilepsy comprises the subtests of the WAIS-R, tests of language, memory, perception and spatial functioning. The Nelson Adult Reading Test is routinely employed to provide an estimate of an individual's premorbid intellectual function. Measures considered sensitive to frontal lobe function are also employed. Additional, more detailed testing of functions is undertaken if specific difficulties are uncovered during the routine neuropsychological screen. The main functions assessed and examples of some of the specific tests used and, where appropriate, the brain regions being evaluated are summarized in Table 3.1. It is recognized that this is a gross over-simplification of the role and interpretation of various test data and it is merely intended to assist the clinician with understanding the role of the range of the tests commonly employed.

### 3.5.3 Interpretation of data in patients with epilepsy

The neuropsychological assessment of patients with epilepsy needs to take into account the possible effects of antiepileptic drug therapy (Ch. 9, 9.5.1), of recent seizures and of ongoing seizure activity. Sometimes this is obvious – for example, the patient who has had a generalized tonic-clonic seizure 2 h previously and who is still drowsy, or the child in whom absences are occurring every few minutes throughout the test session. The possibility of occult disturbance by seizures needs to be considered if performance is less good than expected, and can be assessed by simultaneous video-EEG recording of the patient.

**Table 3.1** Neuropsychological tests used in evaluation of patients with epilepsy

| Function evaluated | Area of brain tested | Test |
|---|---|---|
| Optimal intellectual level | | Nelson Adult Reading Test (Nelson 1982) |
| Current intellectual level | | Wechsler Adult Intelligence Scale – Revised (Wechsler 1981) |
| Mental flexibility, planning | Frontal lobe | Wisconsin Card Sorting Test (Nelson 1976) |
| Verbal memory | Dominant temporal lobe | Recognition memory test (Warrington 1984) |
| | | List learning (Coughlan & Hollows 1985) |
| Non-verbal memory | Non-dominant temporal lobe | Recognition memory test (Warrington 1984) |
| | | Complex Design recall (Coughlan & Hollows 1985) |
| Language | Dominant temporal lobe | McKenna Graded Naming Test (McKenna & Warrington 1983) |
| | | de Renzi Token Test (de Renzi & Vignolo 1962) |
| Literacy skills | Dominant parietal/ occipital lobes | Tests of spelling, reading (Schonell 1971) |
| Calculation | Dominant parietal lobe | Tests of arithmetic (Jackson & Warrington 1986) |
| Visuospatial processing | Non-dominant parietal/ occipital lobes | Dot centre<br>Silhouettes<br>(Warrington & James 1991) |
| Attention and concentration | | Information processing test (Coughlan & Hollows 1985) |

*Relevance to day-to-day functioning*

The relevance of performance on neuropsychological tests to day-to-day functioning is not always evident and this is an area of ongoing research. Measures of general intelligence can be linked to educational attainment and potential to live independently. The finding of even subtle deficits on measures of frontal lobe function can help to explain why an apparently able individual is functioning poorly in daily living situations, for example being dependent on others to structure his or her activities. Language difficulties may have been a hidden deficit over a number of years and may contribute to disturbed behaviour.

*Memory*

Patients with epilepsy frequently complain of difficulties with their memory, but on formal neuropsychological assessment of memory may perform at an average level. It must be noted that memory is an umbrella term and that formal neuropsychological assessment generally focuses on the ability to learn new information in a controlled setting. Important areas that current tests do not adequately evaluate include prospective memory functions, i.e. the ability to remember to carry out tasks in the future, such as to take medication or to attend for an appointment. Subjective memory questionnaires are being developed to identify difficulties in these areas (Corcoran & Thompson 1993).

*Assessment of patients with mental handicap*

At present, there is only a limited range of assessment measures suitable for patients with moderate to severe learning difficulties. The general approach is to employ measures that have been developed for use with children. Unfortunately, such test material may not be entirely appropriate for use with adults. Such assessments, however, do allow consideration of relative strengths and weaknesses of different cognitive functions. The British Ability Scale is one measure that can be employed for this purpose (Elliott et al 1983). Any indication of possible focal deficits in such cases can be valuable as it is now considered, for instance, that a low IQ should not in itself preclude surgical treatment of refractory epilepsy.

*Non-organic impairments*

The pattern of a person's test scores can, on occasion, suggest that there is a functional basis or component to their disorder. Suspicions should be aroused by atypical test profiles, for example if an individual performs extremely poorly on all tests or if they score well below the chance level on a forced choice recognition memory test. It is of note, however, that such a pattern is not commonly seen in patients with non-epileptic attacks that have a psychological basis.

### 3.5.4 Assessment of mood, well-being and behaviour

The measurement of these features, which are very important contributory factors to a patient's perceived quality of life, is less advanced than conventional neuropsychological assessments. Attempts have been made, however, to increase the sophistication beyond that of asking the patients how they are.

At present such measures have little use in the day-to-day management of patients but are used extensively in research protocols that attempt to evaluate the effect of medical and surgical treatment on broader aspects than suppression of seizures (Ch. 9, 9.6.1). Data is usually gathered from patient-compiled questionnaires that result in a single score or a profile of scores (Hermann et al 1992, Vickery et al 1992, McHorney et al 1993).

Behavioural disturbance sometimes accompanies epilepsy, often in the setting of a degree of mental handicap, and may be compounded by some medications such as barbiturates, benzodiazepines and vigabatrin. It can be useful to quantify the extent of this disturbance in order to monitor the effects of changes in medication, environment and behavioural management programmes, with the use of questionnaires and rating scales compiled by relatives, carers and teachers.

### 3.5.5 Presurgical neuropsychological evaluation

Detailed neuropsychological evaluation is fundamental to the consideration of patients for epilepsy surgery (see also Ch. 10, 10.2.3) (Table 3.1), particularly when a temporal lobe resection is contemplated. (See Ch. 10, 10.4.1 for details of neuropsychological changes following epilepsy surgery.) In this setting, evidence is sought for dysfunction of that part of the brain where it is believed seizures are arising, and for the function of the rest of the brain remaining intact. Concordance of neuropsychological deficit with the clinical features and with imaging and EEG data is favourable, as is the lack of widespread cerebral dysfunction. The finding of global or multifocal neuropsychological deficits is an adverse prognostic finding because of the implication of cerebral pathology that would remain after resection of the putative focus. In general, the dominant temporal lobe primarily undertakes verbal memory processing and the non-dominant temporal lobe non-verbal memory processing. Memory test scores and tests of other cognitive functions contribute to the lateralization and localization of disturbed cerebral function.

In patients with temporal lobe epilepsy, it is particularly important to determine the integrity of the memory capacity of the contralateral temporal lobe. There have been cases in which the resection of one temporal lobe led to a profound amnesic state, as the remaining temporal lobe was damaged (by hippocampal sclerosis or a previous surgical procedure) and unable to sustain basic memory function. The carotid amytal (Wada) test (see also Ch. 10, 10.2.3) was introduced to minimize the risk of such catastrophes occurring.

*The carotid amytal (Wada) test*

This test is carried out primarily to determine which cerebral hemisphere is dominant for language and also whether the contralateral hemisphere can sustain basic memory function. If the contralateral hemisphere is not able to support basic memory function, a temporal lobectomy would not be carried out or, in some cases, a more selective procedure would be performed.

A subsidiary role is to find confirmatory evidence of impaired memory function in the temporal lobe proposed for resection. The amytal test is not, however, able to reliably predict the extent of verbal and non-verbal memory impairment that is likely to occur after temporal lobe surgery. Verbal memory impairment is usually worse after a dominant temporal lobe resection, with improvement over the following year. This deterioration is less likely to be noted, however, if the lesion that caused the epilepsy was established early in life, e.g. a prolonged early childhood convulsion, and if the removed hippocampus shows hippocampal sclerosis. The hypothesis proposed to account for this is that in such patients verbal memory functions have been largely transferred to other cerebral areas.

Until recently, and still in some centres, a carotid amytal test was regarded as a mandatory step prior to temporal lobectomy. If, however, a patient is fully right-handed, has a single structural lesion shown on MRI and a concordant psychological deficit, with no suggestion of dysfunction of the contralateral temporal lobe, an amytal test can be omitted. If there is a suggestion of memory dysfunction in the contralateral temporal lobe, or if cerebral dominance is uncertain (80% of left-handers have a left cerebral hemisphere that is language-dominant) an amytal test is necessary. These conditions are particularly likely in a patient who sustained a cerebral insult in early childhood, such as a prolonged convulsion, and in whom cross-lateralization of some functions may have occurred. The determination of language dominance is important in the planning of a temporal lobe resection, as only the anterior 2.5–3 cm of the superior temporal gyrus of the dominant temporal lobe may be resected, whereas on the non-dominant side this may extend for 4.5–5 cm.

Considerable patient co-operation is required and, in general, children under the age of 12 years cannot understand or comply adequately with carotid amytal testing.

Patients need to be alert and to not have any premedication. Testing is conducted in an angiography suite. A catheter is introduced via a femoral artery to the internal carotid. A test injection of 4–5 ml of contrast material is made to ensure accurate placement and determine whether injection results in filling of the posterior communicating cerebral artery or cross flow to the contralateral hemisphere via the anterior communicating cerebral artery. Sodium amytal is injected over 3 s, while the patient counts aloud and holds his/her arms outstretched. Different centres use different doses. It is our practice to inject 75 mg initially, followed by further doses of 50 mg if a hemiparesis does not develop. An excessive dose of amytal results in the patient becoming drowsy and no useful data is obtained. An EEG is recorded throughout and the testing is recorded on videotape, to allow subsequent quantification of scores. The patient is tested for language and memory functions when each cerebral hemisphere is inactivated by the amytal. The exact protocol varies from centre to centre (Loring et al 1992).

The cerebral hemisphere that is proposed for surgery is injected first, the contralateral hemisphere being studied after the patient has fully recovered. An interval of 30 min is usually satisfactory, so the whole procedure takes 90 min and it is feasible to examine two or three patients in a session.

It is the integrity of the non-anaesthetized hemisphere that is assessed. For example if a patient in whom a left temporal lobectomy is planned is amnesic following injection of amytal into the left carotid artery, the implication is that the right cerebral hemisphere cannot support basic memory function. Interpretation of carotid amytal test data is not always straightforward. When the speech-dominant hemisphere receives amytal the subsequent dysphasia may complicate the assessment of whether significant amnesia has occurred or not. If an excessive dose of amytal is given or if there is reflux into the basilar circulation the patient may become too obtunded to co-operate with psychological testing. Sometimes the patient may become very restless and try to get up, resulting in testing having to be abandoned. If a seizure occurs during an examination, the patient may fail the memory tests and it has to be repeated. EEG recording during an amytal test is advisable to detect seizure activity, which might complicate assessment of the results, and to indicate any cross-flow of amytal to the contralateral hemisphere.

If a standard carotid amytal is difficult to interpret because of sedation or behavioural problems it may be possible to undertake a selective amytal examination, with injection of about 30 mg of sodium amytal into the posterior communicating artery. This is not a trivial undertaking as the cannulation may be very difficult and the risks of causing an ischaemic neurological deficit are significantly greater than the 1 in 200 risk associated with internal carotid artery catheterization in patients under the age of 50 years.

It is possible that in the near future cerebral activation studies using $^{15}O$-labelled water and PET, and also functional MRI techniques, will replace carotid amytal testing as tests of the lateralization of language and memory functions in patients in whom surgical treatment of epilepsy is under consideration.

## 3.6 OTHER INVESTIGATIONS

### 3.6.1 At initial diagnostic evaluation

*Biochemistry*

A serum biochemical profile, including assessments of glucose, renal function, liver enzymes and function, and calcium metabolism, is appropriate at the initial diagnostic stage. Further investigation of systemic metabolic or biochemical disturbance may be indicated if there is evidence of abnormalities on screening tests or clinical evaluation. The possibility of hypoglycaemia must always be borne in mind, as episodes of hypoglycaemia may mimic complex partial seizures and may precipitate epileptic seizures. Hypoglycaemia is most commonly the result of hypoglycaemic medication, alcohol abuse, liver impairment and gastrointestinal 'dumping'. If there is any clinical indication that a patient may be having episodes of hypoglycaemia, a 72-h fast should be undertaken under supervision, with blood and urine taken for glucose estimations, and blood for insulin and hydroxybutyrate, at the end of this time and if any symptomatic episodes occur. A blood glucose < 2 mmol/l is abnormal, and if this is found plasma insulin and hydroxybutyrate concentrations should be measured. A low hydroxybutyrate and inappropriately high insulin concentration suggest excessive insulin production and should prompt a search for an insulinoma once it is certain that the patient is not receiving exogenous insulin or oral hypoglycaemic agents.

*Haematology*

A full blood count should be taken at the initial evaluation, principally to detect any intercurrent haematological abnormality before AEDs are prescribed. If there is a suspicion of liver disease or abnormal coagulation, clotting studies should be performed. Measurement of folate concentrations are only indicated if there is a macrocytosis. In this case it is more useful to measure red cell rather than serum folate, as the latter is very labile and affected by recent diet.

*Serology*

It has been traditional to request syphilis serology in patients with new onset of seizures. Unless there are other clinical features to suggest that this is a possibility, the yield in patients presenting with seizures is extremely small and it is not routinely indicated. Patients with HIV infection, however, who have presented solely with the onset of epileptic seizures have been reported recently and this diagnosis should be considered, particularly if the patient has any risk factors for HIV exposure. In patients with HIV infection who develop seizures, the possibility of concurrent CNS pathology such as toxoplasmosis, syphilis lymphoma and cryptococcal infection needs to be considered.

*Serum prolactin*

There is usually a rise in serum prolactin concentration for up to 20 min after a generalized tonic-clonic seizure to above 1000 mU/l, although the rise is not maintained in the event of serial convulsions. It is important to compare postictal prolactin levels with a baseline value, which may be obtained retrospectively, to differentiate between a postictal rise and a persistent elevation of prolactin concentration. Serum prolactin does not elevate after non-epileptic convulsive seizures and this data may be diagnostically useful, in conjunction with video and EEG data (Trimble 1978, Rao et al 1989).

Serum prolactin does not rise as high or as consistently following complex partial seizures. Seizures arising from temporal lobe are more likely to be associated with a rise than those arising from the frontal lobes (Meierkord et al 1992). No consistent rise is seen after simple partial seizures (Pritchard et al 1983). A rise in prolactin, then, may provide confirmatory evidence for a complex partial seizure, but the absence of a rise does not rule this out. In practical terms prolactin estimations are most useful in the differential diagnosis of convulsive seizures, of limited utility in the evaluation of complex partial seizures and unhelpful in the assessment of possible simple partial seizures.

*Cardiac investigations*

If there is a suspicion of arrhythmias or other cardiac disease causing episodes of collapse or loss of awareness, a chest radiograph and ECG are indicated. An ECG should also be requested in all elderly patients and in those with a history of cardiac disease prior to commencing carbamazepine therapy, as the presence of heart block would be a relative contraindication to using this drug.

Further evaluation with echocardiography is indicated if there is suspicion of structural cardiac disease. If there is a possibility of tachy- or bradyarrhythmias causing a patient's attacks, prolonged ambulatory ECG monitoring is needed, ideally to include symptomatic episodes.

Patients with frequent syncopal episodes should be referred for autonomic function testing to assess the integrity of the sympathetic and parasympathetic nervous systems if the basis of the syncope is not readily apparent (Bannister 1988).

*Consideration of inborn errors of metabolism*

Inborn errors of metabolism only rarely give rise to epilepsy. About 160 of 4344 mendelian traits increase the likelihood of seizures and together these conditions account for 1% of patients with epilepsy, most commonly with onset in infancy and childhood (Aicardi 1992). In the majority of cases, epileptic seizures are only part of the phenotype and there is other evidence of neurological disease (see 3.7.4, 3.7.5).

The more common include:

- Pyridoxine dependency, which presents in the neonatal period and responds rapidly to intravenous pyridoxine
- Adrenoleucodystrophy, diagnosed by finding increased very long chain fatty acids in plasma
- Non-ketotic hyperglycinaemia
- D-glyceric acidaemia
- Phenylketonuria
- Porphyria
- Biopterin deficiency
- GABA transaminase deficiency with 4-hydroxybutyric aciduria

The last six conditions may be identified by analysis of urine and plasma organic acid and amino acid profiles.

- *Urea cycle defects*, causing hyperammonaemia, are detected by finding increased plasma ammonia, and orotic acid in urine, particularly after a protein load. It is important to avoid sodium valproate in such patients and to consider the possibility if a patient becomes obtunded after commencing this drug.

- *Mitochondrial cytopathy*: The two principal phenotypes MELAS and MERRF may be diagnosed by finding ragged red fibres on muscle biopsy, lactic acidosis (MELAS), biochemical deficits in muscle biopsy or analysis of leucocyte DNA.

- *Neuronal ceroid lipofuscinosis*: The infantile, juvenile and adult forms can be diagnosed on skin and rectal biopsy.

- *$GM_2$ gangliosidosis*: Leucocyte hexosaminidase A levels are low.

- *Gaucher's disease*: Foam cells are seen on bone marrow examination; Leucocyte beta-glucocerebrosidase activity is deficient.

- *Sialidosis I and II*: Leucocyte enzymes alpha-*N*-acetylneuraminidase and beta-galactosidase are reduced.

- *Lafora body disease*: Characteristic polyglucosan inclusion bodies are evident on skin or liver biopsy.
- *Globoid cell leucodystrophy*: Leucocyte galactocerebroside beta-galactosidase levels are reduced.

*Indications for examination of cerebrospinal fluid*

A lumbar puncture and examination of the cerebrospinal fluid (CSF) is not routinely indicated in the evaluation of patients developing epileptic seizures. This procedure may be necessary if seizures occur in the context of an acute neurological illness, for example meningitis or encephalitis, and in young children developing a febrile convulsion in whom there is a possibility of intracranial infection. In interpretation of results it should be remembered, however, that generalized status epilepticus may itself result in a CSF lymphocyte count of up to 100–200/$mm^3$.

CSF analysis may also be necessary in subacute situations such as chronic infections and autoimmune disorders, e.g. possible tuberculosis, Wegener's granulomatosis or SSPE. In rare patients being investigated for inherited biochemical abnormalities, e.g. tetrahydrofolate reductase deficiency and mitochondrial cytopathy, analysis of the CSF may be valuable.

### 3.6.2 Subsequent monitoring of patients with epilepsy

The indications for repeated EEG, imaging and neuropsychological investigation of patients with epilepsy are discussed above (3.1–3.5). Haematological and biochemical monitoring is primarily aimed at detecting adverse effects of AED treatment (see Ch. 4, 4.5 for details regarding individual AEDs). Monitoring of serum AED concentrations is considered fully in Chapter 4 (4.3). Clearly the development of any clinical features of liver, bone or other metabolic or haematological disorder needs prompt investigation. In general, frequent routine assessments of liver function and full blood counts are unhelpful and do not help to predict the development of rare, idiosyncratic reactions such as hepatic failure or aplastic anaemia. As a routine, in patients taking enzyme-inducing AEDs it is reasonable to assess a full blood count and film, calcium and alkaline phosphatase every 1–2 years. A finding of macrocytosis should be followed up with assay of red cell folate, serum vitamin B12 and liver function tests. A low calcium and elevated alkaline phosphatase raises the possibility of osteomalacia, which should be followed further with measurement of bone isoenzyme determination and vitamin D concentrations. In patients taking valproate, assessment of the full blood count including platelets is reasonable at annual intervals and should be undertaken before any surgical procedure.

## 3.7 INVESTIGATION OF NEUROLOGICAL AND COGNITIVE DECLINE IN PATIENTS WITH EPILEPSY

### 3.7.1 Approach to investigation

As epilepsy often occurs in the context of mental handicap and fixed neurological deficit, it is first important to determine whether a patient with mental and/or neurological dysfunction has a static or progressive deficit. In both situations it is appropriate to seek an aetiology. A static deficit may result from an acquired brain insult or congenital malformation (Table 3.2) (Ch 2). Investigation should be pursued aggressively if there is evidence of progressive deterioration, to determine whether there may be a remediable pathology, to be able to give an estimation of the prognosis so that appropriate care may be arranged, and to ascertain whether there is an inherited condition that may carry genetic implications for the patient's relatives.

*Clinical features*

It is not always straightforward to be certain whether or not a patient is showing progressive decline. A careful history and clinical examination are essential, as is a knowledge of the behaviour and development of normal infants and children. Important aspects of the history are to determine from relatives and carers what social, motor, language and self-care skills a patient had at best, and whether further skills are being acquired, the situation is static, or once-held skills are being lost. This assessment needs to take into account the normal processes of acquisition of skills through the first two decades of life. Normal development may mask the occurrence of gradually progressive dysfunction until the late teens; up to that time it may have been concluded that the patient had slowed mental development but did not have a progressive decline. Further, if a patient is functioning at a low level it may be difficult to

**Table 3.2** Causes of epilepsy and static cognitive and neurological deficit

| Inherited | Acquired |
|---|---|
| *Neurocutaneus Syndromes* | *Prenatal* |
| • Tuberous sclerosis | • Antepartum haemorrhage |
| • Neurofibromatosis | • Toxaemia |
| • Incontinentia pigmenti | • Brain infection (encephalitis, meningitis): esp. CMV, toxoplasmosis, herpes, rubella, Epstein–Barr, influenza, syphilis |
| • Hypomelanosis of Ito | |
| *Neuronal migration defects* | *Perinatal* |
| • Cortical dysplasia (may also result from prenatal, postnatal insult) | • Anoxia |
| | • Hypoglycaemia |
| | • Hypocalcaemia |
| • Aicardi syndrome | |
| • Other cerebral malformations | *Postnatal* |
| *Chromosomal abnormalities* | • Brain infection (encephalitis, meningitis) |
| • Trisomies, | • Hydrocephalus |
| • Deletions, | • Cerebral trauma |
| • Fragile X | • Cerebral ischaemia, infarction |
| *Other* | • Cerebral haemorrhage |
| • Angelman's (happy puppet) syndrome | • Post-immunization encephalopathy |
| | • Malignancy |
| *Non-inherited malformations* | • Radiation |
| • Sturge–Weber syndrome | • Status epilepticus |

detect a progressive deterioration. A careful family history, including enquiries about consanguinuity and more distant relatives than the immediate family, is essential if there is any suggestion that the patient has a genetically determined disorder. In the history and examination particular attention should be paid to identifying any cognitive decline, pyramidal signs, dystonia, myoclonus, other movement disorders, cerebellar ataxia, visual deficit, peripheral neuropathy or myopathy.

*Iatrogenic causes*

It is essential to consider whether apparent cognitive and neurological decline may be iatrogenic, as a result of AEDs or other medication. In patients with pre-existing cognitive and motor impairment, the expected features of dose-related intoxication may not be apparent and serum AED concentrations should be checked. A further complication is that some patients, particularly those with mental handicap, may be intoxicated with AEDs at serum concentrations that are not above the widely quoted 'therapeutic ranges' (Ch. 4, 4.3). If there is a possibility that AEDs may be contributory, the appropriate course is to reduce the dose and then re-evaluate the patient. Although most frequent with barbiturates and phenytoin, this situation may also arise with more modern AEDs, and a 'pseudodementia' in association with sodium valproate is well recognized (Pakalnis et al 1989, Jones et al 1990).

The subsequent parts of this section consider first, conditions in which progressive neurological impairment appears to be secondary to the epilepsy and no other underlying cause can be identified and secondly, conditions in which progressive impairment is the result of intrinsically progressive neurological diseases of which epilepsy is one symptom. It is likely that, with advances in understanding and investigations, more specific causes will be identified and the cryptogenic group will get smaller.

## 3.7.2 Conditions in which progressive neurological impairment is secondary to the epilepsy

These are summarized in Table 3.3. See also Chapters 2 and 6 and Roger et al (1992) for further details.

**Table 3.3** Conditions in which epilepsy is the only evident disorder causing progressive impairment

- *Iatrogenic*: Intoxication with medication
- Cryptogenic infantile spasms (West's syndrome)
- Non-convulsive status epilepticus
  (including some patients with the Lennox–Gastaut syndrome)
- Focal epileptic encephalopathies (e.g. Landau–Kleffner syndrome)
- Electrical status epilepticus in slow wave sleep
- Epileptic encephalopathy: frequent seizures, episodes of status
- Post epileptic damage

*West's syndrome*

This occurs predominantly in first 2 years of life. The most commonly identified aetiology is tuberous sclerosis, but many others include neonatal infection, anoxia, inborn errors of metabolism, cerebral ischaemia and haemorrhage, and a proportion are cryptogenic (Ch. 2, 2.6.2). 80% of affected patients regress and there is a high frequency of autism. Key investigations include an EEG, looking for the characteristic patterns of hypsarrhythmia (see 3.2.5), examination of the skin under UV light to identify tuberous sclerosis, neuroimaging with CT or MRI, and plasma and urine amino acids.

*Non-convulsive status epilepticus*

This is relatively common in childhood. Patients may have prolonged periods of withdrawal, with fluctuation from day to day. A high index of clinical suspicion is necessary. A routine EEG may be confirmatory, but prolonged EEG monitoring may be necessary (see above, 3.2.7 and Ch. 5, 5.2.3).

*Electrical status epilepticus in slow wave sleep (ESES)*

In this syndrome EEG abnormalities occur more or less exclusively during sleep, during which there is continuous or very frequent electrographic seizure activity (see above, 3.2.5 and Ch. 2, 2.6.6).

*Focal epileptic encephalopathies*

Overt seizures may not be clinically identifiable. The EEG, however, is diagnostic. The most well known variety is Landau–Kleffner syndrome, in which there is progressive impairment of language function (Ch. 2, 2.6.7). No specific aetiology has been identified. The syndrome is often cryptogenic, but has also been reported to occur in association with structural lesions and with cerebral vasculitis (Roger et al 1992).

*Epileptic encephalopathy*

Some syndromes with very severe epilepsy, such as severe myoclonic epilepsy in infancy and myoclonic–astatic epilepsy are commonly associated with a progressive impairment of cognitive and locomotor function (Roger et al 1992). In some of these cases the seizures and progressive neurological impairments are probably symptoms of a common aetiology that is as yet undetermined.

*Post epileptic damage*

Following a bout of status epilepticus, patients may acquire fixed cognitive and neurological deficits. If repeated bouts of status epilepticus occur, a progressive decline of function may result (see also Ch. 8, 8.3). A similar cognitive decline may be seen in patients with epilepsy that is poorly controlled over a number of years, particularly if the patient has frequent tonic-clonic seizures, head injuries and high doses of AEDs (Ch. 9, 9.5.1).

### 3.7.3 Investigation of progressive neurological diseases

It is difficult to lay down criteria for when a patient's cognitive deterioration is disproportionate to the severity of their epilepsy and a neurodegenerative condition of which epilepsy is just one manifestation should be sought. The possibility should be considered if a patient is deteriorating, particularly if evidence of other fixed neurological dysfunction becomes apparent.

Identified conditions that give rise to a progressive impairment of higher mental function and epilepsy are mostly, but not exclusively, genetically determined (Table 3.4). There are many common clinical features to diseases causing progressive neurological and cognitive decline and there is a considerable overlap between syndromic groupings and identified aetiologies. It is, however, possible to identify clinical syndromes that have a limited range of aetiologies and necessary investigation can be restricted. One of the most clearly defined syndromes is that of progressive

**Table 3.4** Progressive neurological conditions of which epilepsy may be part

*Structural lesions*

- Hydrocephalus
- Progressive structural lesions, e.g. glioma, lymphoma
- Cerebrovascular disease

*Storage disorders*

- $GM_2$ and $GM_1$ gangliosidosis
- Neuronal ceroid lipofuscinosis
- Niemann–Pick disease
- Gaucher's disease
- Sialidosis
- Lafora body disease

*Leucodystrophies*

- Metachromatic
- Globoid cell (Krabbe's)
- Adrenoleucodystrophy
- Spongiform leucodystrophy (Canavan's)
- Alexander's disease
- Pelizaeus–Merzbacher disease

*Defined neurometabolic disturbance*

- Amino acidurias
- Urea cycle disorders
- Organic acidaemias
- Non-ketotic hyperglycinaemia
- Progressive neuronal degeneration of childhood with liver disease (Alper's Disease)
- Mitochondrial cytopathy (MERRF and MELAS)
- Menkes disease
- Wilson's disease
- Porphyria
- Disorders of folate and cobalamin metabolism
- Lesch–Nyhan disease (and other disorders of purine and pyramidine metabolism)

*Biochemical defect uncertain*

- Rett's syndrome
- Polycystic lipomembranous osteodysplasia with sclerosing leucoencephalopathy
- Neuroacanthocytosis
- Juvenile Huntington's disease

*Infective causes*

- Human immunodeficiency virus
- Creutzfeldt–Jakob disease
- Subacute sclerosing panencephalitis
- Syphilis

*Uncertain aetiology*

- Rasmussen's encephalitis
- Alzheimer's disease

myoclonus epilepsy (see below, 3.7.5). The investigations that may be useful in the investigation of progressive neurological conditions of which epilepsy is a part are summarized in Table 3.5.

### 3.7.4 Conditions causing progressive cognitive impairment and epilepsy

There is overlap between phenotypical and aetiological groupings and not all patients fit neatly into a diagnostic category (see also below, 3.7.5, on progressive myoclonus epilepsy). Epilepsy is often not the presenting or dominant feature of these conditions but is one feature of a clearly progressive condition. The range of conditions is summarized in Table 3.4.

*Structural lesions*

*Progressive structural abnormalities*: Primary and secondary brain tumours, lymphomas, chronic cerebral abscess and granulomata may result in epilepsy and the development of fixed neurological deficit, progressive impairment of mentation and possibly clinical features of raised intracranial pressure. Modern neuroimaging with MRI will reveal the lesions. Biopsy of cerebral or associated systemic lesions may be required to establish the precise diagnosis.

**Table 3.5** Investigations of progressive neurological conditions of which epilepsy may be part. (This list of investigations is included as an aide memoire, from which appropriate investigations may be selected for each patient)

- *Careful history*, including a detailed family history
- *Examination*, including skin with UV light, slit lamp examination of eyes
- *Serum AED concentrations*
- *Neurophysiology*
  EEG: waking, sleep, prolonged monitoring
  Electroretinogram (ERG)
  Visual evoked response (VER)
  Somatosensory evoked response (SER)
- *Imaging*: Brain MRI, X-ray CT scans
- *Haematological indices*
  Full blood count and film
  Vitamin $B_{12}$ and folate
  Lymphocyte vacuolation in peripheral blood
- *Blood chemistry*
  Immunoglobulins
  Electrolytes, glucose, liver function
  Amino acids
  Serum acid phosphatase
  Porphyrins, porphobilinogen
  Leucocyte lysosomal enzymes
  Ammonia: fasting and after protein-containing meal
  Plasma copper, caeruloplasmin
  Very long chain fatty acids
- *Serology*
  Viral: HIV, measles, rubella, Syphilis
- *Urine*
  Amino acids and organic acids
  Porphyrins, porphobilinogen
  Bile salts
  Dolichols (urine sediment)
  Sialyloligosaccharides
- *Genetic analysis*
  Karyotype
  Analysis of DNA in lymphocytes
  Mitochondrial cytopathy
  Prion mutation
  Huntington's disease
- *CSF examination*
  Lactate and amino acids
- *Biopsy*
  Skin
  Muscle
  Bone marrow
  Liver
  Brain

*Hydrocephalus*: If uncompensated, this may result in a progressive impairment of cognitive skills, in addition to focal and false localizing neurological deficits. The diagnosis is usually apparent with MRI or X-ray CT scan.

*Cerebrovascular disease*: Repeated cerebral vascular lesions, on the basis of thrombosis, embolism, haemorrhage or a vasculitis, may result in a progressive deficit of cognitive and other neurological functions and also give rise to intractable epilepsy. The diagnosis of cerebrovascular disease is usually clear from the clinical picture and imaging studies (Schmidley 1991).

*Neuronal storage diseases*

*$GM_2$-gangliosidosis*: The disease is usually evident in the first year of life, with seizures, dementia, blindness, a cherry red spot at the macula and spasticity. Onset in later childhood may be associated with ataxia and lower motor neurone degeneration. Up to 40% of affected children develop a psychosis. The diagnosis is made by finding deficiency of hexosaminidase A activity in leucocytes. EEG abnormalities are minor in the first year of life and then show a rapid deterioration, with irregular slow waves and multifocal discharges. The electroretinogram remains unaffected. Rectal biopsy shows foamy ganglion cells in the submucosa that stain with PAS.

*$GM_1$-gangliosidosis* usually presents with failure to thrive in an infant, hepatosplenomegaly, coarse dysmorphic facial features, kyphosis, mental regression and seizures. A macula cherry red spot may be present. Later-onset forms result in seizures, cognitive decline, spasticity, extrapyramidal rigidity and ataxia. The EEG is abnormal early in the course of the disease and the electroretinogram remains unaffected. The key diagnostic test is reduced leucocyte beta-galactosidase activity. Lymphocytes may show vacuolation. Bone marrow films may show vacuolated cells that can resemble Niemann–Pick and Gaucher cells (Brett & Lake 1991).

*Neuronal ceroid lipofuscinosis*: This condition may result in a picture of progressive myoclonic epilepsy (Ch. 2, 2.8 and below, 3.7.5). The onset of the infantile form is with slowed acquisition and then regression of cognitive skills, ataxia, pyramidal signs, myoclonus, tonic-clonic seizures and visual failure with optic atrophy. The EEG background activity is slowed, usually with irregular generalized spike and wave discharges, and becomes of very low amplitude. The ERG and VER are reduced. Peripheral lymphocytes appear normal on light microscopy, but some have granular inclusions found on EM. Skin biopsies examined with EM show granular inclusions in sweat glands, as do neurones and smooth muscle obtained on rectal biopsy.

The late infantile form presents with loss of skills, dementia, tonic-clonic seizures, myoclonus, ataxia and pyramidal signs. Optic atrophy and retinal pigment changes develop. Neuroimaging shows cerebral atrophy. The ERG is absent and the VER amplitude much larger than normal, in response to light flashes at 1/s. Skin and rectal biopsies examined with EM show characteristic curvilinear bodies in sweat gland epithelial cells and smooth muscle. Curvilinear bodies are often also identifiable with EM in peripheral blood lymphocytes (Brett & Lake 1991).

The juvenile form presents with visual failure, optic atrophy, pigmentary retinopathy and reduced or absent ERG. Tonic-clonic and myoclonic seizures and dementia develop, followed by pyramidal, extrapyramidal and cerebellar signs. Rectal biopsy shows granular PAS-positive material in neurones and smooth muscle that on EM has a fingerprint-like structure. Skin biopsy material is less reliable. 25% of peripheral blood lymphocytes show vacuolation.

In adults onset is with dementia or psychosis and personality change, but no pigmentary retinopathy. Patients may develop the picture of progressive myoclonic epilepsy. Urinary dolichols may be raised. Ultrastructural examination of skin and rectal biopsy material with EM shows inclusion bodies with curvilinear or fingerprint-like structures.

*Niemann–Pick disease*: Type A is characterized by the infant with hepatosplenomegaly, slow development, loss of skills and spasticity as well as seizures. Sphingomyelinase activity in leucocytes is deficient. Type C presents neurologically with tonic-clonic seizures, dementia and ataxia. Half of these patients have failed to thrive and may have hepatosplenomegaly. A vertical supranuclear gaze palsy is common. The bone marrow contains sea-blue histiocytes and dense intracellular inclusions. Peripheral blood lymphocytes are not vacuolated. Sphingomyelinase activity in leucocytes is normal. Liver biopsy shows elevated sphingomyelin, cholesterol and glycolipid.

*Gaucher's disease*: The features of the acute infantile form include seizures, impaired development, spasticity and hepatosplenomegaly. There is also a subacute juvenile form. Adults may present with tonic-clonic seizures, myoclonus, dementia and psychosis. Serum acid phosphatase is increased. The readiest confirmation is by finding reduced beta-glucocerebrosidase activity in leucocytes. The bone marrow contains Gaucher cells, which appear grey-blue with the May–Giemsa–Grunewald stain.

*Sialidosis*: Myoclonic and generalized tonic-clonic seizures, dementia and visual failure occur in this condition (see below, 3.7.5) which is a form of mucolipidosis. The key diagnostic test is finding reduced alpha-*N*-acetylneuraminidase activity in leucocytes. In sialidosis type 1, alpha-*N*-acetylneuraminidase is reduced; in sialidosis type 2, activity of both alpha-*N*-acetylneuraminidase and beta-galactosidase is deficient.

*Lafora body disease*: This condition usually presents with the phenotype of progressive myoclonic epilepsy (see below, 3.7.5). Severe myoclonus, tonic-clonic seizures, cerebellar ataxia, dementia and personality change develop, with death in 10–15 years from onset. Lafora bodies consist of polyglucosans, are found in peripheral nerve, liver, muscle and eccrine sweat gland duct cells, and so may be identified on an axillary skin biopsy.

*Leucodystrophies*

*Metachromatic leucodystrophy*: Presentation is with gait disorder, followed by loss of acquired skills, spasticity, ataxia and dementia. Juveniles and adults usually present with deterioration of personality and dementia. Seizures do not occur in all patients. Tendon reflexes are suppressed and there is often optic atrophy. Nerve conduction studies show a demyelinating neuropathy. Normal background rhythms disappear from the EEG. The ERG is normal. The BSAEP is deranged. MRI and X-ray CT show abnormalities of white matter in the centrum semiovale and frontal and parietal lobes. Metachromatic material is often found in urinary sediment cells. The diagnosis is made by finding reduced arylsulphatase A activity in leucocytes or, in rare cases, deficiency of an activator protein.

*Globoid cell leucodystrophy (Krabbe's)*: Seizures are not a major feature. The infantile form presents with irritability, loss of abilities and spasticity. Juveniles develop spasticity, ataxia and optic atrophy. Peripheral nerve conduction is slowed. The EEG shows abnormal background activity. Brain imaging reveals abnormal white matter, often principally in the parietal lobes and with associated atrophy. The diagnosis is made by finding reduced activity of galactocerebroside beta-galactosidase in leucocytes.

*Adrenoleucodystrophy*: Deterioration in social behaviour is followed by dementia, blindness, spasticity, extrapyramidal signs, peripheral neuropathy and seizures. One in five develops Addison's disease. Nerve conduction studies indicate a demyelinating neuropathy. The EEG shows excessive slow activity, the VER is reduced or absent but the ERG is unaffected. Neuroimaging shows abnormalities of white matter around the trigones and particularly in the parietal and occipital areas. The border of the abnormal area progresses anteriorly and shows contrast enhancement. There may be an impaired adrenal response to Synacthen. This condition is due to the deficiency of the perioxisomal enzyme ligoceroyl CoA. The diagnosis is made by finding elevated plasma concentrations of very long chain fatty acids.

*Spongiform leucodystrophy (Canavan's)*: Onset is before 1 year, with progressive retardation, seizures, optic atrophy, spasticity and enlargement of the head. Nerve conduction studies are normal. The EEG is non-specifically abnormal. Neuroimaging shows widespread abnormalities of central and subcortical white matter. *N*-acetyl aspartic aciduria occurs in some cases. At present cerebral biopsy is still necessary to be certain of the diagnosis.

*Alexander's disease*: There is an insidious dementia, spasticity, seizures and enlargement of the head. Neuroimaging shows large ventricles and dysmyelination of cerebral white matter, particularly frontally. There are no definitive biochemical tests. Appearances on cerebral biopsy are characteristic.

*Pelizaeus–Merzbacher disease*: This condition is usually X-linked, sometimes autosomal recessive. There are several subtypes and onset ranges from the neonatal period to adulthood. Seizures are not invariable but may occur and result in frequent episodes of status epilepticus. A particular clinical feature is gross nystagmus, with dementia, optic atrophy, pyramidal, extrapyramidal and cerebellar deficits. MRI shows dysmyelination of cerebral white matter, without a characteristic pattern. In contrast to metachromatic and globoid cell leucodystrophy, peripheral nerve conduction is not affected. As yet, there is no diagnostic test for Pelizaeus–Merzbacher disease.

*Defined neurometabolic disturbances*

*Amino-acidurias*: The best known is phenylketonuria. Screening tests in the neonatal period should identify affected patients so that dietary restriction is commenced. It should not be assumed when assessing patients, however, that correct screening has taken place. 25% of affected patients develop tonic-clonic seizures. If undetected and untreated there is progressive mental impairment and hyperkinetic behaviour. Diagnosis is made by analysis of the plasma amino acid profile. In about 1% of patients with apparent phenylketonuria, the deficit is not of phenylalanine hydroxylase but of biopterin metabolism (Brett & Smith 1991). This may be diagnosed by assay of urine pterins and blood biopterin activity.

Homocystinuria and other amino acidurias may also be diagnosed by analysis of amino acid profiles in plasma and urine. Epileptic seizures are partial and secondary generalized. Hemiplegia may occur due to arterial thrombosis and embolism. Mental retardation and lens dislocation are common. Skeletal abnormalities, particularly osteoporosis, fractures and the effects of bone infarction, may be diagnosed on plain radiographs.

*Urea cycle disorders*: The presentation may be acute, recurrent or chronic and is manifest by irritability, drowsiness, seizures, vomiting and coma. Focal deficits such as hemiplegia may occur during acute episodes. Sodium valproate therapy may precipitate acute deterioration. The plasma ammonia is raised, usually to greater than 300 μmol/l. The enzyme defect may be characterized by determining the levels of orotic acid in the urine, and of citrulline, alanine and glutamine in plasma. The defect may be precisely diagnosed by determination of enzyme activities in red blood cells (arginosuccinate lyase, arginase) and liver (arginosuccinate synthetase, carbamoyl phosphate synthetase, ornithine carbamoyl transferase) (Leonard 1991). Neuroimaging may reveal cerebral oedema at the time of acute episodes and focal areas of cerebral damage after recovery.

*Organic acidaemias*: The most common forms are propionic, methylmalonic acidaemia, glutaric aciduria and maple syrup urine disease. Severely affected patients present neonatally, but those with mild disease can present much later or even remain asymptomatic. Seizures are resistant to AEDs, and are associated with mental retardation, dystonia, cerebellar ataxia and acute neurological deficits. Neuroimaging during or after acute episodes may show focal areas of brain damage. Metabolic acidosis and hypoglycaemia are common in the acute situation. Plasma ammonia is most raised in methylmalonic and propionic acidaemias, and to a lesser extent in other acidaemias. Leucine, isoleucine, allo-isoleucine and valine in plasma are raised in maple syrup urine disease. Other conditions are not associated with a specific pattern of elevated amino acids. Ketonuria is often found. Organic acids in urine should be examined with high-performance liquid chromatography and mass spectrometry during an acute episode or, if this is not possible, at a time of protein ingestion. The exact enzyme defect may be determined in cultured skin fibroblasts or leucocytes (Leonard 1991).

*Non-ketotic hyperglycinaemia*: Severe epilepsy and mental retardation with a very abnormal EEG are key features. Severe forms present neonatally and milder forms are noted in adolescence. Glycine concentrations are very high in plasma and urine, without ketosis or acidosis. A liver biopsy is necessary to demonstrate reduced activity of glycine cleavage enzyme (Leonard 1991).

*Progressive neuronal degeneration of childhood with liver disease*: In the past this has included a variety of pathologies, under the eponym Alper's disease. Onset may be in childhood or adults. Epilepsy develops explosively with multifocal partial and secondarily generalized seizures, commonly resulting in status epilepticus with subsequent focal neurological deficit and dementia. The EEG shows multifocal derangement of background rhythms, with large slow waves and polyspikes. The ERG is normal, but the VER may become impaired. Neuroimaging shows focal areas of cerebral oedema and damage acutely and, subsequently, focal atrophy. Evidence of liver disease develops later. Liver pathology includes fatty infiltration, subacute hepatitis and cirrhosis. The diagnosis may be made by brain or liver biopsy, but the procedure may be complicated if liver disease has led to abnormalities of coagulation.

*Mitochondrial cytopathy (MELAS and MERRF)*: The MELAS phenotype (myopathy, encephalopathy, lactic acidosis, stroke) often presents acutely, with an encephalopathy associated with a focal neurological deficit and seizures. Dementia and recurrent seizures may occur, along with fixed neurological deficit. Lactate concentrations are increased in blood and CSF, particularly acutely. Neuroimaging shows cerebral oedema acutely and focal atrophy subsequently. EEG changes of abnormal background and epileptiform activity are not specific. Peripheral neurophysiological studies may reveal changes of myopathy and neuropathy. Analysis of leucocyte mitochondrial DNA may reveal causative mutations. Muscle biopsy shows ragged red fibres, which on EM are shown to be due to collections of abnormal mitochondria. Biochemical studies on muscle biopsies can identify the respiratory chain enzyme deficiencies. (See below 3.7.5 for the investigation of patients with the MERRF phenotype.)

*Menkes disease*: This disease is an X-linked disorder of copper metabolism. The onset is with failure to thrive, seizures and hypotonia followed by a progressive deterioration with ataxia and extrapyramidal signs. The hair is characteristically curly. Plasma copper and caeruloplasmin concentrations are low.

*Wilson's disease*: Seizures occur in about 6% of patients with Wilson's disease and may be associated with disorders of movement, psychiatric and behavioural derangement and impaired cognition. Epilepsy is occasionally a major feature and may develop when therapy for the Wilson's disease is initiated. A slit lamp examination of the cornea shows Kayser–Fleischer rings. Plasma caeruloplasmin concentration is low and urine copper excretion is increased. MRI shows lesions in basal ganglia or thalamus. In some cases a liver biopsy may be necessary to confirm the diagnosis.

*Porphyria*: Acute intermittent porphyria, hereditary coproporphyria and variegate porphyria result in intermittent neurological disturbances. Seizures occur in up to 30% of cases. Abdominal pain and vomiting are common. An autonomic neuropathy, causing tachycardia, unstable blood pressure, fever and urinary retention, may occur. A motor neuropathy occurs in 50%. Central features include agitation, psychosis, confusion, seizures and focal neurological deficits. In attacks, delto-amino laevulinic acid and porphobilinogen levels are increased in urine. The precise biochemical defect is characterized by estimation of activities of the specific enzymes: uroporphyrinogen-I synthase, coproporphyrinogen oxidase and protoporphyrinogen oxidase in erythrocytes (Elder 1982). A separate condition is the inhibition of uroporphyrinogen-I synthase by carbamazepine, which occurs only rarely but may result in obtundation and increased seizures (Yeung Laiwah et al 1983).

*Biochemical defect uncertain*

*Rett's syndrome*: Epileptic seizures are often refractory in this condition, which affects females and which usually presents at between 1 and 4 years. Dementia is accompanied by loss of manual skills and development of motor stereotypies and apraxia. There are no diagnostic laboratory investigations. Neuroimaging shows cerebral atrophy and the EEG may contain bursts of spikes and slow waves. Some, but not all, patients have elevated plasma concentrations of ammonia and increased orotic acid in the urine. It has been suggested but not proved that the genetic locus is close to the ornithine carbamoyl transferase gene on the X chromosome. It is likely that over the next decade the genetic basis will be identified and that a probe for the defective gene will become available.

*Polycystic lipomembranous osteodysplasia with sclerosing leucoencephalopathy*: This condition is autosomal recessive and presents with bone pain in the third decade of life. Seizures and dementia develop over the next decade. X-ray CT shows cerebral atrophy and basal ganglia calcification. Hand radiographs show bone cysts. The diagnosis is made on skin or bone biopsy, in which fat cells have folded membranes (Coker 1991).

*Neuroacanthocytosis*: Orofacial dyskinesias, cognitive impairment, generalized chorea, dystonia, parkinsonism and a motor neuropathy occur in this autosomal recessive condition, which progresses at a variable rate (Hardie 1989). In some patients seizures are a prominent feature. The diagnosis is made by the examination of a fresh blood film, which shows that over 10% of red blood cells are in the form of acanthocytes. The serum creatine kinase is elevated and peripheral neurophysiological examination demonstrates a principally motor neuropathy.

*Juvenile Huntington's disease*: A high proportion of patients with the juvenile variant of Huntington's disease develop seizures, in the setting of cognitive decline and an akinetic–rigid syndrome. The diagnosis depends on the family history and on genetic analysis of DNA extracted from peripheral blood leucocytes.

*Infective causes*

Any acute encephalitic or meningitic illness may result in seizures, as may parasitic infection, such as cysticercosis (Ch. 2, 2.5.6). The diagnosis is usually clear from the clinical picture, supplemented by neuroimaging and examination of the cerebrospinal fluid and serological tests. Some conditions, however, merit particular consideration.

*Human immunodeficiency virus*: Seizures may occur in HIV encephalopathy, in the setting of insidious cognitive and mental deterioration, and also in the context of opportunistic infection such as toxoplasmosis, and CNS lymphoma. A high index of suspicion and evaluation of risk factors is necessary and the diagnosis of HIV infection is made serologically.

*Creutzfeldt–Jakob disease*: This rare disorder presents primarily as a rapidly progressive dementia, which may be accompanied by blindness and muscle weakness. Prominent myoclonic jerks are present in 80% of patients and may be localized or general, spontaneous or in response to startle. The background activity of the EEG is slow and a characteristic feature is intermittent sharp wave complexes.

*Subacute sclerosing panencephalitis*: This rare disease is caused by persistent measles virus infection of the brain. Onset is usually in childhood, but may be in adults. Deterioration of behaviour is followed by seizures, cognitive impairment, ataxia, spasticity, myoclonic jerks and finally coma. The EEG shows characteristic periodic complexes and the cerebrospinal fluid contains high concentrations of immunoglobulin. Measles antibodies are found at high titre in blood and cerebrospinal fluid.

*Syphilis*: Paretic neurosyphilis gives rise to a dementia with impairment of personality. Seizures may occur, but are not usually a prominent feature. Diagnosis is by serological testing of serum and cerebrospinal fluid.

*Uncertain aetiology*

*Rasmussen's encephalitis*: A chronic infective aetiology for this condition is suspected and cytomegalovirus has been implicated, but the causal association is unproven. Intractable seizures, often with episodes of epilepsy partialis continua, occur in the setting of a slowly progressive impairment of function of one cerebral hemisphere. This results in varying degrees of hemiparesis, hemisensory loss, hemianopia and, if the dominant hemisphere is affected, dysphasia, but without a global dementia. The onset of the disease is usually in childhood, but it may also develop in adults (McLachlan et al 1993). MRI shows progressive atrophy and areas of increased T2-weighted signal intensity in the affected hemisphere. The diagnosis is confirmed by brain biopsy and the neuropathological appearances of perivascular cuffing, glial nodules, microcystic degeneration and neurone loss (Rasmussen 1978).

*Alzheimer's disease*: Epileptic seizures may occur in the context of the insidious decline of neurological function associated with Alzheimer's disease (Rossor 1991). The nature of the association does not usually give rise to diagnostic difficulties.

## 3.7.5 Progressive myoclonus epilepsy (PME)

The key features of this syndrome are progressive myoclonic seizures, occasional tonic-clonic seizures, ataxia and cognitive impairment (see Ch. 2, 2.8 for clinical details) (Berkovic & Andermann 1986). This syndrome needs to be differentiated from conditions that result in a progressive encephalopathy but in which myoclonic seizures are not usually a prominent feature (Table 3.4).

*Causes of progressive myoclonus epilepsy*

- Unverricht–Lundborg disease
- Lafora body disease
- Sialidosis type I and type II
- Neuronal ceroid lipofuscinosis
- Mitochondrial cytopathy (MERRF: myoclonus epilepsy ragged red fibres)
- Gaucher's disease
- Neuroaxonal dystrophy
- Dentato-rubro-pallido-luysian atrophy
- Biotin-responsive encephalopathy

The most common aetiology is Unverricht–Lundborg disease, which is autosomal recessive and in which no biochemical or pathological abnormality has yet been demonstrated.

*Neurophysiology*

The EEG in PME usually shows generalized spike or polyspike and slow wave discharges and photosensitivity is often present. There is slowing of the background activity, reflecting the underlying progressive disorder. The EEG patterns do not help to distinguish the different aetiologies.

In neuronal ceroid lipofuscinosis, the electroretinogram is usually undetectable. The visual evoked response is enlarged in the late infantile form and the EEG may show a low-frequency photic stimulation response. The VER is reduced in the juvenile form and in sialidosis. Giant cortical responses to somatosensory stimulation are commonly seen in PME but are not specific to the aetiology. Peripheral neuropathy may occur with sialidosis I and mitochondrial cytopathy.

*Neuroimaging*

Variable degrees of atrophy may occur, but the appearances are not specific for the subtypes of PME.

*Urine*

Sedimentary dolichol is often increased in neuronal ceroid lipofuscinosis. Sialyloligosaccharides are increased in sialidoses. Organic acids are increased in biotin-responsive encephalopathy.

*Blood*

Lymphocyte vacuolation may be seen in neuronal ceroid lipofuscinosis and sialidosis. Gaucher's disease is commonly associated with a pancytopenia. Assays of leucocyte enzymes can diagnose the sialidoses (alpha-*N*-acetylneuraminidase, beta-galactosidases) and Gaucher's disease (beta-glucocerebrosidase). In sialidosis type 1 alpha-*N*-acetylneuraminidase is reduced, in sialidosis type 2, activities of both alpha-*N*-acetylneuraminidase and beta-galactosidase are deficient. Analysis of mitochondrial DNA may reveal mutations that underlie mitochondrial cytopathy.

*Biopsies*

Pathological examination of eccrine sweat glands in a skin biopsy for polysaccharide-containing inclusion bodies, using PAS, is a reliable method for diagnosing Lafora body disease. Lafora bodies may also be identified on a liver biopsy. Electron microscopy examination of eccrine secretory cells and other tissues reveals fingerprint profiles, deposits and curvilinear bodies in neuronal ceroid lipofuscinosis. The axon spheroids found in neuroaxonal dystrophy may not be seen in sections of peripheral nerve, but have been reported in autonomic nerve terminals.

A muscle biopsy is currently needed to diagnose mitochondrial cytopathy causing MERRF, but in the future may be obviated by advances in analysis of leucocyte DNA. Gaucher's disease may be diagnosed by finding characteristic foam cells on bone marrow examination. Brain biopsy is only very rarely indicated, when less invasive investigations have not yielded an answer and when there is rapid progression, the possibility of a remediable aetiology, when the patient and family wish to have as precise an explanation as possible, and when the diagnosis has implications for genetic counselling. Currently neuroaxonal dystrophy and atypical inclusion body diseases may only be diagnosed in this way.

REFERENCES

Aicardi J 1992 Epilepsy and inborn errors of metabolism. In: Roger J et al (eds) Epileptic syndromes in infancy, childhood and adolescence, 2nd edn. John Libbey, London, p 97–102

Ajmone Marsan C, Zivin LS 1970 Factors related to the occurrence of typical paroxysmal abnormalities in the EEG records of epileptic patients. Epilepsia 11: 361–381

Andermann F, Robb JP 1972 Absence status. A reappraisal following review of 38 patients. Epilepsia 13: 177–187

Ashtari M, Barr WB, Schaul N, Bogert B 1991 Three dimensional Fast Low Angle Shot Imaging and computerized volume measurements of the hippocampus in patients with chronic epilepsy of the temporal lobe. Am J Neuroradiol 12: 941–947

Babb TL, Brown WJ 1987 Pathological findings in epilepsy. In: Engel J Jr (ed) Surgical treatment of the epilepsies. Raven Press, New York, p 511–540

Bannister R 1988 Autonomic failure. A textbook of disorders of the autonomic nervous system, 2nd edn. Oxford University Press, Oxford

Bartenstein P, Ludolph A, Schober O et al 1991 Benzodiazepine receptors and cerebral blood flow in partial epilepsy. Eur J Nucl Med 18: 111–118

Bergen D, Bleck T, Ramsay R et al 1989 Magnetic resonance imaging as a sensitive and specific predictor of neoplasms removed for intractable epilepsy. Epilepsia 30: 318–331

Bergin PS, Fish DR, Shorvon SD, Oatridge A, de Souza NM, Bydder GM 1995 Magnetic resonance imaging in partial epilepsy: additional abnormalities shown with the fluid attenuated inversion recovery (FLAIR) pulse sequence. J Neurol Neurosurg Psychiat 58: 439-443

Berkovic SF, Andermann F 1986 The progressive myoclonus epilepsies. In Pedley TA, Meldrum BS (eds) Recent advances in epilepsy 3. Churchill Livingstone, Edinburgh, p 157–187

Berkovic SF, So NK, Andermann F 1991a Progressive myoclonus epilepsies: clinical and neurophysiological diagnosis. J Clin Neurophysiol 8: 261–274

Berkovic SF, Andermann F, Olivier A et al 1991b Hippocampal sclerosis in temporal lobe epilepsy demonstrated by magnetic resonance imaging. Ann Neurol 29: 175–182

Brett EM, Lake BD 1991 Progressive neurometabolic brain diseases. In Brett EM (ed) Paediatric neurology. Churchill Livingstone, Edinburgh, p 141–200

Brett EM, Smith I 1991 Phenylketonuria and its variants and some other amino acid disorders. In Brett EM (ed) Paediatric neurology. Churchill Livingstone, Edinburgh, p 201–208

Bronen RA, Cheung G, Charles JT et al 1991 Imaging findings in hippocampal sclerosis: correlation with pathology. Am J Neuroradiol 12: 933–940

Brooks BS, King DW, El Gammal et al 1990 MR imaging in patients with intractable complex partial epileptic seizures. Am J Neuroradiol 11: 93–99

Bruton CJ 1988 The neuropathology of temporal lobe epilepsy. Oxford University Press, Oxford, p 1–158

Cascino GD 1993 Nonconvulsive status in adults and children. Epilepsia 34 (suppl 1): S21–S28

Cascino GD, Jack CR, Parisi JE et al 1991 Magnetic resonance imaging-based volume studies in temporal lobe epilepsy: pathological correlations. Ann Neurol 30: 31–36

Cobb WA, Guiloff RJ, Cast J 1979 Breach rhythm: the EEG related to skull defects. Electroenceph Clin Neurophysiol 47: 251–271

Coker SB 1991 The diagnosis of childhood neurodegenerative disorders presenting as dementia in adults. Neurology 41: 794–798

Connelly A, Duncan JS 1995 Magnetic resonance spectroscopy in epilepsy. In: Pedley TA, Meldrum BS (eds) Recent advances in epilepsy 6. Churchill Livingstone, Edinburgh, p 23-40

Connelly A, Jackson GD, Duncan JS, King MD, Gadian DG 1994 Magnetic resonance spectroscopy in temporal lobe epilepsy. Neurology 44: 1411–1417

Cook MJ, Fish DR, Shorvon SD, Straughan K, Stevens JM 1992 Hippocampal volumetric and morphometric studies in frontal and temporal lobe epilepsy. Brain 115: 1001–1016

Corcoran R, Thompson PJ 1993 Epilepsy and poor memory. Who complains and what do they mean? Br J Clin Psychol 32: 199–208

Coughlan AK, Hollows SE 1985 The adult memory and information processing battery test manual. Coughlan, Leeds

De Renzi E, Vignolo LA 1962 The token test. A sensitive test to detect receptive disturbances in aphasics. Brain 85: 665–678

Dodrill CB 1978 A neuropsychological battery for epilepsy. Epilepsia 19: 611–623

Duncan JS 1993 Positron emission tomography studies in the neuropharmacology of epilepsy. In: Rose FC (ed) Recent advances in neuropharmacology. Gordon & Smith, London, p 97–105

Duncan JS, Jackson GD, Connelly A, Grunewald RA, Gadian DG 1994 Quantitative relaxometry of hippocampal sclerosis. In: Shorvon SD, Fish DR, Andermann F, Bydder G, Stefan H (eds) MRI and epilepsy. New York, Plenum Press, p 67–70

Duvernoy HM 1988 The human hippocampus. Bergmann, Munich, p 1–153

Elder GH 1982 Enzymatic defects in porphyria: an overview. Semin Liv Dis 2: 87–99

Elliott CD, Murray DJ, Pearson LS 1983 British Ability Scales. Windsor, NFER–Nelson

Engel J, Brown WG, Kuhl DE, Phelps ME, Mazziota JC, Crandall PH 1982 Pathological findings underlying focal temporal hypometabolism in partial epilepsy. Ann Neurol 12: 518–528

Engel J, Kuhl DE, Phelps ME, Rausch R, Nuwer M 1983 Local cerebral metabolism during partial seizures. Neurology 33: 400–413

Engel J, Henry TR, Risinger MW et al. 1990 Presurgical evaluation for partial epilepsy: relative contributions of chronic depth-electrode recordings versus FDG-PET and scalp-sphenoidal ictal EEG. Neurology 40: 1670–1677

Fish DR, Quirk J, Smith SJM, Sander JWAS, Shorvon SD, Allen P 1993 The national survey of photosensitivity and electronic screen game seizures. Home and Leisure Accident Research, Department of Trade and Industry. HMSO, London

Franceschi M, Triulzi F, Ferini-Strambi L 1989 Focal cerebral lesions found by magnetic resonance imaging in cryptogenic nonrefractory temporal lobe epilepsy patients. Epilepsia 30: 540–546

Franck G, Sadzot B, Salmon E et al. 1986 Regional cerebral blood flow and metabolic rates in human focal epilepsy and status epilepticus. In: Delgado-Escueta AV, Ward AA, Woodbury DM, Porter RJ (eds) Advances in neurology vol 44. Raven Press, New York, p 935–948

Free SL, Bergin PS, Fish DR, Cook MJ, Shorvon SD, Stevens JM 1995 Proposed methods for normalization of hippocampal volumes measured with MR. Am J Neuroradiology: 16: 637-643

Frey KA, Holthoff VA, Koeppe RA, Jewett DM, Kilbourn MR, Kuhl DE 1991 Parametric in vivo imaging of benzodiazepine receptor distribution in human brain. Ann Neurol 30: 663–672

Frost JJ, Mayberg HS, Fisher RS et al. 1988 Mu-opiate receptors measured by positron emission tomography are increased in temporal lobe epilepsy. Ann Neurol 23: 231–237

Gastaut H, Gomez-Almanzar M, Taury M 1991 The enforced nap: a simple method of inducing sleep activiation in epileptics. Epilepsy Res S2: 31–36

Grand'Maison F, Reiher J, Leduc CP 1991 Retrospective inventory of EEG abnormalities in partial status epilepticus. Electroencephalog Clin Neurophysiol 79: 264–270

Gregory RP, Oates T, Merry RTG 1993 Electroencephalogram epileptiform abnormalities in candidates for aircrew training. Electroencephalog Clin Neurophysiol 86: 75–77

Grunewald RA, Panayiotopoulos CP 1993 Juvenile myoclonic epilepsy. Arch Neurol 50: 594–598

Grunewald RA, Jackson GD, Connelly A, Duncan JS 1994 MRI detection of hippocampal pathology in epilepsy: factors influencing T2 relaxation time. Am J Neuroradiol 15: 1149–1156

Hardie RJ 1989 Acanthocytosis and neurological impairment – a review. Q J Med New series 71: 291–306

Harvey AS, Bowe JM, Hopkins IJ et al 1993a Ictal $^{99m}$Tc-HMPAO single photon emission computed tomography in children with temporal lobe epilepsy. Epilepsia 34: 869–877

Harvey AS, Hopkins IJ, Bowe JM, Cook DJ, Shield LK, Berkovic SF 1993b Frontal lobe epilepsy: clinical seizure characteristics and localization with ictal $^{99m}$Tc-HMPAO SPECT. Neurology 43: 1966–1980

Henry TR, Frey KA, Sackellares JC et al 1993 In vivo cerebral metabolism and central benzodiazepine-receptor binding in temporal lobe epilepsy. Neurology 43: 1998–2006

Hermann B, Wyler A, Somes G 1992 Preoperative psychological adjustment and surgical outcome are determinants of psychosocial status after anterior temporal lobectomy. J Neurol Neurosurg Psychiat 55: 491–496

Hrachovy RA, Frost JD, Kellaway P 1984 Hypsarrythmia: variations on a theme. Epilepsia 25: 688–694

Jabbari B, Gunderson CH, Wippold F et al 1986 Magnetic resonance imaging in partial complex epilepsy. Arch Neurol 43: 869–872

Jack CR, Sharbrough FW, Twomey CK et al 1990 Temporal lobe seizures: Lateralization with MR volume measurements of the hippocampal formation. Radiology 175: 423–429

Jack CR, Sharbrough FW, Cascino GD et al 1992 Magnetic resonance imaging-based hippocampal volumetry: correlation with outcome after temporal lobectomy. Ann Neurol 31: 138–146

Jackson M, Warrington E 1986 Arithmetic studies in patients with unilateral lesions. Cortex 22: 611–620

Jackson GD, Berkovic SF, Tress BM, Kalnins RM, Fabinyi G, Bladin PF 1990 Hippocampal sclerosis can be reliably detected by magnetic resonance imaging. Neurology 40: 1869–1875

Jackson GD, Berkovic SF, Duncan JS, Connelly A 1993a Optimizing the diagnosis of hippocampal sclerosis using magnetic resonance imaging. Am J Neuroradiol 114: 753–762

Jackson GD, Connelly A, Duncan JS, Grunewald RA, Gadian DG 1993b Detection of hippocampal pathology in intractable partial epilepsy: increased sensitivity with quantitative magnetic resonance T2 relaxometry. Neurology 43: 1793–1799

Jackson GD, Connelly A, Cross JH, Gordon I, Gadian DG 1994 Functional magnetic resonance imaging of focal seizures. Neurology 44: 850–856

Jayakar PB, Seshia SS 1991 Electrical status epilepticus during slow-wave sleep: a review. J Clin Neurophysiol 8: 299–311

Johnson EW, de Lanerolle NC, Kim JH et al 1992 'Central' and 'peripheral' benzodiazepine receptors: opposite changes in human epileptogenic tissue. Neurology 42: 811–815

Jones GL, Matsuo F, Baringer JR, Reichert WH 1990 Valproic acid associated encephalopathy. West J Med 153: 199–202

Klass DW, Westmoreland BF 1985 Nonepileptiform epileptiform electroencephalographic activity. Ann Neurol 18: 627–635

Kuzniecky R, de la Sayette V, Ethier R et al 1987 Magnetic resonance imaging in temporal lobe epilepsy: pathological correlations. Ann Neurol 22: 341–347

Leonard JV 1991 Inherited metabolic disease: urea cycle disorders, organic acidaemias and non-ketotic hyperglycinaemia. In Brett EM (ed) Paediatric neurology. Churchill Livingstone, Edinburgh, p 209–222

Lesser RP, Modic MT, Weinstein MA et al 1986 Magnetic resonance imaging (1.5 tesla) in patients with intractable focal seizures. Arch Neurol 43: 367–371

Loiseau P, Beaussart M 1973 The seizures of benign childhood epilepsy with rolandic paroxysmal discharges. Epilepsia 14: 381–389

Loring DW, Meador KJ, Lee GP, King DW 1992 Amobarbital effects and lateralized brain function: the Wada test. Springer-Verlag, New York

McHorney C, Ware J, Raczek A 1993 The MOS 36 Item short-form Health Survey (SF 36): II. Psychometric and clinical tests of validity in measuring physical and mental health constructs. Medical Care 31: 247–263

McKenna P, Warrington E 1983 Graded Naming Test manual. Windsor, NFER–Nelson

McLachlan RS, Nicholson RL, Black S et al 1985 Nuclear magnetic resonance imaging, a new approach to the investigation of refractory temporal lobe epilepsy. Epilepsia 26: 555–562

McLachlan RS, Girvin JP, Blume WT, Reichman H 1993 Rasmussen's chronic encephalitis in adults. Arch Neurol 50: 269–274

Marks DA, Katz A, Booke J, Spencer DD, Spencer SS 1992a Comparison and correlation of surface and sphenoidal electrodes with simultaneous intracranial recordings: an interictal study. Electroencephalog Clin Neurophysiol 82: 23–29

Marks DA, Katz A, Hoffer P, Spencer SS 1992b Localization of extratemporal epileptic foci during ictal single photon emission computed tomography. Ann Neurol 31: 250–255

Mayberg HS, Sadzot B, Meltzer CC et al. 1991 Quantification of Mu and non-Mu opiate receptors in temporal lobe epilepsy using positron emission tomography. Ann Neurol 30: 3–11

Meierkord H, Will RG, Fish D, Shorvon S 1991 The clinical features and prognosis of pseudoseizures diagnosed using video-EEG telemetry. Neurology 41: 1643–1646

Meierkord H, Shorvon S, Lightman S, Trimble M 1992 Comparison of the effects of frontal and temporal lobe partial seizures on prolactin levels. Arch Neurol 49: 225–230

Muller-Gartner HW, Mayberg HS, Fisher RS et al 1993 Decreased hippocampal muscarinic cholinergic receptor binding measured by $^{123}$I-iododexetimide and single-photon emission computed tomography in epilepsy. Ann Neurol 34: 235–238

Nelson H 1976 A modified card sorting test sensitive to frontal lobe deficits. Cortex 12: 313–324

Nelson H 1982 The National Adult Reading Test manual. Windsor, NFER–Nelson

Newton R, Aicardi J 1983 Clinical findings in children with occipital spike-wave complexes suppressed by eye opening. Neurology 33: 1526–1529

Newton MR, Berkovic SF, Austin MC, Rowe CC, McKay WJ, Bladin PF 1992 A postictal switch in blood flow distribution and temporal lobe seizures. J Neurol Neurosurg Psychiat 55: 891–894

Ormson MJ, Kispert DB, Sharbrough FW et al 1986 Cryptic structural lesions in refractory partial epilepsy: MR imaging and CT studies. Radiology 160: 215–219

Pakalnis A, Drake ME, Denio L 1989 Valproate-associated encephalopathy J Epilepsy 2: 41–44

Pritchard JW, Rosen BR 1994 Functional study of the brain by NMR. J Cereb Blood Flow Metab 14: 365–372

Pritchard PB, Wannamaker J, Sagel J, Nair R, DeVillier C 1983 Endocrine findings following complex partial seizures. Ann Neurol 14: 27–32

Rao ML, Stefan H, Bauer J 1989 Epileptic but not psychogenic seizures are accompanied by simultaneous elevation of serum pituitary hormones and cortisol levels. Neuroendocrinology 49: 33–39
Rasmussen T 1978 Further observations on the syndrome of chronic encephalitis with epilepsy. Appl Neurophysiol 41: 1–12
Reilly EL, Peters JF 1973 Relationship of some varieties of electroencephalographic photosensitivity to clinical convulsive disorders. Neurology 23: 1050–1057
Roger J, Bureau M, Dravet C, Dreifuss FE, Perret A, Wolf P 1992 Epileptic syndromes in infancy, childhood and adolescence, 2nd edn. John Libbey, London
Rossor MN 1991 The dementias. In: Bradley WG, Daroff RB, Fenichel GM, Marsden CD (eds) Neurology in clinical practice. Butterworth-Heinemann, Boston, p 1407–1442
Rowe CC, Berkovic SF, Austin MC, McKay WJ, Bladin PF 1991 Patterns of postictal cerebral blood flow in temporal lobe epilepsy: qualitative and quantitative analysis. Neurology 41: 1096–1103
Ryvlin P, Philippon B, Cinotti L, Froment JC, Le Bars D, Maugiere F 1992 Functional neuroimaging strategy in temporal lobe epilepsy: a comparative study of $^{18}$FDG-PET and $^{99m}$Tc-HMPAO-SPECT. Ann Neurol 31: 650–656
Sackellares JC, Abou-Khalil BW, Siegel GJ et al 1986 PET studies of interictal, ictal, and postictal changes in local cerebral blood flow in temporal lobe epilepsy. Neurology 36(suppl 1): 338
Sackellares JC, Siegel JC, Abou-Khalil BW et al 1990 Differences between lateral and mesial temporal metabolism interictally in epilepsy of mesial temporal origin. Neurology 40: 1420–1426
Savic I, Persson A, Roland P, Pauli S, Sedvall G, Widen L 1988 In-vivo demonstration of reduced benzodiazepine receptor binding in human epileptic foci. Lancet 2: 863–866
Schmidley JW 1991 Vascular diseases of the nervous system. In: Bradley WG, Daroff RB, Fenichel GM, Marsden CD (eds) Neurology in clinical practice. Butterworth-Heinemann, Boston, p 907–988
Schomer DL 1993 Focal motor status and epilepsia partialis continua in adults and children. Epilepsia 34(suppl 1): S29–S36
Schonell PJ 1971 Reading and spelling tests. A handbook of instructions. Oliver & Boyd, Edinburgh
Sperling MR, Wilson G, Engel J Jr, et al 1986 Magnetic resonance imaging in intractable partial epilespy: correlative studies. Ann Neurol 20: 57–62
Theodore WH, Dorwart R, Holmes M et al 1986 Neuroimaging in refractory partial seizures: comparison of PET, CT and MRI. Neurology 36: 750–759
Thompson PJ 1991 Integrating computerized and traditional assessment techniques. In: Dodson WE, Kingsbourne M, Hiltbrunner B (eds) The assessment of cognitive function in epilepsy. Demos Publications, New York, p 35–50
Treiman DM, Walton NY, Kendrick C 1990 A progressive sequence of electroencephalographic changes during generalized convulsive status epilepticus. Epilepsy Res 5: 49–60
Trimble MR 1978 Serum prolactin in epilepsy and hysteria. Br Med J 2: 1682
Triulzi F, Franceschi M, Fazio F, Del Maschio A 1988 Nonrefractory temporal lobe epilepsy: 1.5 T MR imaging. Radiology 166: 181–185
Turner R 1994 Magnetic resonance imaging of brain function. Ann Neurol 35: 637–638
Van Isselt JW, van Bentum AME, van Huffelen AC, van Rijk PP 1990 The detection of epileptic foci with $^{123}$I-iomazenil. Eur J Nucl Med 16: 409
Van Paesschen W, Revesz T, Duncan JS et al 1994 Quantitative neuropathology and quantitative MRI of hippocampal sclerosis. Epilepsia 1994; 35(suppl 8): 19
Vickery B, Hays R, Graber J, Rausch R, Engel J, Brook R 1992 A health-related quality of life instrument for patients evaluated for epilepsy surgery. Med Care 30: 299–319
Waltz S, Christen HJ, Doose H 1992 The different patterns of the photoparoxysmal response – a genetic study. Electroencephalog Clin Neurophysiol 83: 138–145
Warrington E 1984 Recognition memory test manual. Windsor NFER-Nelson
Warrington E, James M 1991 The visual object and space perception battery. Thames Valley Test Company. Bury St Edmonds
Wechsler D 1981 WAIS-R manual. Psychological Corporation, New York
Wilkus RJ, Vossler DG, Thompson PM 1993 Comparison of EEG derived from sphenoidal, infrazygomatic, anterior temporal and midtemporal electrodes during complex partial seizures. J Epilepsy 6: 152–161
Yaqub BA 1993 Electroclinical seizures in Lennox–Gastaut syndrome. Epilepsia 34: 120–127
Yeung Laiwah AAC, Rapeport WG, Thompson GG et al 1983 Carbamazepine-induced non-hereditary acute porphyria. Lancet 1: 790–792.

# 4 Medical treatment of epilepsy

## 4.1 WHEN SHOULD ANTIEPILEPTIC DRUG TREATMENT BE STARTED?

The decision to treat seizures with antiepileptic drugs (AEDs) should not be taken lightly. It usually leads to regular medication for long periods of time, a risk of toxic side-effects (some serious or even fatal), it may have social repercussions and can confirm illness status at a psychological level. While the need for treatment is clear-cut in many cases, in a minority – perhaps 20% of the total – it may be difficult to decide whether treatment is appropriate (Table 4.1). The knee-jerk reaction of advising drug treatment after two seizures, in disregard of any other factors, is to be deprecated. For some patients, if there is a high risk of recurrence, it is appropriate to commence AEDs after a single seizure. In other cases, it may be the right course to defer starting treatment. In all cases, initial counselling is helpful about such aspects as the role of treatment, the length of time it will be continued, its effectiveness and its drawbacks. The patient may only just have received a diagnosis of epilepsy and may need time to adjust to this as well as to the prospects for treatment. Drug treatment is given to lower the risk of seizure recurrence; it is justified only when these risks outweigh the risks, medical and psychosocial, of medication. A number of factors influence the decision.

**Table 4.1** The initiation of antiepileptic drug treatment

- Is the diagnosis of epilepsy certain?
- What are the risks of recurrence of seizures without treatment?
- What are the risks of recurrence of seizures with treatment?
- Are the presence of precipitating factors relevent?
- Are the seizure characteristics relevent?
- Are personal factors relevent?
- What are the risks of side-effects to treatment?

### 4.1.1 The diagnosis of epilepsy

The diagnosis should be certain before treatment is started. Syncope and non-epileptic attacks (pseudoseizures) are not infrequently mistaken for epileptic attacks (Ch. 1), and many patients with these conditions receive inappropriate AED treatment over many years. If the diagnosis of epilepsy is uncertain, it should be kept under review and is often clarified with the passage of time. There is very little place for a 'trial of treatment' in a suspected but unconfirmed case, as the evaluation of such a trial is almost invariably inconclusive. Tentative treatment almost always complicates assessment, lengthening the time taken to make a firm diagnosis.

Until recently there was a vogue for prescribing AEDs prophylactically to patients who were perceived to be at significant risk of developing seizures, for example after supratentorial neurosurgical procedures or head injury. Recognition of the adverse effects of AEDs and of problems with compliance in patients with no history of epileptic seizures has led this practice to being largely abandoned, although it still has some advocates (Temkin et al 1990, Foy et al 1992).

### 4.1.2 The risks of seizure recurrence (with or without treatment)

A knowledge of the risks of seizure recurrence in untreated patients is essential to determine the need for drug treatment. The salient points regarding the prognosis of epilepsy are summarized here (see Ch. 8, 8.1 for more details). The risk of recurrence after a first seizure has been calculated in a prospective population-based study of 564 newly diagnosed patients (Hart et al 1990, Sander et al 1990a). The risk of recurrence is highest in the days or weeks after the first attack and then falls with time. In about 30% of cases, a second attack will have occurred within 3 months of the first, in 67% in the first 12 months and in 78% within 36 months. The risk is higher in those with pre-existing long-standing neurological disorder (100%), those whose first seizure is partial in nature (94%), young children and the elderly. The risk is lower in those with seizures occurring during acute illnesses or with acute precipitants (40%). A recommendation about treatment should therefore take into account the period that has elapsed since the seizure. EEG has proved disappointing in predicting recurrence: minor changes are of little prognostic value, although frank epileptic EEG changes such as generalized spike-wave activity are usually associated with a greater risk.

After two or more attacks, the risks of recurrence are higher, but data in this area are scarce. Most patients in whom a diagnosis is made are treated at this stage and, because of this, there is little information about the course of the untreated condition. Clinical factors associated with a higher risk of seizure recurrence are shown in Table 4.2.

Most patients suffer only a small total number of attacks once established on treatment. In a survey of a population of 6000 persons, over half the patients with firmly diagnosed epileptic seizures had less than 10 attacks in all (Goodridge & Shorvon 1983a, b). Similarly, in 1628

**Table 4.2** Features associated with an increased risk of seizure recurrence

- Certain seizure types (e.g. partial seizures, tonic seizures, absence seizures, etc)
- High previous seizure frequency
- Long duration of epilepsy
- Structural or diffuse cerebral disorders
- Certain epileptic syndromes (e.g. juvenile myoclonic epilepsy, Lennox–Gastaut syndrome)
- Additional neurological, psychiatric handicap or intellectual deficit
- No immediate precipitant

patients on therapy, randomly identified at a population level, 1026 (63%) had had less than 10 attacks in total and 384 (24%) less than five (Hart 1992). It is not clear to what extent treatment is responsible for this good prognosis. In studies of patients with chronic epilepsy who have not received medication, the commencement of AEDs is associated with more than 50% becoming seizure-free, suggesting that AED therapy suppresses seizures but does not affect the long-term prognosis (Sander 1993). There is, however, some circumstantial evidence to suggest that, in some patients, the ultimate prognosis may be worsened if treatment is delayed (Shorvon & Reynolds 1982, Shorvon 1984). If this is so, the case for early effective treatment would be overwhelming. This question is being addressed by ongoing randomized studies of the early and late initiation of treatment (Musicco et al 1994).

Whatever the effects of drug treatment on long-term prognosis, there is no doubt that AEDs reduce the immediate risks of seizure recurrence in all situations. In the population-based survey referred to above (Sander et al 1990a, Hart et al 1990), 86 patients were treated after a first attack (presumably the cases thought more likely to have further seizures) and recurrence occurred in 50% by 12 months compared with over 70% in 478 untreated cases. In hospital-based studies of initial treatment in drug-naive patients after two or more seizures, with appropriate antiepileptic drug monotherapy, complete seizure control was obtained in between 50% and 90% of cases. An estimate of how effective drug treatment is can be gauged from a study of 73 patients with tonic-clonic and 42 with partial seizures treated with either carbamazepine or phenytoin (Shorvon 1982); seizure frequencies were reduced from 0.7 tonic-clonic attacks/month before treatment to 0.09 attacks/month at suboptimal and 0.02 attacks/month at optimal levels and from 11.6 partial attacks/month to 1.8 attacks/month at suboptimal and 0.73 attacks/month at optimal serum concentrations (followed up for a mean of nearly 2 years). See Chapter 8, 8.1 for more details on the factors influencing response to treatment.

### 4.1.3 Avoidance of epileptogenic stimuli

*Fever*

In children, particularly those with a history of febrile convulsions, fever should be treated with paracetamol as an antipyretic and removal of excessive coverings. There is no evidence that tepid sponging confers additional benefit, but it helps the parents to feel positively involved. Patients with a prior history of febrile convulsions may be given prophylactic rectal diazepam solution, 5 mg if the child is under 3 years and 7.5 mg if older than this, in the event of a fever in excess of 38.5°C, repeated after 12 h if the child is still febrile (see also below, 4.4.3). Prophylactic sodium valproate and phenobarbitone reduce the recurrence rate of febrile convulsions. Phenobarbitone, however, has been associated with a high risk of behaviour disturbance (Wolf & Forsythe 1978) and valproate has been associated with a significant risk of hepatotoxicity in young children (Dreifuss et al 1989). The adverse effects of these therapies in young children are generally felt to outweigh the benefits, but they may be useful if rectal diazepam has failed to be effective, or administration proves impossible.

*Alcohol, sedatives, drugs of abuse*

Patients should be counselled to avoid excessive alcohol and to seek medical advice for controlled detoxification after a period of heavy drinking, particularly if other alcohol-withdrawal symptoms become apparent. Prophylactic AEDs are not indicated for patients who only have seizures in the context of alcohol withdrawal. In this population, compliance is likely to be very erratic and to lead to a greater, rather than lesser risk of seizures on alcohol withdrawal (Duncan 1988). Excessive fatigue often accompanies alcohol excess and may in itself increase the tendency towards seizures; so far as it is possible, this should be avoided. Withdrawal of barbiturates, benzodiazepines and other sedatives needs to be very gradual, over weeks or even months, if there is a history of a withdrawal seizure or other significant reaction. Almost all drugs of abuse, particularly amphetamines and cocaine, and organic solvents, have been associated with precipitation of epileptic seizures. Complete avoidance is to be recommended and, as with alcohol abuse, prophylactic AEDs are likely to cause more problems than they solve.

*Medications*

Iatrogenic hypoglycaemia in patients receiving insulin or oral hypoglycaemic agents may produce epileptic seizures. This possibility should always be considered and evaluated by checking the blood glucose concentration at the time of seizures. Other medications that are associated with an increased risk of seizures include isoniazid, chloroquine, aminophylline, lignocaine, antidepressant and neuroleptic medication. In the event of seizures occurring in this context the dose and nature of the medication, possible alternative agents and the risk–benefit ratio of continued therapy should be reviewed.

*Photosensitivity*

Photosensitivity is a potent precipitant of epileptic seizures in susceptible persons. Patients who are known to be photo- or pattern-sensitive should take precautions when using televisions and VDUs or playing computer games (Fish et al 1994). Principally these are:

- Using a small screen relative to the viewing distance
- Using a remote control for changing channels, etc
- Using a 100 Hz television screen or a non-interlaced computer screen with a high refresh rate or liquid crystal display
- Closing one eye or using polarizing glasses
- Keeping the screen contrast and brightness low
- Avoiding exposure when sleep-deprived
- Avoiding looking at a fixed flickering pattern

*Fatigue*

Fatigue can exacerbate the tendency for seizures to occur, particularly in patients with idiopathic generalized epilepsy and if fatigue is accompanied by alcohol abuse. The role of excitement and emotional upset is less certain and is difficult to evaluate, but does seem to be a relevant factor in certain individuals.

### 4.1.4 Seizure characteristics

Patients with minor attacks that do not interfere with normal activities may not require treatment, although this is often an individual decision. Similarly, those who only experience nocturnal attacks may well prefer not to receive medication, even if the attacks are generalized convulsions; although in many such cases, daytime seizures will develop (Janz 1974). If seizures are very infrequent, it is reasonable to consider not prescribing AEDs, although how long a period between seizures should be to allow therapy to be deferred is arbitrary.

Before withholding therapy in active epilepsy, however, it should be remembered that seizure type and frequency may change, and that seizures, even if infrequent, may result in serious injury or death (Ch. 8, 8.3, 8.4).

### 4.1.5 Personal factors

The activities and aspirations of the patient are important factors in the decision to start therapy. These are individual matters, and should be considered in all patients prior to the initiation of treatment. Areas of importance include the need to drive, schooling, leisure activities, employment and plans to conceive. A balance needs to be struck between the psychological and domestic implications of treatment and of seizures.

It is important to counsel all patients carefully about their epilepsy and its treatment, as misconceptions, resentment or ignorance may compromise treatment. Good compliance is essential for successful therapy but will not be achieved unless the patient fully accepts the need for treatment and understands its role in a realistic fashion. The prescription of long-term antiepileptic drug treatment without explanation will often fail, and may result in hostility and loss of trust.

### 4.1.6 Toxic side-effects

If AED treatment was entirely innocuous, the decision to initiate therapy would be easy. There are of course adverse effects, which may be serious and even fatal, and the decision to treat should be taken in the light of these risks. Side-effects may be categorized as acute idiosyncratic, acute dose-related, chronic and teratogenetic and are discussed elsewhere in this book. Suffice to say here that although toxic side-effects are usually minor and reversible, occasional severe or fatal reactions do occur (see below, 4.5 and Ch. 6, 6.3.3).

## 4.2 DRUG TREATMENT STRATEGIES

This section considers the stepwise approach to treating a patient with newly diagnosed epilepsy, the need to recognize the limits of the efficacy of currently available AEDs, the introduction and tapering of drugs; followed by strategies for treating patients with chronic epilepsy.

Precise diagnosis and classification of the types of seizure (Commission on Classification and Terminology of the International League Against Epilepsy 1981) and type of epilepsy (Commission on Classification and Terminology of the International League Against Epilepsy 1989) (Ch. 2, 2.2, 2.3), using clinical and EEG data, careful recording of seizure frequency and severity, and monitoring side-effects of AEDs are essential if rational management decisions are to be made.

### 4.2.1 Stepwise AED plan for newly diagnosed patient

The goal of therapy is to achieve complete seizure control with a single drug taken once or twice a day, without side-effects. Approximately 70–80% of patients who develop epilepsy may expect to have their seizures controlled with optimal AED therapy. Monotherapy with AEDs was popularized in the 1980s and about 80% of patients developing seizure disorders will achieve the best control with a single drug. For the remainder, combination therapy provides improved seizure control (see below, 4.2.4).

It is most useful to formulate a treatment plan at the time of a patient's initial evaluation. This is particularly useful when treatment is being shared between the family practitioner and hospital consultant, and in busy clinics at which many different junior doctors may be involved. The plan may then be followed as far as necessary, although it is clearly important to retain flexibility if the clinical situation changes.

*Step 1*: Any precipitating factors, such as fever in young children, excessive fatigue, alcohol and drug abuse, iatrogenic hypoglycaemia and photosensitivity, should be identified and the patient and relatives counselled about their avoidance (see above, 4.1.3).

*Step 2*: The reasons for instituting AED treatment, the expectations, limitations and likely duration of therapy, and the need for regular tablet taking, should be explained. Time taken with the patient at this stage will pay dividends later in terms of easier management and greater patient satisfaction. In particular, it needs to be explained that AEDs do not provide a cure for epilepsy and have to be taken for a long time, usually years; that 70–80% of patients may expect to have their seizures controlled by medication; and that AEDs need to be taken regularly, usually once or twice a day, and that omitting doses raises the likelihood of further seizures occurring.

*Step 3*: Patients should be commenced on a small dose of one of the first-line AEDs recommended for their type(s) of seizure (Tables 4.3 and 4.4). Dose increments should then be made if seizures continue and side-effects do not occur. The strategy should be gradually to increase the dose of the chosen agent up to the maximum tolerated dose, if necessary.

When employed as a guide to dosing, measurement of the serum concentrations of phenytoin are particularly useful; assay of concentrations of carbamazepine, phenobarbitone and ethosuximide are moderately helpful. It is not yet established whether measuring serum concentrations of gabapentin and lamotrigine are useful or not. Knowing serum concentrations

**Table 4.3** AEDs for different seizure types (The sequence of AEDs to use is controversial and individual patient factors need consideration. In many cases there is not a clear consensus between the present authors!)

| Seizure Type | First-choice | Second-choice |
|---|---|---|
| *Partial seizures* | | |
| Simple partial,<br>complex partial,<br>secondarily generalized | Carbamazepine<br>Valproate | Vigabatrin<br>Phenytoin<br>Lamotrigine<br>Clobazam<br>Gabapentin<br>Acetazolamide<br>Phenobarbitone<br>Felbamate* |
| *Generalized seizures* | | |
| Tonic-clonic, clonic | Valproate<br>Carbamazepine | Phenytoin<br>Lamotrigine*<br>Clobazam<br>Vigabatrin<br>Phenobarbitone<br>Acetazolamide<br>Felbamate* |
| Absence | Ethosuximide<br>Valproate | Lamotrigine*<br>Clonazepam<br>Acetazolamide |
| Atypical absences,<br>atonic, tonic | Valproate | Lamotrigine*<br>Clobazam<br>Clonazepam<br>Acetazolamide<br>Phenobarbitone<br>Felbamate*<br>Phenytoin<br>Gabapentin* |
| Myoclonic | Valproate | Clonazepam<br>Piracetam<br>Phenobarbitone<br>Acetazolamide |
| Infantile spasms | ACTH | Vigabatrin<br>Nitrazepam<br>Clonazepam |

*Not a licensed indication in UK (1995)

of valproate, vigabatrin and primidone is of very little utility in this regard. Rigorous adherence to quoted 'therapeutic ranges' of serum AED concentrations is inappropriate (see below, 4.3). These data should always be of secondary importance to the clinical situation of whether or not the patient continues to have seizures and/or dose-related adverse effects from AEDs.

*Step 4*: If seizures continue despite a maximally tolerated dose of a first-line AED, the diagnosis of epilepsy and its putative aetiology should be reconsidered. It may be that the patient's attacks do not have an epileptic basis (Chs 1 and 9, 9.1), or may be the result of an underlying structural lesion. Imaging of the brain should be reviewed at this time (Ch. 3, 3.3). It should also be determined whether or not the patient is taking the

**Table 4.4** Commonly used starting and maintenance doses of AEDs for adults

| AED | Starting dose (mg) | Average maintenance dose (total mg/day) | Doses/day |
|---|---|---|---|
| Acetazolamide | 250 | 500–1000 | 2 |
| Carbamazepine | 100 | 600–1800 | 2–4 (Retard: 2) |
| Clobazam | 10 | 10–30 | 1–2 |
| Clonazepam | 0.5 | 0.5–3 | 1–2 |
| Ethosuximide | 250 | 500–1500 | 1–2 |
| Felbamate | 1200 | 2400–3600 | 2 |
| Gabapentin | 300 | 900–2400 | 3 |
| Lamotrigine | 50* | 200–400* | 2 |
| Oxcarbazepine | 300 | 900–2400 | 2–3 |
| Phenobarbitone | 60 | 60–180 | 1 |
| Phenytoin | 200–300 | 200–400 | 1–2 |
| Piracetam | 7200 | 12 000–24 000 | 3 |
| Valproate | 500 | 1000–2500 | 1–2 |
| Vigabatrin | 500 | 2000–3000 | 1–2 |

*Reduce by 75% if on valproate

prescribed medication by non-confrontational enquiry of the patient and carers (see also below, 4.2.5). Counting the number of tablets remaining after an interval may indicate discrepancies. Measurement of serum drug concentrations may show inappropriately low serum AED levels that suggest non-compliance. When used to assess compliance, serum AED concentrations are particularly useful if the patient is not expecting a sample to be taken. If patients know that a blood sample is usually drawn at a clinic visit, most will take their prescribed medication for the previous day or two, lessening the value of the measure as a check on compliance.

*Step 5*: Another first-line drug for that patient's seizure type (Table 4.3) should then be commenced and built up to an optimal dose, and the initial agent should then be withdrawn. It is generally best to make such a changeover of AED treatment in two sequential steps, rather than simultaneously decreasing the dose of one AED while increasing the dose of another. Although a sequential approach may take longer it is more satisfactory because it can be established that the new therapy is reasonably well tolerated before the first drug is tapered. Further, if there is an adverse effect, such as an acute psychiatric disturbance or an increase in seizures, it is much easier to identify the cause and correct the situation if only one drug change has been made at a time. During such a changeover of therapy it is necessary to be alert to the possibility of pharmacokinetic interactions between AEDs developing (see Table 4.5).

**Table 4.5** Principal pharmacokinetic interactions with AEDs (with grateful acknowledgements to Dr P.N. Patsalos) Key: ▼ = decrease in serum concentrations expected; ▲ = increase in serum concentrations expected; N.E. = no significant pharmacokinetic interaction expected; ? = unknown at present; CBZ = carbamazepine; CBZ-E = carbamazepine epoxide; VPA = valproate; PHT = phenytoin; PB = phenobarbitone; PMD = primidone; GVG = vigabatrin; LTG = lamotrigine; ESM = ethosuximide; GBP = gabapentin; FBM = felbamate. Converse changes expected if AED withdrawn

| | **Existing drug** | | | | | | | | | |
|---|---|---|---|---|---|---|---|---|---|---|
| **AED added** | CBZ | VPA | PHT | PB | PMD | GVG | LTG | ESM | GBP | FBM |
| CBZ | Auto induction | ▼VPA | ▼▲ PHT | N.E. | ▼ PMD<br>▲ PB | N.E. | ▼ LTG | ▼ ESM | N.E. | ▼ FBM |
| VPA | ▲ CBZ-E | | ▼▲ PHT | ▲ PB | ▲ PMD<br>▲ PB | N.E. | ▲ LTG | ▲ ESM | N.E. | N.E. |
| PHT | ▼ CBZ | ▼ VPA | | ▲ PB | ▲▼ PMD<br>▲ PB | N.E. | ▼ LTG | ▼ ESM | N.E. | ▼ FBM |
| PB | ▼ CBZ | ▼ VPA | ▼▲ PHT | | Not used together | N.E. | ▼ LTG | ▼ ESM | N.E. | ▼ FBM |
| PMD | ▼ CBZ | ▼ VPA | ▼▲ PHT | Not used together | | N.E. | ▼ LTG | ▼ ESM | N.E. | ▼ FBM |
| GVG | N.E. | N.E. | ▼ PHT | ▼ PB | ▼ PMD<br>▼PB | N.E. | N.E. | N.E. | N.E. | N.E. |
| LTG | ▲ CBZ-E | N.E. | N.E. | N.E. | N.E. | N.E. | Auto induction? | N.E. | N.E. | N.E. |
| ESM | N.E. | N.E. | ▲ PHT | N.E. | N.E. | N.E. | N.E. | | N.E. | N.E. |
| GBP | N.E. | N.E. | N.E. | N.E. | N.E. | N.E. | N.E. | N.E. | | N.E. |
| FBM | ▼ CBZ<br>▲ CBZ-E | ▲ VPA | ▲ PHT | ▲ PB | ▲ PB | N.E. | ? | ? | N.E. | |

*Step 6*: The dose of the second drug, taken alone, should then be adjusted to optimum, as with the initial agent.

*Step 7*: If seizures continue despite a maximally tolerated dose of all individual first-line drugs, the next step is to try a combination of two first-line drugs for that seizure type (e.g. ethosuximide and sodium valproate for generalized absences; valproate and carbamazepine for partial seizures). There is a 10–15% chance of duotherapy controlling seizures when monotherapy has been unsuccessful (Reynolds & Shorvon 1981, Schmidt 1982, Mattson et al 1985).

*Step 8*: If a combination of two first-line agents is not helpful, the drug which has been most beneficial and has the least toxicity should be continued, and the other AED replaced by a second-line drug (see Table 4.3).

*Step 9*: If the addition of a second-line drug provides effective seizure control, withdrawal of the initial agent should be considered. Similarly, an unhelpful second-line agent should not be continued.

*Step 10*: If seizures are still not adequately controlled, the use of a novel AED may be considered. In general, such drugs should only be used as part of a formal, organized trial with very accurate documentation of efficacy and tolerability.

The above scheme will generally take a number of months, or even years to work through. It is important to follow a treatment plan expeditiously and if satisfactory control cannot be obtained with AEDs within 2–3 years and the patient has partial seizures, consideration should be given to surgical treatment (Ch. 10).

### 4.2.2 Recognition of the limits of AED efficacy

The emphasis of the above scheme is to try each appropriate AED in turn, up to a maximum tolerated dose, singly and as duotherapy. Occasional patients, about 5% in our practice, often those with a combination of intractable seizure types, have their best possible seizure control on a combination of three AEDs. It is important carefully to review these patients for evidence of adverse effects from AEDs.

If seizures continue or if the patient suffers adverse effects from AEDs it is appropriate to review the aims of therapy and to modify these to the prescription of the minimum dose of one AED, or combination of AEDs, that can be taken without a marked increase in seizure frequency. In this situation there is usually a trade-off between the beneficial effects of AEDs in terms of seizure control, and dose-related adverse effects. The views of the patient are paramount when deciding what is the best compromise and what are acceptable adverse effects of medication (Duncan 1993).

In a few patients, no AEDs, singly or in combination, appear to have any beneficial effect on the seizure disorder and some patients wish to discontinue their medication altogether. There is a substantial risk of a deterioration in seizure control when this course is taken, and of status epilepticus. It is not, therefore, a course of action that we would advocate, particularly in those patients with tonic-clonic or secondarily generalized seizures. If a patient with active epilepsy is insistent on stopping their medication this should be carried out in small decrements every 1–2 weeks, and every month for barbiturates, so that tapering is completed over 6–12 months. The patients should be strongly advised that, should there be a significant increase in seizures, the drug should be restarted immediately at a higher dose than that which was being taken when seizure control deteriorated.

## 4.2.3 Introduction and tapering of AEDs

*Introduction of AEDs*

In the emergency situation, when a full and rapid antiepileptic effect is required (Ch. 5, 5.3), commencement of the full dose, and for phenytoin and barbiturates a loading dose, is necessary. In the non-acute situation it is generally best to introduce an AED at low dose and to increase over several weeks to the anticipated maintenance dose. A slow rate of introduction is generally better tolerated and results in less adverse effects. If seizures continue it is appropriate to increase doses gradually up to the maximum tolerated.

If the patient does not have further seizures during the phase of drug introduction it is customary to continue treatment at a low dose. It may, however, be difficult to decide how high to build up the dose. At the extremes, there are the *maximalist* and *minimalist* approaches. In the former the AED is increased up to the maximum tolerated. In the latter the planned dose is low, with increments only being made if further seizures occur. It is important to discuss the different possible treatment strategies with the patient and to modify the plans according to the patient's individual circumstances. Schedules for the introduction of individual AEDs are discussed below (4.5) and in Table 4.4.

*Tapering of AEDs in patients with active epilepsy*

It is advisable to make only one drug change at a time. Although simultaneous tapering and introduction of different AEDs may seem attractive and quicker, it can make it very difficult to determine the cause of any adverse effect that may develop.

The ideal rate of AED reduction and withdrawal when making a planned changeover in drug therapy is controversial. A common situation is that an AED that is not thought to be contributing greatly to seizure control is reduced, and the patient is also taking an AED that is thought to be efficacious. In clinical practice, there are several advantages to tapering the AED to be withdrawn as quickly as possible, so long as there is no increased risk of an exacerbation of seizures from so doing. These are principally:

- The patient may be supervised closely over a short time
- The strategy is more likely to be followed through
- The effect of the drug change on seizures, side-effects of medication and concomitant AED concentrations may be determined quickly
- Potentially beneficial drug treatments may be rapidly explored and the patient established on optimal therapy sooner

Determination of the longer-term effects on seizure control, however, of course require more prolonged observation. In this situation phenytoin and sodium valproate can probably be safely withdrawn over 1–2 weeks, but carbamazepine, barbiturate and benzodiazepine withdrawal should probably occur over several weeks (Duncan et al 1990a). If barbiturates and benzodiazepines have been taken at a high dose or for many months, even slower tapering, over months, may be needed. Clinical experience with vigabatrin and lamotrigine suggests that reduction over 2–3 weeks is usually reasonable. In the event of a significant idiosyncratic adverse effect, however, such as a drug rash, it will generally be appropriate to discontinue the suspected agent abruptly or over a few days.

More rapid AED reductions may be reasonable if the patient is under in-patient supervision than if he/she is an out-patient. It is quite inappropriate, however, to admit a patient to withdraw phenobarbitone or primidone and to discharge them at the end of the tapering. With the 96 h half-life of phenobarbitone, it is 3 weeks before the drug is cleared completely and the high risk period of a marked increase in seizures continues through this time.

Stopping an AED will often result in a pharmacokinetic interaction and change in the concentration of concomitant AEDs (Duncan et al 1991) (Table 4.5). The serum concentrations of remaining AEDs should be checked if there is an increase in seizures or development of symptoms of toxicity. If there is an increase in seizures, there may be scope to increase the dose of the retained AED. It must be recognized that sometimes an AED that was contributing more to seizure control than had been appreciated is withdrawn. In this situation the drug should be re-introduced. It is appropriate to make allowance for spontaneous seizure clustering, but if there is a marked or sustained increase in seizures, the AED being tapered should be returned to its original dose and its role should be reviewed. It may be that a larger dose of that drug can result in improved seizure control. Conversely, it may be that a lower dose confers as much antiepileptic effect as the full dose, with fewer adverse effects.

If there is a serious increase in seizures on withdrawal of an AED, a benzodiazepine may be needed acutely (Ch. 5, 5.1) for immediate antiepileptic effect while maintenance therapy is reintroduced. Should there be an increase in seizure frequency on withdrawal of an AED, this invariably resolves when that drug is reinstated. Although there have been some anecdotal reports of a persistent worsening of seizure control in this situation, controlled studies have not shown this.

If withdrawal of an AED fails because of increased seizures, it is reasonable to consider a further attempt, after optimization of other AED therapy and perhaps after introduction of a new agent that appears to confer benefit, and at a slower rate of tapering.

Withdrawal symptoms from AEDs other than benzodiazepines are not to be expected at clinically used doses and rates. A flurry of seizures, however, may be associated with an organic brain syndrome, with postictal psychotic symptoms and anxiety. These symptoms may be expected to resolve rapidly after reintroduction of the AED being tapered and restoration of seizure control (Duncan et al 1988, Ketter et al 1992).

### 4.2.4 Monotherapy and polytherapy with AEDs

Combination therapy was in vogue in the 1950s and 1960s. In the 1970s and 1980s evidence accrued for the advantages of monotherapy (Shorvon & Reynolds 1977, Reynolds & Shorvon 1981). Studies of the tapering of polytherapy to monotherapy, of the initiation of monotherapy and of the effects of duotherapy have indicated that monotherapy is associated with complete or optimal seizure control in 80% of patients and that 10–15% have improved seizure control on a combination of two AEDs (Reynolds & Shorvon 1981, Schmidt 1982, Thompson & Trimble MR 1982, Theodore & Porter 1983, Callaghan et al 1984, 1985, Albright & Bruni 1985, Mattson et al 1985).

The advantages of monotherapy over polytherapy may be summarized as:

- Patients are likely to tolerate higher doses of a single AED, which may be more effective, and have less adverse effects
- A simpler regimen: compliance easier, less intrusive
- Minimizes long-term toxicity
- No interactions between AEDs and less risk of interactions with other drugs
- Less teratogenic risk (Ch. 6, 6.3.3)

The advantage of polytherapy is that a combination of AEDs may be helpful for some patients, giving improved seizure control without adverse effects.

When two or more AEDs are combined, the likelihood of pharmacokinetic interactions that may affect drug efficacy or result in adverse effects needs consideration (Table 4.5). An attractive possibility is that there may be a pharmacodynamic interaction that results in a synergistic antiepileptic effect without a concomitant increase in adverse effects, so giving rise to a useful increase in therapeutic index of the medication.

There has been some work on the possibility of a synergistic antiepileptic effect of some combinations of AEDs, leading to an enhanced therapeutic index. It has, for example, been suggested that a combination of carbamazepine and valproate leads to an increase in therapeutic index, whereas combining carbamazepine and phenobarbitone does not (Bourgeois & Wad 1988). The findings, however, are only based on a single rodent model and it is by no means certain how relevant the results are to the human epilepsies.

There have been many fashions for particular drug combinations, such as phenytoin and phenobarbitone in the past and carbamazepine and vigabatrin at present. It may be argued that, on a theoretical basis, it is likely to be more helpful to combine two AEDs that have differing modes of action rather than two agents that act in similar ways. There have not been adequate scientific studies to guide practice, however, and a reasonable approach at present is to combine two first-line AEDs for the patient's seizure types or to prescribe a first- and a second-line AED. The situation with regard to absences and myoclonic seizures is clearer than for other seizure types. There is a reasonable body of evidence that a combination of valproate and ethosuximide controls absences in some patients that are not controlled by either drug alone. Similarly, myoclonic seizures may respond to a combination of valproate and clonazepam.

Patients need to be advised carefully about the implications of polytherapy, especially compliance, the potential for drug interactions and risks of teratogenesis. Specific combinations of AEDs for different seizure types are considered below (see also 4.4).

### 4.2.5 Treatment of patients with chronic epilepsy

Patients with chronic epilepsy should generally be treated with a single AED, or at most two AEDs, shown to have some efficacy, at doses that do not give rise to intolerable side-effects. This is a difficult area and a specialist evaluation is appropriate (Duncan 1991, Shorvon 1991). The general principles are as follows.

*Review diagnosis and aetiology*

The diagnosis and history of epilepsy should be critically reviewed by interviewing the patient and a witness to the seizures, and by inspection of previous clinical records. It should be asked whether the diagnosis of epilepsy is secure and whether there is any evidence for non-epileptic attacks. In many series of patients with supposed chronic epilepsy, 10–15% have non-epileptic attacks (Chs 1 and 9, 9.1).

The types of seizure and type of epilepsy should then be classified. The aetiology of a seizure disorder may be identified in up to 80% of patients and it is appropriate to obtain imaging of the brain with magnetic resonance imaging (MRI). MRI is more sensitive than X-ray CT, detecting a relevant underlying lesion in 30–80% of patients in whom no lesion is visualized by X-ray CT scans (Ch. 3, 3.3).

*Review compliance*

Many patients with chronic epilepsy comply poorly with their prescribed medication, particularly if seizures are uncontrolled and if dosing is complicated, involving many doses per day, or causing adverse effects. It is necessary to establish a positive rapport with the patient, to explain the rationale, expectations and limitations of treatment, and the need to take medication regularly.

It should be made clear to the patient that it is understood that it is hard to take medication that appears ineffective and causes problems, and that the aim is to improve control of the epilepsy with a simplified regimen and minimum adverse effects. Patients should be encouraged to report any dissatisfaction with their therapy (Cramer 1991) (Table 4.6).

Prescribing more than two doses of medication per day strains compliance, particularly for the middle-of-the-day doses, and polytherapy is less likely to be taken accurately. Poor memory is often a contributory factor to poor compliance. A written summary of dosing instructions, a preset alarm and a drug wallet in which the doses for an entire week may be placed in individual compartments, so that it is clear to the patient and their carers whether a particular dose has been taken or not, are frequently useful.

In addition to asking the patient and his/her carers, compliance can be checked by tablet-counting, if dispensing is from one source. It is helpful to check serum concentrations of AEDs unexpectedly, to determine whether there are inappropriately low serum concentrations for the

**Table 4.6** Methods to improve compliance

*Educate patient and carers*
- Basis of diagnosis and rationale of treatment
- Expectations and limitations of treatment
- Drug doses and schedule of administration
- Use of cues, clock-alarm

*Dosing*
- Reduce to monotherapy
- Reduce to one or two doses per day
- Provide a summary of treatment doses and times
- Provide a drug wallet

*Review in clinic*
- Continuity of follow up
- Discuss with patient how to improve treatment

prescribed doses. A microchip device built into the tops of drug containers, which registers when medication has been taken, has been developed and used in clinical trials and can also be useful in assessing compliance (Cramer & Mattson 1991).

*Review drug history*

Time spent ascertaining what AEDs have been used in the past, in what doses, and the evidence for beneficial and adverse effects often pays dividends. As a result of such a review, it should be possible to identify a list of AEDs that have not been used to their full potential, which may be appropriate to try. This process requires a history from patient and relatives and careful inspection of previous medical records. It may, for example, be a patient's understanding that he is allergic to carbamazepine, whereas review of records may indicate that the starting dose was 200 mg thrice daily (much too high) and that the drug was discontinued after 2 days because of nausea.

*Form treatment strategy*

A treatment plan should be made, based on the types of seizure and epilepsy and by review of all the AEDs that have and have not been used to their maximum tolerated doses, those that may have shown some benefit, those that have not been used at all, and those that it would be appropriate to try. It is then possible to select the AED that is most likely to be efficacious and to have the fewest side-effects, and to adjust the dose of this drug to the optimum. This drug will usually be chosen on the grounds that it has previously not been used to its full potential and/or appears to have had a definite beneficial effect.

*Taper unhelpful AEDs*

AEDs that have not aided seizure control and have produced adverse effects should then be gradually tapered and discontinued. Seizures may worsen at this time and the strategy may need revision (see above, 4.2.3). Frequently, however, reduction of the number of AEDs results in fewer adverse effects, improved seizure control and better compliance (Shorvon & Reynolds 1979, Thompson & Trimble 1982, Theodore & Porter 1983, Callaghan et al 1984, Albright & Bruni 1985, Duncan et al 1990a, b).

*Subsequent strategy*

If seizures remain uncontrolled, other first-line and second-line drugs that have been identified as being possibly helpful, and surgical treatment (Ch. 10), should be considered, as for newly diagnosed patients. It is important, however, to recognize the limits of the efficacy of currently available AEDs and the need to avoid intoxication (see above, 4.2.2).

## 4.3 SERUM ANTIEPILEPTIC DRUG CONCENTRATION MONITORING

### 4.3.1 Which AEDs, timing of samples

Total serum concentrations of phenytoin, carbamazepine, phenobarbitone, primidone, valproate and ethosuximide may be readily measured in most clinical biochemistry laboratories. Some centres also have assays for lamotrigine, vigabatrin, oxcarbazepine, benzodiazepines, gabapentin and the active metabolites 10,11-carbamazepine epoxide and 10,11-dihydro-10-hydroxy carbamazepine (DHC).

*Rapid assay service*

Rapid assays of serum AED concentrations are useful in clinics so that the patient may be seen with a current result. This facilitates interpretation of the data and appropriate action in the light of the current clinical situation. This is only feasible if the laboratory can provide immediate results, ideally with the facility in close physical proximity to the clinic. It is not an efficient use of resources to have serum AED concentrations measured in all patients on all visits. Some patients may be identified on their prior visit or on a preclinic notes review as needing an AED concentration measurement. Blood may then be taken on arrival and the patient can be seen with the result. Other patients may have their need for serum AED concentration assay identified at the time of consultation, have blood drawn and then be seen again, or have the result and action communicated by letter to the patient and family doctor. A rapid serum AED concentration assay service has been shown to be efficient and cost-effective in terms of the time taken to establish patients on optimal therapy, and the numbers of letters written (Patsalos et al 1987, Larkin et al 1990).

Rapid AED concentration assays are also useful in emergency situations, particularly in accident and emergency departments and intensive care units, for evaluation of patients who have taken an overdose or are in status epilepticus. If clinical biochemistry laboratories with 24 h rapid AED concentration assays are not available there are two alternatives being developed.

*Acculevel tests* employ enzyme immunochromatography and consist of a paper strip in a plastic cassette that is placed in a mixture of the patient's blood and reagent. These are available for phenytoin, carbamazepine and phenobarbitone. Results are available in 25 min and cost approximately £12, compared with £7 for a standard laboratory estimation.

*The biotrack device* is a photometric instrument that is extremely easy to use. A drop of blood, as from a fingerstick, is placed in a single-use cassette in the instrument. The result is available in 3 min. Analyses are currently available for phenytoin, carbamazepine and phenobarbitone, with a comparable cost to standard techniques.

*Optimal timing of samples*

In a non-emergency setting it is useful to standardize the timing of blood sampling and drug ingestion. In in-patients and early morning clinics this is easiest by taking trough levels, but this is generally not feasible for late morning or afternoon clinics. It is possible to standardize samples to peak levels, but these show greater variability. This is a particular issue with respect to carbamazepine and carbamazepine epoxide, which may show a 50% variation between peak and trough concentrations. Serum valproate concentrations vary markedly through the day and do not correlate well with therapeutic effect; standardized trough concentrations are needed to interpret changes in concentrations. For phenobarbitone and phenytoin, the longer half-life results in a smaller peak–trough concentration variation, so timing of samples is much less of an issue. At present there is little experience with the interpretation of serum concentrations of lamotrigine.

In the non-acute situation it is generally most helpful to assay serum AED concentrations when the patient has reached a stable steady-state after a change in therapy. A steady-state serum AED concentration is reached after five half-lives of the drug. This depends on the elimination half-life of the drug and the effect of the index drug and concomitant medication on hepatic enzyme induction. In practical terms, phenytoin has an average half-life of 30 h in an adult, so a steady-state will not be reached until 1 week after initiation of treatment or a change in dose, unless a loading dose has been used. Serum phenobarbitone concentrations will take about 3 weeks to reach a new steady-state, reflecting the average 96 h half-life of that drug in adults.

After commencement, or significant dose increase, of an enzyme-inducing drug it takes 2–3 weeks for hepatic enzyme induction to develop, which may lead to a lowering of serum drug concentrations over this time. In contrast, inhibition of hepatic enzymes occurs and resolves immediately following introduction and withdrawal of an enzyme inhibitor.

Carbamazepine shows the phenomenon of autoinduction, and serum concentrations may fall by 25% in the 34 weeks after starting the drug, necessitating a further dose increase (see below, 4.5.2). Lamotrigine is thought to show a degree of autoinduction but the clinical significance of this is presently uncertain. In general, serum concentrations of oxcarbazepine, its primary metabolite, DHC, valproate and ethosuximide are likely to represent the new steady-state 1 week after a change in dose.

Conversely, when an AED is withdrawn the new steady-state of serum concentrations of the remaining drugs is, for practical purposes, achieved 1 week after completion of tapering (Duncan et al 1991). Enzyme deinduction may not be complete for 2–3 weeks after stopping an inducing agent, but the residual effects are not of clinical significance. The exceptions are phenobarbitone and primidone. By virtue of the long elimination half-life of phenobarbitone, the new steady-state is not reached until 4 weeks after withdrawal.

## 4.3.2 Use and abuse of AED concentration measurements

The major indications for assaying serum AED concentrations may be summarized as:

- To check on compliance with prescribed therapy
- To determine whether symptoms or signs are likely or not to be dose-related adverse effects of prescribed therapy
- To guide dosing of the AEDs
- To monitor pharmacokinetic interactions
- To monitor patients who are acutely unwell, pregnant or planning to become pregnant, and those with mental handicap

*Compliance*

The measurement of serum AED concentrations may be a useful adjunct to patient counselling in assessment of compliance with prescribed therapy (see above, 4.2.5). Generally, a result will only determine whether AEDs have been taken in the preceding 2–3 days or not, and does not assess the long-term level of compliance. If a patient is expecting a measurement, he/she is more likely to take doses immediately prior to the visit. Accordingly, there is benefit from unexpected sampling at the time of a clinic visit, or by a primary health care worker. Interpretation of AED concentrations must be cautious, and it needs to be recognized that some patients are quick metabolizers and that trough levels of some AEDs, e.g. carbamazepine and valproate, will be much lower than peak levels.

Further information may be available from interpretation of concentrations of AEDs that have a primary metabolite, e.g. primidone, carbamazepine and oxcarbazepine. Inappropriately high ratios *for that patient* of primidone/phenobarbitone suggest the possibility that the patient was not normally compliant and took a larger dose on the day prior to sampling. Pilot work has been carried out on the measurement of AED concentrations in hair, and these levels may give an indication of compliance over prolonged periods.

*Is an AED causing symptoms and signs?*

Measurement of serum AED concentrations can help to decide whether a patient's symptoms or signs are likely or not to be dose-related adverse effects of AEDs. Drug concentrations are not diagnostically helpful in the assessment of possible idiosyncratic side-effects.

It is important to recognize the limitations of quoted therapeutic ranges. These ranges were defined on a small number of patients and the 'upper limit' is only an indication of a concentration above which dose-related adverse effects are more likely to be noted. There is no clear cut-off between toxic and non-toxic concentrations in the population, nor when applied to individual patients. For example, the commonly quoted top of the 'therapeutic range' for phenytoin is 80 μmol/l (20 μg/l) and if a patient with nystagmus and ataxia has a serum phenytoin concentration of 73 μmol/l it would be erroneous to discount phenytoin as the cause. Conversely, some patients tolerate phenytoin concentrations of 100–110 μmol/l without adverse effects and for them, these values are within the 'therapeutic range'.

It is more difficult to ascribe cause to symptoms if a patient is taking two or more AEDs. In that situation it is generally appropriate to reduce the dose of one AED and to then review the clinical situation and repeat the serum AED concentration measurement.

If serum concentrations are very low it is less likely that a patient's symptoms and signs are due to that medication, and it is necessary to look elsewhere for a cause. This is not an absolute rule and some patients, for example, may complain bitterly of headache and diplopia that is temporally related to taking carbamazepine even when serum concentrations are low. This is particularly likely to occur when the drug is commenced. The best approach is either to switch to another AED, if there is one that is likely to be equally effective, or to reduce the dose of the drug and to then build it up even more slowly.

*Serum AED concentrations as a guide to dosing*

The ready availability of serum concentrations of phenytoin is essential if that drug is to be used safely and effectively. This is because of the zero order kinetics of phenytoin metabolism, the great interpersonal variability in the rate of metabolism and the effect of other drugs on this. If phenytoin is being increased, knowledge of the serum concentration on a certain dose is necessary to guide the size of the next dose increment (see below, 4.5.11).

The serum concentration/dose response curves for carbamazepine, phenobarbitone, ethosuximide and DHC (the primary metabolite of oxcarbazepine) are approximately linear in the range of clinically used doses. Serum concentrations of these AEDs are of moderate use in guiding dosing of these drugs and determining whether serum drug concentrations are altering as expected in response to a change in dose. This may be a very useful means of identifying those patients who are rapid or slow metabolizers of AEDs. In general, serum concentrations do not contribute greatly to defining the optimal dose of a particular AED for individual patients, which is better determined by the clinical situation.

Serum concentrations of vigabatrin, valproate, clonazepam and primidone are generally of no utility in making decisions about dosing. The therapeutic effects of vigabatrin and valproate do not correlate well with their serum concentrations, and the latter are very variable. The role of measuring lamotrigine and gabapentin serum concentrations, other than as a check on recent compliance, is not yet defined. As a guide to dosing, the measurement of primidone is superfluous to the assay of phenobarbitone concentrations.

*Monitoring of pharmacokinetic interactions*

AEDs are subject to, and give rise to, many clinically significant pharmacokinetic interactions on the addition and withdrawal of another drug (Brodie 1992, Patsalos & Duncan 1993). The principal interactions between AEDs are summarized in Table 4.5. If a pharmacokinetic interaction is anticipated it is a good principle to check serum AED concentrations before another drug is withdrawn or commenced. This value then provides a baseline against which a further measurement after the intervention can be judged. Should there be an interaction of clinical significance, it is then relatively straightforward to predict the dose adjustment needed to restore the original concentration. However, a corrective dose adjustment is not always necessary in the event of pharmacokinetic interactions. This is only appropriate if there is a deleterious effect such as worsened seizure control or emergence of adverse effects.

*Routine 'prophylactic' monitoring*

The routine measurement of serum AED concentrations in patients whose epilepsy control and medication is stable and who are not experiencing adverse effects is not necessary. In the absence of any clinical concerns or changes in therapy there is no benefit to measuring AED concentrations more often than every 12–24 months. It is more useful to identify patients in whom there is a need to ascertain AED concentrations, as and when that occurs.

*Special categories of patient*

Patients who are acutely unwell, those who are pregnant and mentally and physically handicapped patients require special consideration.

*Patients who are acutely unwell*: Patients with epilepsy in intensive care units receiving multiple drug treatments, with risk of dysfunction of liver and/or kidneys, malabsorption and metabolic disturbance should have their serum AED concentrations measured every 24 h, or even more frequently if seizures are uncontrolled and loading doses of AEDs are required.

*Pregnancy*: Serum AED concentrations frequently fall during pregnancy, often as a result of a combination of factors including poor compliance, changes in absorption, increased metabolism by maternal and fetal liver, haemodilution and changes in clearance (Ch. 6, 6.3.6). It is advisable to determine, preconception, the AED concentration that gives the optimal seizure control and to repeat measurements every 1–3 months, according to circumstances. The merit of repeating assays is that it is then straightforward immediately to recommend an appropriate dose alteration without delay, should clinical need arise, such as an increase in seizures.

*Mental handicap*: Management of epilepsy is frequently more difficult in patients with mental handicap. It is often hard to assess compliance and seizure control is commonly very brittle. Further, the patients may be unable to report troublesome adverse effects such as dizziness and diplopia and it may not be possible reliably to identify signs of intoxication such as nystagmus and increased ataxia. In this setting it is reasonable, without ignoring clinical features that may be discerned, to place greater reliance on serum AED concentrations to check on compliance, guide dosing and avoid over-medication.

### 4.3.3 Limitations of the utility of 'therapeutic range' of AEDs

The concept of the therapeutic range, or target range, of serum concentrations of AEDs is often abused. The quoted ranges simply give an indication of the concentrations at which the majority of patients have optimal seizure control from that drug, and above which dose-related adverse effects are more likely. Zealous adherence to quoted ranges is inappropriate and AED concentration data should always be subordinate to, and interpreted in the light of, clinical data. Approximately 20% of patients attending our clinics have optimal seizure control with serum AED concentrations outside quoted ranges. Further, these ranges usually apply to trough concentrations and for some AEDs, such as carbamazepine, the peak concentrations may be considerably higher.

It is a reasonable rule of thumb that if a patient has no adverse effects from an AED the dose is not too high, and that if seizures are controlled the dose is high enough. Conversely, if the patient has adverse effects a reduction of dose should be considered and, if seizures continue, an increase should be entertained.

### 4.3.4 Salivary and 'free' serum AED concentrations

*Salivary AED concentrations*

AEDs enter saliva in a concentration that approximates to free, (i.e. non-protein-bound) serum concentrations. Saliva may be collected and AED concentrations assayed (Knott 1983). It is important to avoid contamination of the sample with medication that has remained in the mouth. This technique is a useful alternative for patients, particularly children, for whom venepuncture is difficult or traumatic. Obtaining a satisfactory sample requires a co-operative patient and some practice, however, and most patients generally find venepuncture quicker and more convenient.

*'Free' serum AED concentrations*

Varying proportions (10–50%) of total AED concentrations in serum are bound to plasma proteins (see below, 4.5 for individual AEDs). Laboratories usually measure the total (protein-bound and free) AED concentrations. The free drug may be separated by ultrafiltration and assayed. The measurement of free concentrations costs approximately twice as much as total concentration measurement and, because the amounts are 50–90% lower, the measurement inaccuracy is greater.

Measurement of free concentrations of AEDs is not indicated in routine clinical practice but may be useful in particular circumstances in which plasma protein binding may be affected, such as: co-prescription of other drugs that have a major effect on binding of AEDs to plasma proteins; hypoalbuminaemia, as after severe burns; in liver and renal disease; and in pregnancy.

## 4.4 ANTIEPILEPTIC DRUGS FOR DIFFERENT SEIZURE TYPES AND SYNDROMES

### 4.4.1 Partial and secondarily generalized seizures

Table 4.3 summarizes these data. For the purposes of selecting an AED, simple partial, complex partial and secondarily generalized seizures may be regarded together and there is no evidence that AEDs have differential efficacy against partial seizures arising from different parts of the brain or caused by different aetiologies.

Many comparative studies have not shown significantly different efficacy among barbiturates, carbamazepine, phenytoin and valproate (Turnbull et al 1982, Callaghan et al 1985, Mattson et al 1985, Heller et al 1995). In a recent Veterans' Administration study, carbamazepine showed some benefits over valproate in the treatment of complex partial seizures, but no difference against secondarily generalized seizures, and had fewer long-term side-effects (Mattson et al 1992). The choice of AED is determined more by known adverse effects, individual patient factors, pharmacokinetics, experience of use and cost. The studies from King's

College Hospital (Heller et al 1995) and the first Veterans' Administration study (Mattson et al 1985) showed that barbiturates resulted in more adverse effects than did the other AEDs.

Carbamazepine would generally be favoured over phenytoin because of the latter's adverse dental, cosmetic and greater cognitive effects (see also Ch. 9, 9.5.1). A potential advantage of phenytoin is that once a day medication is usually possible, making supervision of administration and compliance as easy as possible. Valproate has the advantage of not inducing hepatic enzymes, and so of not causing a pharmacokinetic interaction with the oral contraceptive pill, but does give rise to greater concern about neural tube defects if taken during pregnancy (Ch. 6 6.3.3). Phenobarbitone is no longer regarded as a first-line drug in most developed countries because of its adverse cognitive and behavioural effects. As an AED, primidone has nothing to commend it over phenobarbitone (Duncan 1990).

Vigabatrin, lamotrigine and gabapentin are recently developed AEDs and currently licensed, in most countries, for refractory seizures only. Comparative monotherapy studies in newly diagnosed patients are in progress. In 1995 lamotrigine was approved for use as monotherapy in several countries and it is likely that vigabatrin and gabapentin will be approved for use as first-line drugs in the next 5 years. At present, many neurologists consider it reasonable to regard vigabatrin as a second-line drug for partial seizures in preference to phenytoin, unless there is a significant psychiatric or conduct disorder. The sequence of second-line AEDs to employ, however, is controversial and there is no uniform consensus, even among the authors of this book.

*Combination AED therapy for partial seizures*

There is no good scientific evidence on which to make logical decisions about which combinations are likely to be most effective (see above, 4.2.4). Practice has been largely determined by fashion, such as that for phenytoin and phenobarbitone in the past, and more recently for carbamazepine and vigabatrin. There have also been recent anecdotal reports of benefit from combining vigabatrin and lamotrigine, but there have not been any controlled studies to evaluate this. There is a theoretical argument that a combination of two AEDs that have differing modes of action, rather than two agents that act in similar ways, is more likely to be beneficial. There have not, however, been any satisfactory scientific studies to guide practice. A reasonable approach at present is to try the most effective first-line AED and to add a second-line agent or to combine two first-line AEDs for that patient's seizure types.

## 4.4.2 Generalized seizures

*Tonic-clonic, clonic*

Valproate is the drug of choice if absences or myoclonic seizures co-exist, as in the syndromes of idiopathic generalized epilepsy (Ch. 2, 2.7). Carbamazepine and phenytoin are alternatives. Clobazam may be useful and phenobarbitone still has a role in the refractory case. The role of vigabatrin, lamotrigine and gabapentin in this seizure type is not yet clear. If vigabatrin is used the possibility of worsening co-existent absences and myoclonic seizures should be borne in mind.

*Typical absences*

The typical absences found in some forms of idiopathic generalized epilepsy, e.g. childhood absence epilepsy, respond equally well to etho-suximide and valproate (Bourgeois 1995). A point in favour of etho-suximide is the concern about severe valproate-related hepatic reactions. It is important to consider the epilepsy syndrome and not just the seizure type (Duncan 1995). An advantage of valproate is that it is also effective against tonic-clonic and myoclonic seizures, which may also affect the patient. 30% of patients with juvenile myoclonic epilepsy have absences as their first seizure type, subsequently developing myoclonic jerks and then tonic-clonic seizures (Grunewald et al 1992), and overall 30% of children presenting with typical absences will subsequently develop tonic-clonic and/or myoclonic seizures. If valproate or etho-suximide do not provide adequate control of absences it is appropriate to try the other, and then the two agents in combination (Sato et al 1982, Rowan et al 1983). Some subtypes of idiopathic generalized epilepsy, for example, eyelid myoclonia with typical absences (Appleton et al 1993), appear to respond poorly to valproate or ethosuximide in isolation but well to the combination.

Second-line medications for intractable absences include clonazepam, acetazolamide and lamotrigine. There is, however, a dearth of good clinical studies of the effect of these drugs on absences (Gram 1995). The use of the first two is often complicated by the development of tolerance, and clonazepam use is frequently limited by drowsiness. There is anecdotal experience of lamotrigine benefiting otherwise intractable absences, especially when given with valproate (Timmings & Richens 1992, Panayiotopoulos et al 1993). Gabapentin appears to be ineffective against absences (Chadwick 1995) and vigabatrin in liable to exacerbate the occurrence of absences.

*Atypical absences, atonic, tonic*

These types of seizure are often very refractory to AEDs. Valproate is appropriate as an initial choice, followed by a benzodiazepine such as clonazepam. Uncontrolled observations have suggested that lamotrigine may be extremely useful against this group of seizures, particularly when used in combination with valproate (Sander et al 1991a). Felbamate has been reported to be useful in a recent study (Felbamate Study Group in Lennox–Gastaut Syndrome 1993) (see below, 4.5.6 for details of the current status of felbamate). Barbiturates are worthy of consideration if other AEDs have not helped, as are carbamazepine and phenytoin for tonic and atonic seizures, although atypical absences may be exacerbated.

*Myoclonic*

Myoclonic seizures may occur in a variety of epileptic syndromes (Ch. 2). Myoclonic seizures that occur in the setting of idiopathic generalized epilepsy, e.g. juvenile myoclonic epilepsy, generally respond very well to valproate (Grunewald et al 1992). Myoclonic seizures that occur in association with progressive myoclonic epilepsy, severe myoclonic epilepsy and Lennox–Gastaut syndrome are more resistant to treatment. If myoclonic seizures continue on a maximum dose of valproate the addition of a benzodiazepine, such as clonazepam, is appropriate (Browne 1978, Mireles & Leppik 1985). Principal limitations are sedation and development of tolerance. Piracetam is effective against myoclonic seizures, the main limitation to use being the bulk of the dose the patient is required to take (Brown et al 1993). A reasonable strategy for treating myoclonic seizures is to start with valproate, add clonazepam if necessary, and then add piracetam if troublesome seizures continue.

Barbiturates have antimyoclonic activity, but adverse effects generally limit their use to patients with severe and refractory myoclonic seizures. Acetazolamide may be a useful therapy for myoclonic seizures (Resor & Resor 1990). The role of lamotrigine is uncertain and not yet established. Vigabatrin may exacerbate myoclonic seizures and should be avoided in these patients. A developmental drug, zonisamide, has been reported to be effective against myoclonic seizures (Henry et al 1988), but its position is not established.

### 4.4.3 Particular syndromes

*Neonatal seizures*

Drug therapy should be in concert with treating any correctable disorder, such as hypoglycaemia, hypocalcaemia, hypoxia, acidosis, meningitis or pyridoxine dependency. Pyridoxine dependency responds rapidly to 100 mg of intravenous pyridoxine and this needs to be continued orally.

Phenobarbitone is regarded as the drug of choice for seizures occurring in the neonatal period, particularly in cases of hypoxic–ischaemic encephalopathy. Parenteral administration is recommended in sick infants, to ensure bioavailability. A loading dose of 15–20 mg/kg and daily maintenance doses of 2–4 mg/kg usually give plasma concentrations of the order of 100 μmol/l. Plasma concentrations need to be measured frequently as the rate of metabolism is very variable and alters with age, being slow in neonates (half-life of up to 140 h), and then accelerating. Respiratory depression and sedation are common dose-related side-effects. If phenobarbitone does not control seizures adequately, phenytoin at a loading dose of 15–20 mg/kg and daily maintenance doses of 2–4 mg/kg are appropriate. Clobazam and clonazepam may also be useful. Experience with carbamazepine, sodium valproate and the newer AEDs is very limited in the neonatal period.

*Infantile spasms*

Therapy should be directed against the underlying cause when this is possible (e.g. infection, hypoglycaemia, metabolic and endocrine disorders). Infantile spasms do not respond to phenytoin, carbamazepine or phenobarbitone and poor results have been reported with valproate. ACTH has been used since the 1950s. An average dose is 20–40 IU/d initially (150 U/m$^2$/d in two divided doses), reducing over subsequent weeks. Therapy is usually continued for 5–8 weeks. Higher steroid doses may be required for resistant spasms in some children, and may need to be continued for 4–6 months). Prednisolone 2–3 mg/kg/d has been suggested as an alternative, but there is doubt as to whether this is as effective. The prognosis of patients with infantile spasms is not good, particularly if there is a history of antecedent neurological or developmental deficit. Nevertheless, there is good evidence that, if infantile spasms occur in the setting of normal neurological development, control of spasms by ACTH improves the chance of a good outcome. Careful attention needs to be paid to the possible development of adverse effects from steroids (Kellaway et al 1983, Velez et al 1990, Snead 1990).

Clonazepam and nitrazepam may be effective, but adverse effects and development of tolerance are often problematic (Schmidt 1983). Experience with vigabatrin is limited, but early reports are encouraging and some advocate vigabatrin as a first-line treatment for infantile spasms. (Chiron et al 1990, Appleton & Montiel-Viesca 1993). Resective neurosurgery can be considered in refractory cases in whom focal lesions are demonstrable (Chugani et al 1990) (see also Ch. 10).

*Febrile convulsions*

The mainstays of treatment are antipyretics, and prophylactic rectal diazepam in patients with a prior history of febrile convulsions: 5 mg if the child is under 3 years and 7.5 mg if older than this, in the event of a fever in excess of 38.5°C repeated after 12 h if necessary (see above, 4.1.3). Prophylactic sodium valproate and phenobarbitone have been shown to reduce the recurrence rate of febrile convulsions. Phenobarbitone, however, has been associated with a high risk of behaviour disturbance (Wolf & Forsythe 1978) and valproate with a significant risk of hepatotoxicity in young children (Dreifuss et al 1989). In consequence, it is not surprising that compliance with prolonged therapy is generally poor (McKinlay & Newton 1989). The adverse effects of these therapies in young children are generally felt to outweigh the benefits, but they may be useful if rectal diazepam has failed to be effective or administration proves impossible.

In the acute situation of a continuing febrile convulsion, diazepam 0.2–0.3 mg/kg should be given intravenously or as the rectal solution, with a careful watch kept on the patient for the development of cardiorespiratory depression (see Ch. 5, 5.3 for further details on the treatment of status epilepticus).

*Lennox–Gastaut syndrome*

Patients with the Lennox–Gastaut syndrome often respond poorly to treatment and it is important to recognize the limits of drug efficacy and to avoid intoxication. They frequently have a combination of different seizure types (Ch. 2, 2.6.8) and optimal seizure control may require treatment with a combinations of AEDs. Valproate and benzodiazepines (clobazam or clonazepam) may help myoclonic and atonic seizures. Benefit has been noted from lamotrigine in combination with valproate in this setting (Panayiotopoulos et al 1993). Felbamate has been reported to be useful against atonic seizures and atypical absences (Felbamate Study Group in Lennox–Gastaut Syndrome 1993), but the future use of this agent is currently in question. Carbamazepine and vigabatrin can have a useful action against partial and secondarily generalized seizures, but may exacerbate atypical absences, atonic and myoclonic seizures (see below, 4.5.2, 4.5.15).

Prednisolone and ACTH have been used, but are associated with a high incidence of adverse effects and only a short-lived benefit. A ketogenic diet (see below, 4.7.4) helps some children, but is generally poorly tolerated and the response is unpredictable.

*Electrical status epilepticus during slow wave sleep (ESES) and acquired epileptic aphasia (Landau–Kleffner syndrome)*

The electrographic status in these conditions does not usually require urgent therapy. It is uncertain to what extent it is worthwhile attempting to abolish the abnormal electrical activity by oral AEDs. Clonazepam or valproate therapy are usually tried initially (Yasuhara et al 1991), and ACTH and steroids have been given. In the Landau--Kleffner syndrome, there have been reports of benefit from immunosuppressant and corticosteroid therapy (Lerman et al 1991). There is, however, a lack of sound evidence on which to base rational management decisions.

## 4.5 THE INDIVIDUAL ANTIEPILEPTIC DRUGS

In this section licensed individual AEDs are considered in alphabetical order, followed by promising developmental agents. For further details about the AEDs discussed in this section the reader is referred to Levy et al 1995. Data on principal indications, starting and average maintenance doses, and pharmacokinetic interactions are summarized in Tables 4.3–4.5.

### 4.5.1 Acetazolamide

(Resor et al 1995)

*Action*

Acetazolamide inhibits carbonic anhydrase in glia and myelin, resulting in accumulation of $CO_2$ in the brain, and this appears to be the mechanism of the antiepileptic effect. The effects on neurotransmitters are uncertain. Tolerance often develops, and this is in parallel to increased synthesis and activation of carbonic anhydrase in glia.

*Indications*

Acetazolamide can have a marked effect against partial, secondary generalized, tonic-clonic, absence and myoclonic seizures, when used as an adjunct to a first-line drug. In view of the frequent development of tolerance, short-term treatment, for example in catamenial exacerbations of seizures, may be useful.

*Dosing and pharmacokinetics*

Acetazolamide is rapidly absorbed from the gastrointestinal tract. Excretion is renal and the elimination half-life is about 12 h. The usual adult starting dose is 250 mg a day, increasing up to 750 mg twice daily. Higher doses inhibit red blood cell carbonic anhydrase and result in increased toxicity without increased efficacy.

*Drug interactions*

Clinically significant pharmacokinetic interactions with other AEDs do not usually occur, although some elevation of concomitant carbamazepine concentrations may occur.

*Adverse effects*

While acetazolamide is generally well tolerated, tingling in the extremities, sedation, alteration of taste and nausea may occur. Allergic skin rashes occur rarely. Some patients treated with acetazolamide have an increased tendency to develop renal calculi.

## 4.5.2 Carbamazepine

*Action*

The principal antiepileptic action of carbamazepine is by stabilization of neuronal membranes pre- and postsynaptically by use and frequency-dependent blockade of sodium channels. Blockade of NMDA-receptor-activated sodium and calcium flux may also be contributory.

*Indications*

Carbamazepine is a drug of first choice in tonic-clonic, tonic, clonic, partial and secondarily generalized seizures, and may be of benefit in all other types except absences and myoclonic seizures. Myoclonic, atypical absence and atonic seizures may actually worsen with carbamazepine therapy (Shields & Saslow 1983, Johnsen et al 1984, Snead & Hosey 1985).

In patients with idiopathic generalized epilepsy, who frequently have co-existent myoclonic seizures and absences, valproate is clearly preferred. In a population of patients the efficacy of carbamazepine against partial seizures is equivalent to that of phenytoin and valproate (Troupin et al 1977, Turnbull et al 1982, Ramsay et al 1983, Callaghan et al 1985, Mattson et al 1985, Richens et al 1994, Verity et al 1995, Heller et al 1995). One study showed superiority of carbamazepine over valproate on some measures of control of complex partial seizures and adverse effects (Mattson et al 1992). Tolerance to the antiepileptic effect does not usually develop.

Carbamazepine has been claimed to have positive psychotropic effects in its own right (Post 1982), in addition to beneficial psychological effects by virtue of improved seizure control and substitution for AEDs with more side-effects. This argues in favour of using carbamazepine in patients with psychopathology.

*Pharmacokinetics and dosing*

Absorption from the gastrointestinal tract is slow and variable. Peak concentrations usually develop at 4–8 h, but may not occur until as late as 24 h. Administration with food may result in faster absorption. Absorption is fast in neonates, with peak concentrations at 3–6 h. The bioavailability of the slow-release formulation Tegretol Retard is about 85–90% of the regular preparation. Carbamazepine is poorly soluble in water and no parenteral formulation is available. 75–80% is protein-bound in plasma. Concentations in cerebrospinal fluid and saliva are similar to the free plasma concentrations.

Carbamazepine is metabolized in the liver and less than 1% is excreted unchanged. The elimination half-life on starting treatment is 20–50 h, shortening to 6–30 h after hepatic enzyme autoinduction has developed, which takes 3–4 weeks if no other enzyme-inducing drugs are being taken and probably less if the patient's liver enzymes are already induced. Clearance is more rapid in infants and children. The principal metabolite, carbamazepine epoxide, contributes to efficacy and adverse effects, having a total plasma concentration of the order of 20–50% of that of the parent carbamazepine and, as it is only about 45% protein-bound, is proportionately more biologically active than carbamazepine.

Carbamazepine should, if possible, be introduced at very low doses and built up over many weeks as autoinduction and tolerance develop. This is particularly important if the patient is not already taking enzyme-inducing medication and minimizes the risk of acute dose-related adverse effects. Rapid introduction is less likely to be tolerated. For an adult, 100 mg at night is a reasonable starting dose. When changing doses, increments and decrements of 200 mg are generally appropriate for adult patients, with changes made every 7–14 days in outpatients.

Few adults can tolerate more than 400 mg of the regular release preparation of carbamazepine at a single dose, with the consequence that, if large doses of carbamazepine are needed, this will have to be divided into three or four doses, which strains compliance (see above, 4.2.5). The slow release formulation is to be preferred, particularly if large doses of carbamazepine are needed, as peak concentrations are minimized and twice daily dosing is feasible (Kramer et al 1985, McKee et al 1991). As the bioavailability of the slow-release formulation is less than preparations of ordinary carbamazepine a higher dose of the latter needs to be prescribed and it is useful to check trough serum concentrations of carbamazepine when changing to this formulation. Many adults tolerate 800–1000 mg twice a day of slow-release carbamazepine, and children 10–30 mg/kg/d. Dose-related adverse effects are more likely to occur at serum concentrations in excess of 50 μmol/l, but many patients can tolerate higher levels than this, with beneficial effects on seizure control.

*Drug interactions*

A number of clinically important pharmacokinetic interactions may occur (Duncan et al 1991, Brodie 1992, Patsalos & Duncan 1993) (Table 4.5).

*Effects of other drugs on carbamazepine*: Phenytoin and barbiturates induce the metabolism of carbamazepine to carbamazepine epoxide, resulting in lower carbamazepine concentrations with little change in epoxide levels. Felbamate results in lower carbamazepine levels with elevation of the epoxide. Valproate usually has little effect on carbamazepine itself but inhibits onward metabolism of the epoxide, raising concentrations. Lamotrigine may result in symptoms suggestive of carbamazepine intoxication if it is added to a maximally tolerated dose of carbamazepine. It was noted in one study that lamotrigine appears to inhibit metabolism of the epoxide (Warner et al 1992), but this has not been a universal finding.

Cimetidine, verapamil, diltiazem, propoxyphene, nafimidone, viloxazine, isoniazid and erythromycin all inhibit carbamazepine metabolism and may precipitate intoxication.

*Effects of carbamazepine on other drugs*: Carbamazepine induces hepatic enzymes and reduces plasma concentrations of valproate, ethosuximide, benzodiazepines, felbamate, haloperidol, oral contraceptives, theophylline, steroids and warfarin. The interaction with phenytoin is complex as carbamazepine is also an inhibitor of phenytoin metabolism and if a patient already has a phenytoin concentration that approaches enzyme saturation, phenytoin intoxication may develop if carbamazepine is added.

*Acute adverse effects*

Common, predictable dose-related symptoms include blurring of vision, diplopia, sedation, nausea, anorexia, dizziness, ataxia and headache. These symptoms frequently show a diurnal variation, coinciding with peak serum concentrations, although this pattern may be less obvious when the slow-release formulation is used. Acute adverse effects are most common in the first days and weeks after initiation of therapy and can be largely avoided by introducing the drug slowly over several weeks.

*Idiosyncratic adverse effects*

About 5% of patients develop a skin rash. This may be serious, resulting in an exfoliative dermatitis or Stevens–Johnson syndrome. Other serious adverse events, including hepatic failure and severe bone marrow depression, are extremely uncommon. The incidence of agranulocytosis has been estimated at 2/100 000 treatment years, and for aplastic anaemia 0.7/100 000 treatment years, compared with background risks of 0.47 and 0.2/100 000 treatment years respectively. There is no evidence that routine monitoring of blood counts is useful for anticipating this problem. A mild leucopenia, however, occurs in about 10% of patients, is usually transient and is not clearly dose-related. Generally a white count above $2 \times 10^9$/l, and a neutrophil count above $1 \times 10^9$/l, and platelet count over $100 \times 10^9$/l are acceptable. If a total white cell count of less than $3 \times 10^9$/l or a platelet count under $125 \times 10^9$/l is found, the full blood count should be monitored to ensure that there is not a progressive fall of the white count or platelets.

*Chronic adverse effects*

Carbamazepine results in some motor slowing and appears to have fewer adverse cognitive effects than barbiturates and phenytoin (Thompson & Trimble 1982, Duncan et al 1990b).

Hyponatraemia and water retention are not uncommon. The mechanism appears to be by stimulation of antidiuretic hormone release and potentiation of its action on the kidney. Carbamazepine-related hyponatraemia does not affect all patients and is dose-related, and serum sodium concentrations of 120–130 mmol/l are not unusual. If this is asymptomatic, no action needs to be taken. If, however, oedema, headache, confusion or an increase in seizures occur, electrolytes should be measured and the dose of carbamazepine reduced. Hepatic enzyme induction may result in reduced sex hormone concentrations. Inhibition of haem biosynthesis may result in a clinical picture that resembles acute porphyria (Ch. 3, 3.7.4).

Atrio-ventricular conduction block may occur, particularly in the elderly. An electrocardiogram should be obtained before prescribing carbamazepine to such patients and the drug should be avoided if there is evidence of heart block. If a patient develops syncopal attacks while taking carbamazepine the possibility of carbamazepine-induced heart block should be considered and an electrocardiogram carried out.

## 4.5.3 Clobazam

(Shorvon 1995)

*Action*

Clobazam, a 1,5-benzodiazepine, binds to alpha subunits of the pentameric $GABA_A$ receptor complex and enhances the inhibitory effects of GABA on the post-synaptic membrane. As with other benzodiazepines, the development of tolerance is often a problem, resulting in loss of efficacy and difficult withdrawal.

*Indications*

This is as an adjunctive second-line drug for the treatment of partial, secondary generalized, tonic, clonic, atonic and atypical absence seizures. Some good results have been reported in patients with the Lennox–Gastaut syndrome. Up to 50% of patients with partial and secondarily generalized seizures have a 50% or more reduction in seizures and 10–20% become seizure-free. Different studies have reported that in 40–77% of patients who have a useful therapeutic effect from clobazam there is loss of efficacy, with the development of tolerance over weeks or months. However, about 10–30% of patients commenced on clobazam derive significant and sustained benefit from it. If seizures recur after an initial beneficial effect, there is usually little benefit from increasing the dose and it is best to withdraw the medication. Clobazam is often particularly useful as a short-term treatment, either prophylactically over special occasions such as a wedding or during anticipated times of high risk such as menses in women with catamenial exacerbation of seizures (Ch. 6, 6.1), and is also useful in response to spontaneous clusters of seizures.

*Dosing and pharmacokinetics*

Clobazam is well absorbed from the gastrointestinal tract, with peak plasma levels in 1–4 h. Clobazam is 85% protein-bound in plasma and the elimination half-life is about 18 h. Metabolism is to the less potent *N*-desmethylclobazam, which has a half-life of about 40 h. As a result the steady-state plasma levels of *N*-desmethylclobazam are usually about 10 times that of clobazam. For adults 10 mg clobazam at night, increasing as tolerated to 30 mg/d would be usual, given as a single or two daily doses. When used in response to a cluster of seizures, 10 mg twice a day for 3 days is generally suitable. When tapering clobazam that has been taken continuously for months or more, reductions of 10 mg per week are satisfactory for most patients. Apart from increased seizures, withdrawal symptoms include insomnia, anxiety, agitation, sweating, tremor and nausea (Duncan 1988). If there is a marked increase in seizures on tapering at this rate, a subsequent attempt could be made with reductions of 5 mg every 2 weeks.

*Drug interactions*

Clinically significant interactions are not common. Some studies have found the addition of clobazam to increase the plasma concentrations of other AEDs. The metabolism of clobazam is increased by the concomitant administration of enzyme-inducing AEDs, but this is not usually clinically significant. There have been reports of elevation of valproate, carbamazepine, phenytoin and phenobarbitone concentrations on co-administration of clobazam, but these are rarely of clinical significance.

*Acute adverse effects*

It has been suggested that sedation, impairment of memory and psychomotor retardation are less of a problem with clobazam than with the 1, 4-benzodiazepines. Other acute dose-related adverse effects include dizziness, nystagmus, ataxia, headache, depression, aggression and irritability. These may lessen with the development of tolerance.

*Idiosyncratic adverse effects*

Allergic reactions are very rare.

*Chronic adverse effects*

Behaviour disturbance, sedation and psychomotor retardation may develop.

## 4.5.4 Clonazepam

*Action*

Clonazepam is a 1,4-benzodiazepine and a potent agonist at the alpha subunit of the $GABA_A$ receptor complex.

*Indications*

Myoclonic seizures that do not respond to valproate, or in patients who are intolerant of valproate, are the prime indication for clonazepam (Browne 1978). It may also be used as a second-line drug against intractable absences and atonic seizures and markedly reduces photosensitivity. Efficacy against tonic-clonic seizures is controversial. Some good effects have been reported in patients with the Lennox–Gastaut syndrome. Parenteral clonazepam is useful in status epilepticus (Sato & Malow 1995) (Ch. 5, 5.3).

*Dosing and pharmacokinetics*

Clonazepam is rapidly absorbed from the gastrointestinal tract, with peak plasma concentrations in 1–4 h and metabolism to inactive derivatives, with an elimination half-life of 20–60 h. 85% is protein-bound and clonazepam does not induce liver enzymes. Once-daily dosing is feasible for most patients. As tolerance frequently develops, measurement of plasma concentrations as a guide to dosing or causation of adverse effects is not helpful. Tolerance to the antiepileptic effect often occurs without the development of tolerance to the adverse effects.

Starting at a low dose, e.g. 0.5 mg/d for an adult, and increasing in 0.5 mg steps every 1–2 weeks as tolerated reduces the risk of acute adverse effects. The usual adult dose range is 2–8 mg/d. Withdrawal of chronic clonazepam therapy should be slow and gradual, and may not be possible because of increased seizures and other symptoms of benzodiazepine withdrawal (Duncan 1988). Abrupt cessation carries a significant risk of a marked deterioration in seizure control. A reduction rate of 1 mg per week is possible in about 70% of adult patients. If this fails, a further attempt at a rate of 0.5 mg per fortnight is worth trying (Chataway et al 1993).

*Drug interactions*

Enzyme-inducing AEDs increase the metabolism of clonazepam, resulting in lower plasma concentrations. There may be a synergistic pharmacodynamic interaction with barbiturates, resulting in marked sedation.

*Adverse effects*

These are qualitatively similar to those of clobazam (see above), but clonazepam is thought to cause greater sedation, motor retardation, ataxia, memory impairment and behavioural disturbance and to cause more problems with tolerance and dependence.

Acute administration of clonazepam may result in cardiorespiratory depression, particularly if combined with other depressants such as alcohol or barbiturates. There have been reports of the co-administration of clonazepam and valproate being associated with the occasional development of absence status, but this combination is frequently of benefit against absences and myoclonic seizures.

## 4.5.5 Ethosuximide

(Sherwin 1995)

*Action*

Ethosuximide inhibits low-threshold calcium currents in the thalamus that are thought to underlie the generation of generalized spike-wave discharges (Coulter et al 1989), and reduces excitatory transmitter release.

*Indications*

In a population of patients, typical absence seizures respond to ethosuximide as well as they do to valproate. Valproate is preferred if the patient also has myoclonic jerks and/or tonic-clonic seizures. A combination of valproate and ethosuximide is indicated if either provides inadequate seizure control when given alone. A combination is often particularly helpful for patients with eyelid myoclonia and typical absences and those with myoclonic absences.

*Dosing and pharmacokinetics*

Peak plasma levels occur 1–4 h after ingestion and absorption from the gastrointestinal tract is complete. Excretion is mainly by hepatic metabolism and about 20% is excreted unchanged in the urine. Although the elimination half-life of 20–40 h in children and 40–70 h in adults suggests that once-daily administration should be feasible, gastrointestinal intolerance of large doses results in twice-daily dosing being preferred for most patients. Steady-state plasma concentrations are achieved in 6 days in children and in 12 days in adults. For an adult, 250 mg at night, increasing in 250 mg steps up to 750 mg twice a day, as tolerated. For children, maintenance doses are 10–30 mg/kg/d. In most patients optimal control of absences is achieved with plasma concentrations of 200–800 μmol/l. When discontinuing the drug in patients with active absences, tapering over 2–3 weeks is reasonable.

*Drug interactions*

Ethosuximide does not have clinically significant effects on other medications. Enzyme-inducing drugs hasten metabolism of ethosuximide and result in lower concentrations. Valproate may cause significant inhibition of ethosuximide metabolism and increased plasma concentrations.

*Acute adverse effects*

Nausea, abdominal discomfort, hiccough, sedation, headache and ataxia all occur if doses are excessive and usually respond to dose reduction.

*Idiosyncratic adverse effects* Allergic skin rashes occur in up to 5% of patients. Immunologically mediated adverse effects including a systemic-lupus-erythematosis-like syndrome, pericarditis, myocarditis and thyroiditis may occur. Significant blood dyscrasias are very rare, but a mild leucopenia is a common occurrence. Bradykinesia and parkinsonism have been reported.

*Other adverse effects* Behaviour disturbance, depression, confusion, irritability, aggression, anxiety, cognitive impairment and psychotic symptoms have been reported within weeks or months of commencing ethosuximide. Although the causal relationship of these symptoms to ethosuximide is often unclear, the drug should be used with caution in patients with a history of psychiatric disturbance.

## 4.5.6 Felbamate

*Action* Felbamate is structurally similar to meprobamate. Its mode of action is not certain. A current hypothesis is that it has an inhibitory action at the NMDA receptor and a facilitatory effect at the $GABA_A$ receptor (Rho et al 1994).

*Indications* Experience with this drug is limited (Brodie 1993). A licence was issued in the United States in 1993. A European Union product licence was granted in 1994, and implementation was under consideration by member States. Later in 1994, however, the prescription of felbamate was suspended after the reporting of several cases of aplastic anaemia and of hepatic failure in patients taking the drug and, at present, its long-term future is uncertain.

Five clinical trials have shown efficacy against partial and secondarily generalized seizures (Leppik et al 1991, Theodore et al 1991, Sachdeo et al 1992, Bourgeois et al 1993, Faught et al 1993). A further study has shown benefit against atonic seizures and atypical absences in children with Lennox–Gastaut syndrome (Felbamate Study Group in Lennox–Gastaut Syndrome 1993). Open studies for more than 6 months do not suggest that the development of tolerance is a problem. If felbamate is reinstated, the indications for its use are likely to be as a second-line drug for partial and secondarily generalized seizures and for the Lennox–Gastaut syndrome.

*Dosing and pharmacokinetics* Absorption from the gastrointestinal tract is good. 40% of the administered drug is metabolized in the liver to inactive metabolites and the drug is renally excreted. The elimination half-life is 15–23 h. Children should be started on 15 mg/kg/d in divided doses, and adults on 600 mg twice daily, with increments of 600–1200 mg/d at weekly intervals. Doses of up to 3600 mg/d have been used, divided into three to four doses in clinical trials. Twice-daily dosing should be feasible. The measurement of felbamate plasma concentrations does not appear to be a useful guide to dosing.

*Drug interactions* *Effect of other drugs on felbamate:* Enzyme-inducing drugs, such as carbamazepine and phenytoin, result in enhanced metabolism of felbamate and lower felbamate concentrations by approximately 30%. Valproate does not appear to have a significant effect.

*Effect of felbamate on other drugs*: Phenytoin and valproate concentrations rise by an average of 30%. There is a similar rise in phenobarbitone concentrations. Carbamazepine concentrations fall by a similar degree, with a concomitant 50% rise in carbamazepine epoxide. In consequence of these pharmacokinetic interactions, the doses of phenytoin, carbamazepine, valproate and barbiturates should be reduced by 10–30% on initiation of felbamate therapy, with further reductions of a similar magnitude when the dose of felbamate is increased to 2400 mg. Patients need to be followed closely if felbamate is being added to or withdrawn from treatment with other AEDs and monitoring AED concentrations will assist decisions to make optimal dose adjustments.

The effect of felbamate on oral contraceptives, anticoagulants and steroids is unknown at present.

*Adverse effects*

Experience currently extends to about 150 000 patients. Dose-related symptoms include insomnia, nausea, anorexia, weight loss, headache, sedation, ataxia and dizziness. In patients receiving other AEDs, the possibility that the adverse effects are the result of elevated serum concentrations of these agents needs to be borne in mind. Insomnia, anorexia and weight loss appear to be adverse effects that are specifically related to felbamate.

Hypersensitivity reactions have been noted in approximately 3%, typically 2–3 weeks after starting treatment. Features include rash, fever, myalgia, pharyngitis, arthralgia, leucopenia, thrombocytopenia and elevated liver enzymes. Adverse psychiatric effects are rare, although aggression, depression and paranoia have been reported. By November 1994, however, 20 cases of aplastic anaemia had been reported in patients who had received felbamate for up to 7 months, and there had also been several reports of liver failure. Preliminary analysis indicates that the level of risk is about 50 times the baseline incidence of aplastic anaemia. In consequence the prescription of felbamate has been restricted in Europe and has a restricted use in the United States, pending further investigation, and the long-term future of the drug is uncertain.

## 4.5.7 Gabapentin

*Action*

Although gabapentin was designed as a structural analogue of GABA, the drug does not bind to GABA receptors. Gabapentin does, however, bind to specific cerebral sites that have not yet been characterized, and the mode of action is unclear.

*Indications*

Double-blind studies have shown efficacy against refractory partial and secondarily generalized seizures, with a > 50% seizure reduction in 13–29% of patients (Crawford et al 1987, UK Gabapentin Study Group 1990, Bruni et al 1991, Oommen et al 1993). Open follow-up studies have not suggested a loss of efficacy over 12–18 months. Gabapentin appears to have little efficacy against absences and primary generalized tonic-clonic seizures (Chadwick 1995). Monotherapy studies comparing gabapentin to established AEDs are in progress. At this time gabapentin is a second-line agent for refractory partial and secondarily generalized seizures.

*Dosing and pharmacokinetics*

Gabapentin is rapidly absorbed, with a peak plasma concentration in 2–3 h, is not protein-bound and is excreted unchanged, 80% in the urine. The elimination half-life is 5–7 h if renal function is normal. Thrice-daily dosing is currently felt to be necessary. If evidence of a prolonged pharmacodynamic effect emerges, twice-daily administration may be feasible.

The recommended starting dose is 300 mg once on the first day, twice on the second day and thrice daily on the third day, increasing to 400 mg thrice daily. In our experience, however, introducing the drug so rapidly is often not tolerated by patients and 300 mg increments at weekly rather than daily intervals is more suitable. Subsequent dose adjustments may be made, in 300 mg increments, up to 800 mg thrice daily. Withdrawal of gabapentin should be over a minimum of 1 week.

*Drug interactions*

No clinically significant interactions have been noted between gabapentin and other AEDs.

*Adverse effects*

Predictable dose-related adverse effects include diplopia, nystagmus, dizziness, tremor and sedation. Some patients have a paradoxical increase in seizures, particularly myoclonic jerks. Serious idiosyncratic adverse effects, hypersensitivity reactions and chronic adverse effects have not been identified, although experience is necessarily very limited at present. One early potential concern was that male rats receiving large doses of gabapentin had an increased incidence of pancreatic neoplasms, which delayed the development of the drug. There has not been any suggestion, however, that gabapentin is associated with an increased risk of neoplasia in humans.

### 4.5.8 Lamotrigine

*Action*

Lamotrigine is a phenyltriazine that was developed as a folate antagonist. It has a phenytoin-like action on neuronal membranes, inhibiting voltage-dependent sodium channels, and is thought to reduce the release of the excitatory amino acids aspartate and glutamate (Lees & Leach 1993).

*Indications*

Lamotrigine is modestly effective against partial seizures, with about 30% of patients having a 50% or more reduction in seizures in controlled trials (Binnie et al 1989, Jawad et al 1989, Sander et al 1990b, c, Loiseau et al 1990, Matsuo et al 1993, Schapel et al 1993, Messenheimer et al 1994). Recent anecdotal reports, however, suggest that it may be more effective in generalized seizures, particularly in atypical absences and tonic seizures and against the Lennox–Gastaut syndrome (Oller et al 1991, Sander et al 1991a, Timmings & Richens 1992). Lamotrigine was recently approved, in the UK, as a drug of first-use in patients with partial, secondary generalized and primary generalized tonic-clonic seizures.

*Dosing and pharmacokinetics*

Lamotrigine is well absorbed from the gastrointestinal tract with peak plasma levels in 3 h. Elimination is by conjugation in the liver to inactive metabolites. Lamotrigine appears to be a weak enzyme inducer and to be subject to a minor degree of autoinduction. Dosing is generally twice-daily. In healthy adults the elimination half-life is about 24 h, reducing to 15 h if enzyme-inducing AEDs are being taken and increasing to 59 h if valproate, but no enzyme-inducing medication, is taken. Doses are influenced by the nature of concomitant medication. If enzyme-inducing AEDs are being taken, 50 mg once daily is a usual starting dose, increasing in 50 mg steps every 1–2 weeks to the maximal tolerated dose, which is often 400–600 mg/d. If valproate is being taken without any inducing AEDs, the starting dose for an adult would be 25 mg on alternate days, increasing to 25 mg daily after 2 weeks, with subsequent increments every 2 weeks up to 100–150 mg/d. Dosing is intermediate if both valproate and an enzyme-inducing AED, or neither, are being taken. There is little data on the optimal rate of withdrawal: over 2–3 weeks would be usual unless the reason is an acute adverse effect, in which case withdrawal would be abrupt. At present there is inadequate data on plasma lamotrigine concentrations to comment on their clinical utility.

*Drug interactions*

*Effect of other drugs on lamotrigine*: Lamotrigine metabolism is strongly inhibited by sodium valproate. Other drugs do not appear to have a significant pharmacokinetic or pharmacodynamic effect on lamotrigine. There have been anecdotal reports of synergistic efficacy with vigabatrin and also with valproate, but there is no controlled data to substantiate this.

*Effect of lamotrigine on other drugs*: Some studies have found that lamotrigine inhibits the metabolism of carbamazepine epoxide, resulting in raised concentrations of the epoxide without change in the concentration of parent carbamazepine (Warner et al 1992), although other investigations have not found this effect. In practical terms this interaction is likely to be clinically significant if a patient has lamotrigine added to a maximum tolerated dose of carbamazepine. A high index of suspicion is necessary if symptoms suggestive of carbamazepine intoxication develop, as carbamazepine epoxide concentrations are not measured routinely by most laboratories.

*Acute adverse effects*

Drowsiness, headache and diplopia are amongst the most common adverse effects reported and usually respond to a dose reduction of lamotrigine. If a patient is taking carbamazepine the possibility of the adverse effects being due to the latter needs to be considered.

*Idiosyncratic adverse effects*

An allergic skin rash occurs in about 3% of cases. The risk appears to be higher if valproate is a co-medication, possibly because higher plasma concentrations of lamotrigine result. There are suggestions that very slow introduction of lamotrigine results in a lower incidence of rash. Out of about 20 000 patients who have taken lamotrigine for more than 1 month there has been one case of an allergic drug rash being complicated by fatal liver failure. There have been a few reports of disseminated intravascular coagulation and sudden death occurring in patients taking lamotrigine, but the incidence has not been higher than expected and the significance of the drug in these cases is uncertain.

*Chronic adverse effects*

In the time that lamotrigine has been available no significant chronic adverse effects have become apparent.

## 4.5.9 Oxcarbazepine

(Anonymous 1989, Dam & Ostergaard 1995)

*Action*

Oxcarbazepine is the 10-keto analogue of carbamazepine, with a similar mode of action.

*Indications*

These are as for carbamazepine. At present oxcarbazepine is licensed only in Scandinavia, the Netherlands and Argentina, and is under development elsewhere. The principal advantage of oxcarbazepine over carbamazepine is that the former appears to cause little, if any, induction of hepatic enzymes, with a consequent lack of autoinduction of the drug's metabolism and fewer pharmacokinetic interactions. Furthermore, as oxcarbazepine is not converted to carbamazepine or carbamazepine epoxide in vivo, two-thirds of patients who are allergic to carbamazepine can tolerate oxcarbazepine.

*Dosing and pharmacokinetics*

Oxcarbazepine is an inactive prodrug and is converted in the liver to the active metabolite dihydro-hydroxycarbamazepine (DHC), bypassing the 10, 11-epoxide that is the primary metabolite of carbamazepine. The half-life of oxcarbazepine is very short, and that of DHC is 10–15 h.

A dose of 300 mg of oxcarbazepine is approximately equivalent to 200 mg of carbamazepine. An adult starting dose would be 300 mg at night, increasing to twice daily, with subsequent increments of 300 mg in the total daily dose. Average daily doses are 600–1200 mg/d as monotherapy and 900–3000 mg/d when given as part of polytherapy, with larger doses being divided into thrice-daily administration. Serum concentrations of DHC that have been therapeutic have usually been in the range 30–120 μmol/l.

*Adverse effects*

The adverse effects of oxcarbazepine are broadly comparable to those of carbamazepine. Allergic skin rashes occur less frequently than with carbamazepine. Hyponatraemia appears to occur more frequently than with carbamazepine for doses of equivalent efficacy. This is not usually symptomatic, but if it is temporary fluid restriction and reduction of the dose of oxcarbazepine is necessary.

## 4.5.10 Phenobarbitone

*Action*

Barbiturates have an allosteric effect at the $GABA_A$ receptor, enhancing the inhibitory effects of GABA.

*Indications* (Painter & Gaus 1995)

Phenobarbitone was developed in 1912 and is the oldest and cheapest AED in regular clinical use. In developed countries phenobarbitone is now considered to be a second-line AED. The risk of adverse effects is greater than that associated with other agents, although its efficacy against partial and generalized seizures is similar to phenytoin, valproate and carbamazepine and the drug also has activity against myoclonic seizures. Phenobarbitone may be given intravenously and has an important role in the treatment of status epilepticus (Ch. 5, 5.3.4). Phenobarbitone is still widely used in developing countries, where the cost of more modern AEDs is prohibitive.

*Dosing and pharmacokinetics*

Phenobarbitone is well absorbed from the gastrointestinal tract, with peak plasma concentrations up to 6 h later. It is 40–50% protein-bound. 10–40% is excreted unchanged in the urine and the remainder is metabolized in the liver to inactive metabolites. The elimination half-life is 50–140 h in adults, even longer in neonates and 30–80 h in children. After a change in dose, it takes approximately 3 weeks for the new steady-state to be established. The plasma concentration–dose response curve is virtually linear over the clinically used range of doses.

In children, the usual starting dose is 3 mg/kg/d, with maintenance doses in the range 3–6 mg/kg/d. Adults will normally tolerate a starting dose of 30–60 mg daily, with maintenance doses of 60–240 mg/d. A small starting dose, with increments every 2–3 weeks, improves tolerability. Tolerance to the antiepileptic effect may also develop. In an acute situation a loading dose may be necessary: 10 mg/kg by slow intravenous infusion over 10 min, and a further 5 mg/kg if necessary. Careful cardiorespiratory monitoring is essential and this should be undertaken in an ITU.

Once-daily administration is usually satisfactory in adults; twice-daily may be necessary in children on account of the shorter half-life.

The widely quoted therapeutic range is 70–170 μmol/l, although many patients develop dose-related adverse effects at concentrations over 100 μmol/l.

Barbiturate withdrawal is a slow process with a risk of exacerbation of seizures. Optimal rates have not been defined; in a seizure free patient tapering over 6–12 months would be usual. In a patient with active epilepsy, on other AEDs, 60 mg decrements every 4 weeks is a reasonable schedule, with final steps of 30 mg daily and then 15 mg daily for the last month.

*Drug interactions* (Brodie 1992, Patsalos & Duncan 1993)

*Effect of other drugs on phenobarbitone*: Valproate, felbamate and dextropropoxyphene inhibit phenobarbitone metabolism, leading to raised levels. Phenytoin may also inhibit phenobarbitone metabolism. The magnitude of these reactions varies greatly from person to person, depending on genetic factors and concomitant medication. Rifampicin is a powerful enzyme inducer and may lower phenobarbitone levels.

*Effect of phenobarbitone on other drugs*: Phenobarbitone is a potent inducer of hepatic enzyme activity and hastens the metabolism of other drugs such as oestrogen in the oral contraceptive pill, steroids, warfarin, aminophylline and valproate. The conversion of carbamazepine, diazepam and clobazam to active metabolites is accelerated by phenobarbitone. The effect on phenytoin is complex and not reliably predictable in an individual patient, due to the combined effects of inhibition and induction.

In some patients combination therapy with phenobarbitone and valproate results in profound obtundation.

*Acute adverse effects* (Cramer & Mattson 1995)

Sedation, unsteadiness, nystagmus, giddiness, nausea and vomiting are common, especially on introduction of treatment. Tolerance to these effects usually develops if the dose is built up slowly, over many weeks.

*Idiosyncratic adverse effects*

Allergic skin reactions occur in approximately 3% of patients. Hepatotoxicity and serious haematological effects develop rarely.

*Other adverse effects*

Sedation, poor memory, cognitive impairment and depression are the most common long-term adverse effects. Conduct disorder may develop in nearly 50% of children and many become hyperkinetic. Other potential problems include folate deficiency leading to megaloblastic anaemia, osteomalacia, coarsening of the features, hirsutism, connective tissue disorders such as frozen shoulder, Dupuytren's contractures, impotence and reduced libido.

## 4.5.11 Phenytoin

*Action*

The principal antiepileptic action of phenytoin is by stabilization of neuronal membranes by virtue of inhibition of sodium channels. A further relevant mechanism is the inhibition of calcium channels and sequestration of calcium in nerve terminals.

*Indications*

In most developed countries, phenytoin is now regarded as a second-line drug for partial and tonic-clonic, tonic, clonic and atonic seizures. It is not effective against typical absences and myoclonic seizures. Phenytoin is very useful in the emergency treatment of status epilepticus (Ch.5, 5.3.4).

*Pharmacokinetics and dosing*

The sodium salt of phenytoin is well absorbed from the gastrointestinal tract with peak serum concentrations 4–12 h later. The acidic parent compound is less well absorbed. Absorption may be inhibited by antacid medications. If a patient is unable to take medication by mouth or is not absorbing ingested drugs, phenytoin may be given by intravenous infusion. The intravenous route is also appropriate for emergency situations (Ch.5, 5.3.4). Phenytoin should never be given by intramuscular administration as absorption is slow and erratic and sterile abscess formation is a risk.

Phenytoin is about 90% bound to plasma proteins and the concentrations in saliva and CSF are similar to the free concentrations in plasma. Less than 5% of administered phenytoin is excreted unchanged in the urine. The principal metabolite of phenytoin is the biologically inactive 5-*p*-hydroxyphenyl-5-phenylhydantoin. The enzymes responsible for this step show saturation kinetics at therapeutic concentrations of phenytoin. In the clinically used range of doses, equal increments of phenytoin result in progressively greater increases in serum concentration of the drug. Further, there is considerable interindividual variation in rates of phenytoin metabolism (Fig. 4.1). In adults the elimination half-life ranges from 10–140 h. In neonates the rate of metabolism is very slow, unless there has been exposure in utero. The rate of metabolism increases over subsequent months to be greater than adult values, and then gradually decreases through childhood. Once-daily dosing is usually satisfactory for adults. Tolerance to its antiepileptic action does not usually occur. As children metabolize phenytoin faster they may need twice-daily dosing.

Because of the pharmacokinetic properties and the low therapeutic index of phenytoin it is not an easy drug to use. It most patients serum concentration measurements are essential to obtain optimal doses.

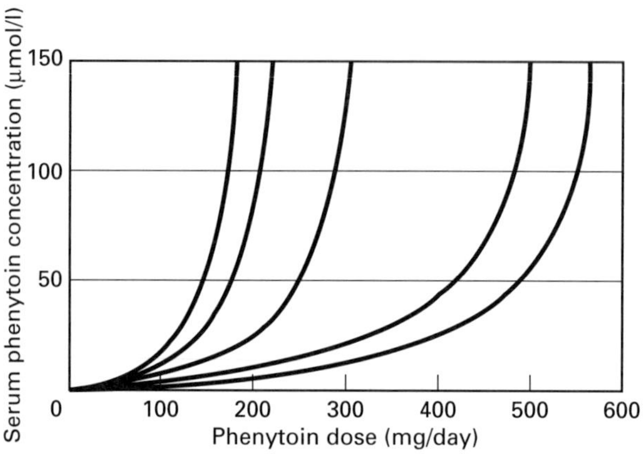


**Fig. 4.1** Representation of phenytoin serum concentration–dose response curves for five patients, showing interindividual variability and zero-order kinetics. An increment of 50 mg would have markedly different effects on the serum con-centration in different patients receiving the same dose and also have different effects in the same patient at different dose levels

A typical starting dose in an adult would be 200–300 mg, and in children 5 mg/kg/d. In the acute situation a loading dose of 15–18 mg/kg may be given (Ch. 5, 5.3.4). If phenytoin is being increased it is generally reasonable, in adults, to increase the daily dose by 100 mg if the serum concentration is less than 20 µmol/l, by 50 mg if it is 20–50 µmol/l and by 25 mg if it is greater than 50 µmol/l. Such increments are unlikely to precipitate serious intoxication. Serum concentrations take approximately one week to reach steady-state after a change in dose, but in slow metabolizers this may take as long as 4 weeks. When tapering phenytoin, small decrements will result in a large fall in concentration if metabolizing enzymes are saturated and smaller falls will occur with the same decrement at lower levels. In patients with active epilepsy who are having their medication changed, reductions of 50 mg every 2–7 days is generally reasonable for an adult.

Generic formulations of phenytoin may contain different excipients that materially affect bioavailability. In some patients, a change in preparation can result in clinically significant changes in serum concentration that may result in toxicity or impaired seizure control. In patients with a low tolerance for changes in serum concentration it is best to restrict prescription to the brand name preparation, as generic preparations will often be obtained from a number of different suppliers.

The widely quoted 'therapeutic range' of serum phenytoin concentrations of 40–80 μmol/l is only an estimation of the concentration range within which the majority of patients have optimal control of seizures, without dose-related adverse effects. Many patients are optimally treated at concentrations outside of this range (see above, 4.3.3). Phenytoin in plasma is approximately 90% bound to plasma proteins and only free phenytoin is biologically active and metabolized. Free phenytoin levels may be measured but in these are only indicated in particular clinical situations (see above, 4.3.4).

*Drug interactions*

Pharmacokinetic interactions are common, as phenytoin metabolism is very susceptible to inhibition by other drugs and it may itself enhance the metabolism of other drugs. The extent of interactions is determined by genetic factors and the doses of drugs taken. The best clinical management is to monitor plasma phenytoin levels and adjust doses if there are clinically significant alterations.

*Effects of other drugs on phenytoin*: At therapeutic concentrations, with the saturable metabolism of phenytoin, the addition of an inhibitor may result in a clinically significant rise in concentrations (Duncan et al 1991, Brodie 1992, Patsalos & Duncan 1993) (Table 4.3). Phenytoin metabolism is inhibited by phenobarbitone and carbamazepine but as these are also enzyme-inducers the end result depends on the relative doses of the drugs and genetic factors. Valproate inhibits phenytoin metabolism and also displaces phenytoin from plasma protein binding sites; the end result is often a rise in free phenytoin levels and a fall in the total concentration. Felbamate, amiodarone, isoniazid, fluconazole, chloramphenicol, propoxyphene, sulthiame and cimetidine may all inhibit phenytoin metabolism. A displacement of phenytoin from plasma protein binding sites, such as by tolbutamide and valproate, only necessitates a reduction of phenytoin dose if metabolism is close to saturation.

Antacids impair the absorption of phenytoin. Vigabatrin may result in a 20–30% fall in serum phenytoin concentrations. This interaction is usually noted approximately 1 month after vigabatrin has been started and the mechanism is unclear.

Chronic ethanol usage and rifampicin can lower phenytoin levels by virtue of liver enzyme induction.

*Effects of phenytoin on other drugs:* Phenytoin, being an inducer of liver microsomal enzymes, results in lowered concentrations of other antiepileptic drugs that are metabolized: carbamazepine, valproate, lamotrigine, felbamate, benzodiazepines and other drugs such as oestradiol, steroids, cyclosporin, theophylline, chloramphenicol, quinidine and warfarin. Phenytoin may also competitively inhibit phenobarbitone metabolism.

*Acute adverse effects*

Acute dose-related adverse reactions are common and include nystagmus, ataxia, lethargy and headache. These are more likely to occur at serum concentrations in excess of 80–100 μmol/l, but may also be noted at lower concentrations. Other dose-related symptoms include confusional states, involuntary movements including dystonia, orofacial dyskinesia and chorea, similar to those seen in association with neuroleptics, and occasionally exacerbation of seizures.

*Idiosyncratic adverse effects*

Hypersensitivity reactions causing skin rash occur in up to 5%, are most common in the first 4 weeks of treatment and may be associated with fever, lymphadenopathy and eosinophilia. A mild leucopenia may occur. Serious agranulocytosis, thrombocytopenia and red cell aplasia is very rare.

Hepatitis occurs rarely, is usually associated with a skin rash and fever and is fatal in one-third of cases. This is to be distinguished from the asymptomatic elevation of liver enzymes that is commonly seen in patients taking phenytoin. An illness very similar to systemic lupus erythematosus is sometimes due to phenytoin and is reversible.

*Chronic adverse effects*

Phenytoin, as with other AEDs, causes a degree of motor slowing and, in addition, may adversely effect concentration and attention. It is controversial whether the latter effects are greater for phenytoin than for other AEDs (Thompson & Trimble 1982, Dodrill & Temkin 1989, Duncan et al 1990b, Meador et al 1990).

Cosmetic effects such as gum hypertrophy, hirsutism and acne are well recognized adverse effects and should be taken into account, particularly when prescribing for children and young women. Folate deficiency causing a macrocytosis occurs in up to 50% of patients, but an overt megaloblastic anaemia develops in under 1%. Lowered concentrations of IgA, and less commonly IgG and IgM, may occur. Drug-induced vitamin D deficiency may result in rickets or osteomalacia. In the UK this is particularly likely to occur in females of Asian extraction, because of dietary factors and their lack of exposure to sunlight. Impotence and reduced libido may be related to changes in free testosterone concentrations. In some susceptible patients, hyperglycaemia may be precipitated. Attacks of acute hepatic porphyria may be induced in patients at risk. Other chronic adverse effects include mild peripheral neuropathy and cerebellar atrophy. Lymphoma and impaired cellular and humoral immune responses have been ascribed to phenytoin but the causal relationship is unclear.

## 4.5.12 Piracetam

*Action*

Piracetam (2-oxo-1 pyrrolidine acetamide) was developed as a cyclic analogue of GABA. However, despite evaluation in many seizure models, and studies of serotonergic and GABAergic function, the mode of action of piracetam is unknown (Vial et al 1974, Copani et al 1992).

*Indications*

Piracetam has been marketed for many years in several countries as a memory enhancer, although evidence of sustained effects on memory is slight. More recently, considerable efficacy against cortical myoclonus has been demonstrated in about 75% of patients, and its main indication in epilepsy is for myoclonus that persists despite therapy with valproate and clonazepam (Obeso et al 1988, Brown et al 1993).

*Dosing and pharmacokinetics*

Absorption from the gastrointestinal tract is rapid and complete. Piracetam is not protein-bound and is excreted unchanged in the urine, with an elimination half-life of about 5 h. Large doses need to be taken. A usual starting dose for an adult would be three 800 mg tablets three times a day, increasing to seven tablets three times daily. Some patients appear to benefit from even higher doses; 38 g a day has been used without evident adverse effects. Withdrawal needs to be gradual; abrupt cessation has been associated with an increase in seizures (Brown et al 1993).

*Drug interactions*

No clinically significant interactions with other AEDs or other medications appear to occur.

*Adverse effects*

Apart from its bulk, piracetam is generally well tolerated. One to 3% of patients have reported hyperkinesia, dizziness, insomnia, depression or nervousness, nausea or weight gain.

## 4.5.13 Primidone

*Action*

This is predominantly via the primary metabolite, phenobarbitone, although the other metabolite, phenylethylmalonamide, is contributory.

*Indications*

The spectrum of activity of primidone is similar to phenobarbitone, which is the principal metabolite of primidone in vivo. As an AED, primidone has nothing to recommend it over phenobarbitone (Duncan 1990).

*Dosing and pharmacokinetics*

250 mg of primidone has similar efficacy to 60 mg phenobarbitone. Primidone is well absorbed from the gastrointestinal tract, with peak plasma concentrations in about 3 h. Primidone is metabolized in the liver to phenobarbitone and phenylethylmalonamide, which are both pharmacologically active. The half-life of primidone is 4–12 h, which is overshadowed by the much longer half-life of phenobarbitone. The average ratio of phenobarbitone to primidone is 1.4 : 1. If phenytoin or carbamazepine are also taken, this ratio increases to 4 : 1.

If plasma concentration monitoring is wanted, measurement of phenobarbitone is generally sufficient. Inappropriately high levels of primidone suggest recent non-compliance (see above, 4.3.2).

An average starting dose for an adult would be 62.5–125 mg at night, with increments every 2–4 weeks, if tolerated.

*Drug interactions*

*Effect of other drugs on primidone:* Phenytoin and carbamazepine increase the rate at which primidone is converted to phenobarbitone. Valproate also raises the phenobarbitone to primidone ratio, by virtue of inhibition of onward metabolism of phenobarbitone.

*Effect of primidone on other drugs*: The enzyme-inducing effects of primidone and phenobarbitone result in reduced plasma concentrations of other AEDs and medications.

*Adverse effects*

These are as for phenobarbitone, although primidone is tolerated less well, particularly when first introduced. Some patients have a severe reaction comprising dizziness, nausea and sedation when commenced on primidone and it is advisable to start at a very low dose: 62.5 mg at night, and to slowly increase this over the following weeks. If the patient develops an acute adverse reaction it may be necessary to start with an even smaller dose, such as 15 mg, and to only increase the dose when this amount is tolerated.

## 4.5.14 Valproate

*Action*

The dominant mechanisms of action of clinically used doses of valproate in vivo are not certain. Possibilities include an elevation of GABA concentrations, an indirect modulatory effect on GABAergic transmission and membrane stabilization.

*Indications*

Sodium valproate is a drug of first choice for the treatment of typical absences, myoclonic seizures and generalized tonic-clonic seizures, especially if these occur as part of the syndrome of idiopathic generalized epilepsy. Sodium valproate is also used in all other seizure types (Table 4.3). The recent Veterans' Administration comparison between carbamazepine and valproate for complex partial and secondarily generalized tonic-clonic seizures reported a modest superiority of carbamazepine over valproate in terms of control of complex partial seizures and adverse effects (Mattson et al 1992). Studies in the UK have found no significant difference in efficacy of valproate, carbamazepine and phenytoin against partial and tonic-clonic seizures (Richens et al 1994, Verity et al 1995, Heller et al 1995). Valproate is effective at reducing the risk of recurrence of febrile convulsions, although the place of regular prophylactic therapy in this situation is very limited (see above, 4.1.2).

*Pharmacokinetics and dosing*

Valproate is completely absorbed from the gastrointestinal tract, with peak serum levels after 1–4 h if syrup is taken and 4–8 h after taking enteric-coated tablets. An intravenous formulation of valproate is most useful for patients who are unable to take medication by mouth or who are malabsorbing.

Valproate is metabolized in the liver with an elimination half-life of 10–20 h in adults and 20–60 h in infants. Twice-daily dosing is most satisfactory for the majority of patients. More frequent fractionation of doses may reduce the risks of teratogenesis (Ch. 6, 6.3.3). There is evidence that the antiepileptic effect of valproate lags behind serum concentrations, taking a longer time to develop when treatment is initiated and persisting after withdrawal. As a result, once-daily dosing has been evaluated and shown to have as good results as more frequent administration. This being the case, there is probably only a limited role for slow-release formulations of valproate, unless it can be shown that adverse effects, such as teratogenicity, may be reduced by achieving lower peak valproate concentrations.

Adults may generally be started on 500 mg of valproate, with 500 mg dose increments up to a ceiling of 3000 mg/d, if tolerated. Maintenance doses for children are 10–40 mg/kg/d. Plasma concentrations of valproate vary by more than 100% through a 24-h period, even with thrice-daily dosing, and monitoring of plasma valproate concentrations as a guide to dosing is of very little utility. Acute dose-related adverse effects are more likely to be noted at plasma concentrations in excess of 700 μmol/l (see above, 4.3).

A slow-release formulation of valproate has recently become available and has significant advantages for patients with side-effects from valproate, particularly dose-related neurotoxic effects. The slow release formulation may also have a role in pregnancy, by virtue of minimizing the peaks of valproate concentrations that occur after ingestion (Ch. 6, 6.3.3).

*Drug interactions* (Brodie 1992, Patsalos & Duncan 1993)

*Effect of valproate on other drugs:* Valproate does not induce the activity of hepatic enzymes and so does not enhance the metabolism of other agents, but does inhibit the oxidative metabolism of other drugs. Phenobarbitone levels increase with co-medication with valproate, and a combination of these two drugs may result in severe sedation. Sodium valproate may also inhibit the metabolism of lamotrigine, phenytoin, carbamazepine, primidone and ethosuximide, resulting in an elevation of concentrations. The interaction with phenytoin is particularly complex, because of the displacement of phenytoin from plasma protein binding sites by valproate and the fact that the inhibitory effects of valproate depend on the degree of saturation of the enzymes metabolizing phenytoin (see above, 4.5.11).

*Effect of other drugs on valproate:* Enzyme-inducing drugs (phenytoin, carbamazepine and barbiturates) enhance the metabolism of sodium valproate, resulting in lower concentrations. Conversely, valproate concentrations will rise if enzyme-inducing co-medication is tapered (Duncan et al 1991). Felbamate inhibits the metabolism of valproate. Salicylates may displace valproate from plasma proteins.

*Acute adverse effects*

Anorexia, nausea, vomiting and diarrhoea are most common. These are less common with the enteric-coated preparation. Predictable neurotoxicity includes sedation and dizziness, which may be reduced by using the slow-release formulation.

*Idiosyncratic adverse effects*

Rashes occur rarely. The risk of serious adverse effects, including fatal hepatic failure, with a histological picture of microvesicular steatosis, is 1/500 in children under 2 years of age who are on other AEDs and who have pre-existing neurological deficit; the risk of fatal hepatotoxicity to adults on valproate monotherapy is 1/45 000 (Dreifuss et al 1989). Severe hepatic reactions generally occur within 90 days of commencing therapy. Routine monitoring of liver enzymes does not help to avert severe reactions and the benign asymptomatic modest elevation of liver enzymes that is commonly seen in association with valproate therapy is not a forerunner of a severe hepatic reaction. Initial symptoms include nausea, vomiting and drowsiness, sometimes accompanied by bruising, jaundice and increased seizures. If there is a suspicion of a severe hepatic reaction the valproate should be stopped and liver function evaluated.

Patients with defects of urea cycle enzymes should not be given valproate, as they have a high risk of developing severe hyper-ammonaemia.

If possible, valproate should be avoided in patients with pre-existing liver disease and a family history of hepatic disease in child-hood. In some patients an encephalopathy may develop in patients treated with valproate, and be associated with low concentrations of carnitine (Triggs et al 1990, Coulter 1991).

Acute haemorrhagic pancreatitis, which is commonly fatal, has been reported and should be considered if the patient develops abdominal pain and vomiting.

*Other adverse effects*

Occasional patients become obtunded and confused, often in association with prominent delta waves on the EEG (Ch. 3, 3.6.1).

Significant weight gain affects about 15% of patients, is most probably due to stimulation of appetite and can be a severe problem, with weight gains in excess of 20 kg. Postural tremor and mild hyperammonaemia are usually dose-related. Alopecia occurs unpredictably. This effect is usually predominantly transient and dose-related, and hair often regrows curly. A dose-related thrombocytopenia is common. This is not usually clinically significant. It is advisable to check platelet counts before any surgical procedure in patients taking valproate, and platelet function tests if there is any concern about excessive bruising and bleeding. Occasionally, amenorrhoea develops in association with valproate therapy.

## 4.5.15 Vigabatrin

*Action*

Vigabatrin is an irreversible inhibitor of GABA transaminase, the principal enzyme that metabolizes GABA in glia and neurones. Vigabatrin forms a covalent bond with this enzyme and activity is only restored by synthesis of new enzyme. The consequence is elevation of brain GABA concentrations by approximately 150%, resulting in augmented GABAergic inhibitory transmission. Magnetic resonance spectroscopy (MRS) can demonstrate this elevated concentration of GABA in the brain in vivo (Rothman et al 1993, Preece et al 1994).

*Indications*

Vigabatrin is a second-line drug for partial seizures and secondary generalized tonic-clonic seizures. Controlled studies have shown that about 50% of patients with refractory partial seizures show more than a 50% reduction in seizure frequency, and up to 10% may attain complete seizure control (Mumford & Dam 1989, Reynolds et al 1991, McKee et al 1993, Grunewald et al 1994). Vigabatrin may also be useful against other seizure types, with the exception of generalized absences and myoclonus, which may be markedly exacerbated. There have been uncontrolled reports of benefit against infantile spasms (Chiron et al 1990, Appleton & Montiel-Viesca 1993). In general a beneficial effect of vigabatrin is usually maintained but tolerance may develop in some patients who show an initial response (Sander et al 1990d, Sivenius et al 1991).

*Dosing and pharmacokinetics*

Absorption from the gastrointestinal tract is rapid and almost total, with peak plasma concentrations in 2 h. Vigabatrin is not significantly bound to plasma proteins and excretion is mainly renal.

In view of the mode of action, plasma concentrations of vigabatrin do not relate well to clinical efficacy or the development of adverse effects. As a result, measurement of plasma concentrations is not useful, other than as a check on recent compliance.

A usual starting dose for an adult is 500 mg, once or twice a day, increasing in 500 mg steps every 1–2 weeks. Average maintenance doses are 1–1.5 g twice daily. About 25% of patients have better control on 3 g than on 2 g. Conversely, some patients seem to be better controlled on the lower dose (McKee et al 1993). In general, there appears to be no benefit from increasing doses beyond 3–4 g per day. In children, 40–80 mg/kg/d is a usual dose. Abrupt cessation of vigabatrin has been associated with a marked increase in seizures (Ring et al 1990) and tapering over 2–3 weeks is recommended.

*Drug interactions*

*Effect of other drugs on vigabatrin:* Other drugs do not appear to have a significant pharmacokinetic or pharmacodynamic effect on vigabatrin. There have been anecdotal reports of synergism with lamotrigine, but there is no controlled data to substantiate this.

*Effect of vigabatrin on other drugs*: Plasma phenytoin concentrations may fall by up to 30% about 1 month after the addition of vigabatrin to phenytoin. The mechanism of this interaction is not established; one possibility is that the absorption of phenytoin is impaired. A corrective increase in phenytoin dose may be necessary if there is a loss of seizure control at this time. Clinically significant pharmacokinetic interactions with other AEDs are not likely to occur.

*Acute adverse effects*

Sedation and dizziness are most common, particularly when doses are being increased. Headache, ataxia and tremor also occur. However, tolerance often develops and these symptoms are frequently self-limiting.

*Idiosyncratic adverse effects*

Allergic skin rashes and other hypersensitivity reactions are extremely rare.

*Neuropsychiatric adverse effects*

Up to one patient in 10 treated with vigabatrin develops a change in mood, commonly depression, or agitation, ill-temper and disturbed behaviour. Overall, up to 4% may develop paranoid and psychotic symptoms (Sander et al 1990d, 1991b) although other groups have found a lower incidence (Betts & Thomas 1990, Dam 1990).

Depression has been noted to develop in 4–9% of patients receiving vigabatrin in double-blind studies (Rimmer & Richens 1984, Gram et al 1985, Loiseau et al 1986, Remy et al 1986, Tartara et al 1986, 1989, Tassinari et al 1987, Grunewald et al 1994). Depression has generally been noted when the drug dosage is being introduced or following a subsequent dose increase. A past history of psychiatric disturbance appears to increase the risk of developing depression (Ring et al 1993) and such patients should be kept under close review.

The incidence of psychiatric adverse effects appears to have reduced since the recognition of this problem in 1990, most probably because of the trend towards slower introduction of the drug, awareness of the initial symptoms of psychiatric disturbance that will resolve on dose reduction, and greater caution when considering the treatment of patients with a history of psychiatric disturbance. A psychosis may develop abruptly, but in most patients in whom psychiatric adverse effects occur the symptoms usually evolve over several days and serious problems may generally be averted if the drug is tapered and stopped at this time.

*Chronic adverse effects*

Weight gain of 10 kg or more occurs in about 15% of adults. Effects on cognitive function have been assessed by several studies with the conclusion that there is no adverse effect (Mumford et al 1990, McGuire et al 1992, Gillham et al 1993), or a slowing of motor function and slight impairment of visual memory (Grunewald et al 1994). Neuropathological studies in animal models raised a concern about intramyelinic oedema and reactive astrocytosis related to administration of vigabatrin (Butler et al 1987, Gibson et al 1990). Human data, however, have been reassuring in that examination of patients by evoked responses (Hammond et al 1985, Ylinen et al 1992), quantitative MRI (Jackson et al 1994) and pathological examination of biopsy and autopsy material (Cannon et al 1991) have not suggested that this phenomenon occurs with clinically used doses in patients over 18 months of continuous treatment.

### 4.5.16 Developmental antiepileptic drugs (Patsalos & Duncan 1994)

Several novel AEDs are in the course of clinical development and evaluation, and many more candidate compounds are undergoing preclinical development. This is a rapidly changing field, with new agents emerging and others being withdrawn.

*Tiagabine*

Tiagabine blocks the re-uptake of GABA into glia and neurones, resulting in increased GABA concentrations at the synaptic cleft.

*Indications*: Tiagabine is a developmental drug that has demonstrable efficacy against complex partial seizures when added to conventional therapy in patients with refractory epilepsy, with about 30% of patients having complex partial seizures reduced by 50% or more (Rowan et al 1993, Richens et al 1995). Monotherapy studies comparing tiagabine with carbamazepine in newly diagnosed patients with partial seizures and generalized seizures are in progress.

*Dosing and pharmacokinetics*: Tiagabine is rapidly absorbed from the gastrointestinal tract, with peak plasma concentrations in 1 h. Metabolism is in the liver with an elimination half-life of 5–8 h, and this appears to be induced by phenytoin, carbamazepine and barbiturates. Twice- or thrice-daily administration is necessary. In double-blind add-on studies, initial dosing was 2 mg thrice daily, and the median maximum tolerated dose was 10 mg thrice daily. In other studies up to 80 mg/d have been used.

*Drug interactions*: Tiagabine does not affect other AEDs. The metabolism of tiagabine is accelerated by concomitant administration of enzyme-inducing AEDs, leading to an elimination half-life of 2–4 h.

*Adverse effects*: Predictable dose-related CNS effects include fatigue, tremor, nausea, headache and dizziness. As yet, serious or idiosyncratic adverse effects have not been noted and there appears to be a low incidence of associated behavioural disorders.

*Topiramate*

*Action:* Topiramate is a weak carbonic anhydrase inhibitor. It is uncertain whether this is related to its antiepileptic properties. Topiramate's profile of action in animal models is similar to that of phenytoin.

*Indications*: Topiramate is under development and has been shown so far to be active against partial and generalized seizures.

*Dosing and pharmacokinetics*: Maximum plasma concentrations are reached in 1–4 h after oral administration. The unchanged compound is renally excreted, with an elimination half-life of 19–23 h. Initial dosing is with 100 mg daily, increasing by 100 mg steps. Average maintenance doses are about 600 mg. Some patients have taken up to 1600 mg daily, divided into two or three doses per day.

*Drug interactions*: These have not yet been fully investigated. Concomitant administration of enzyme-inducing drugs results in lower plasma concentrations of topiramate.

*Adverse effects*: Mild dose-related neurotoxicity occurs. Other reported adverse effects include renal calculi, weight loss and depression.

*Remacemide*

This is an acetamide derivative that is metabolized to desglycine, which functions as a non-competitive NMDA-receptor antagonist. The drug is in the early stages of development and appears to be efficacious against partial and secondary generalized seizures. Concomitant enzyme-inducing drugs hasten its metabolism and remacemide results in an increase in phenytoin and carbamazepine concentrations.

*Other NMDA receptor antagonists*

Development of the NMDA-linked calcium channel blocker MK-801 as a potential AED was ceased because of significant adverse motor and behavioural effects (Troupin et al 1986). The only clinical trial of a competitive NMDA-receptor antagonist in patients with epilepsy, D-CPP-ene, had to be terminated prematurely because of adverse effects – principally sedation, impaired motor control and amnesia – at doses that did not have significant antiepileptic effect (Sveinbjornsdóttir et al 1993). It remains to be seen whether less potent NMDA-receptor antagonists, and antagonists at other excitatory amino acid receptors, may have useful antiepileptic effects without severe toxicity.

*Zonisamide*

Zonisamide appears to act by blocking sodium channels and T-type calcium channels. It is well absorbed from the gastrointestinal tract and concentrated in red blood cells. Development in Europe and the USA was suspended in 1988 after the finding of renal calculi in some patients who had received the drug, but continued in Japan, where this problem was not noted. Further development is now planned. Add-on studies suggested efficacy against partial, secondarily generalized, atonic, atypical absence and myoclonic seizures (Leppik et al 1993, Schmidt et al 1993, Patsalos & Duncan 1994).

*Other developmental agents*

$GABA_B$-receptor antagonists have been shown to be effective in some animal models of typical absence seizures and may well be effective against absences in man. Drugs in this class are being evaluated as a treatment for dementia, but are not being developed as anti-absence drugs at the present time, primarily for commercial reasons.

LO-59, a derivative of piracetam, shows promise against partial and secondarily generalized seizures. Eterobarb is a barbiturate that appears to be relatively non-sedating and is under consideration.

### 4.5.17 Last-ditch agents

In some patients with chronic and refractory epilepsy there is great pressure to 'do something', even after all appropriate currently available and developmental agents have been tried. It is important to explain to these unfortunate patients and their families that there is a limit to the efficacy of currently available medication and that it is necessary to avoid over-medication and prescription of drugs that do not improve seizure control but which give rise to adverse effects. In this situation patients may prefer to try non-medical treatments for their epilepsy (see below, 4.7). Other medications that may be considered in this situation include: allopurinol, up to 600 mg/d; vitamin E, up to 3200 U/d; oral chlormethiazole; methsuximide, up to 1200 mg/d, which is widely available in the USA, but in the UK may only be prescribed on a named patient basis from the manufacturers (Parke-Davis).

## 4.6 STOPPING ANTIEPILEPTIC DRUG THERAPY IN PATIENTS WHOSE EPILEPSY IS IN REMISSION

In the majority of patients with epilepsy, seizures remit on treatment (Ch. 8, 8.1). For this reason the questions of whether and when to withdraw therapy are common and important clinical issues. A balance has to be drawn between the risk of inducing a relapse of the epilepsy and the inconvenience and risks of unnecessary therapy. Advice is difficult to give and is often contradictory (Pedley 1988, Chadwick 1994). Adult neurologists tend to recommend withdrawal of therapy to their patients less willingly than do paediatricians, among the reasons for which are the complicating factors of driving and employment and the anxiety about the retarding effects of medication on learning and cerebral development. It is also clear that many patients withdraw from medication without medical advice (Hauser & Kurland 1975, Annegers et al 1979, Goodridge & Shorvon 1983a, b).

### 4.6.1 Overall risks of relapse of seizures after withdrawal of medication

The first point to make is that, while there is statistical data on which to base risk assessment, no guarantee of seizure freedom can ever be given when a drug is withdrawn (or even indeed when doses are lowered).

A most important contribution was that of Chadwick and colleagues (MRC Antiepileptic Drug Withdrawal Study Group 1991), who carried out a prospective multicentre study comparing the risks of withdrawal and non-withdrawal in 1013 patients in remission for a period of at least 2 years. Overall risks of relapse following withdrawal of medication were 43% after 2 years, compared with an annual risk of about 10% in those maintaining therapy. There are criticisms that can be levelled at this study: no checks were made on compliance with medication; the group was selected (e.g. few children, few patients with driving licences, etc); many patients who had successfully discontinued therapy on their own account would not be included (such hospital-based studies will therefore over-estimate the risks of withdrawal). Nevertheless, this study provides the best figures available for assessing the risks of stopping medication, at least for the average patient presenting to a largely adult neurological out-patients.

A Cox's proportional hazard model was developed from this trial in which seven factors were identified that predicted an increased risk of recurrence (Table 4.7): age over 16 years (relative risk 1.75); taking more than one antiepileptic drug (1.83); a history of seizures after starting antiepileptic drug therapy (1.56); a history of tonic-clonic seizures (1.56); a history of myoclonic seizures (1.84); and an abnormal EEG in the previous year (1.32). The risk of seizures also declined the longer the seizure-free period. Personal clinical practice also suggests that the longer the history of active epilepsy prior to remission the less likely is withdrawal to be successful (Shorvon 1991).

The problem has also been the subject of several paediatric surveys. In a recent prospective study of 264 children, there was a 36% recurrence rate following withdrawal of drug after a mean seizure-free period of 2.9 years (Shinnar et al 1994). Factors associated with a higher risk of seizures included symptomatic epilepsy (relative risk 1.81) and, in the idiopathic group, age of onset above 12 years (5.4), a family history of seizures (2.4), the presence of EEG slowing (2.4) and a history of atypical febrile seizures (2.8). This investigation also emphasized the importance of syndromic diagnosis in predicting outcome, which will prove a much more fruitful approach than one based simply on seizure type. Certain childhood syndromes carry a particularly good prognosis after

**Table 4.7** The risks of relapse by 1 and 2 years after withdrawing medication (prognostic model) ((Calculations made sequentially, from MRC Antiepileptic Drug Withdrawal Study Group 1993)

| | | |
|---|---|---|
| 1. Starting score for all patients | | – 175 |
| 2. Age of 16 years or older | | + 45 |
| 3. Taking more than one AED | | + 50 |
| 4. Seizures after starting AEDs | | + 35 |
| 5. History of tonic-clonic seizures | | + 35 |
| 6. History of myoclonic seizures | | + 50 |
| 7. EEG in past year – not available | | + 15 |
| – abnormal | | + 20 |
| 8. Period seizure free (*t* years) | | + 200/t |
| 9. **Total score** | | $=T$ |
| 10 Divide T by 100 and exponentiate ($e^x$) | | $z = e^{T/100}$ |
| *Probability of seizure recurrence:* | By year 1 | By year 2 |
| On continued treatment | $1 - 0.89^z$ | $1 - 0.79^z$ |
| On slow withdrawal | $1 - 0.69^z$ | $1 - 0.60^z$ |

*Sample calculations:*
In an adult with no adverse prognostic factors, the risk of recurrence on withdrawal of treatment at 1 year is 21% and 28% at 2 years. For a child the risks are 14% and 19% respectively. At the other extreme, for an adult seizure-free for 2 years on one drug with all the other risk factors, the risks are 84% and 92%.

cessation of seizures, such as childhood absence epilepsy, benign rolandic epilepsy and uncomplicated febrile convulsions. A meta-analysis of 25 studies (excluding the reports of the MRC Antiepileptic Drug Study Group) showed an overall risk of relapse in the first 12 months after withdrawal of 25%, and 29% at 2 years. The risk was increased in childhood-onset seizures, symptomatic seizures and in those with an abnormal EEG (Berg & Shinnar 1994). The role of EEG in predicting relapse after withdrawal has proved controversial, although frank epileptic activity (especially of the spike/wave discharges) does carry a worse prognosis, and the EEG seems to be of more prognostic value in children than in adults.

Another approach to assessing risk, which avoids the problems of selection bias, is to use epidemiological data, comparing the proportion of patients on and off medication in a population. Two such studies show that within 10–15 years after onset of epilepsy about 70% of patients are in at least 5-year remission and 50% are off therapy (Hauser & Kurland 1975, Annegers et al 1979, Goodridge & Shorvon 1983), demonstrating the good overall outcome of epilepsy.

### 4.6.2 Risks of relapse during withdrawal of therapy

There is general agreement that the risks of relapse are at their greatest during the withdrawal phase, a period when about 50% of relapses occur, and 70–80% within a year of withdrawal. Only, occasionally do relapses occur after long periods of freedom from seizures, as demonstrated by Thurston and colleagues (1982), who found a relapse rate of 24% in a group of 148 children studied first at 5–12 years of follow-up, and a further 4% in the subsequent 10 years. The corollary of this is that, if a patient remains seizure free after withdrawal for a prolonged period, the subsequent risk of relapse is greatly reduced. Occasionally, status epilepticus results from precipitate withdrawal, and in this instance the withdrawn drug should be restored as rapidly as possible, ideally parenterally (Ch. 5, 5.3.2). Finally, it should not be forgotten that if further seizures do occur when drugs are withdrawn or reduced, full control may not be regained even if the previous drug regimen is restored (Todt 1984) – an eventuality about which the patient should be warned.

### 4.6.3 Speed of withdrawal of medication

Too fast a rate of withdrawal of many antiepileptic drugs (especially of barbiturates, benzodiazepines, carbamazepine or vigabatrin) may result in withdrawal seizures. The fastest safe rate of reduction probably depends upon a number of individual factors, and it is difficult to give adequate guidelines, but typical rates of staged dosage reduction are given in Table 4.8. In patients on combination therapy, one drug should be tapered at a time.

There is usually no urgency when withdrawing medication and the period of withdrawal of course can be considerably lengthened. This clinical situation is quite different from the withdrawal of AEDs from the treatment of patients with active epilepsy who are taking more than one drug and in whom changes in medication are being made (see above, 4.2.3).

**Table 4.8** Fastest recommended rates of drug reduction when withdrawing therapy in a seizure-free patient

| Drug withdrawn | Decremental dose reduction every 4 weeks (mg) |
|---|---|
| Carbamazepine | 200 |
| Clonazepam | 1 |
| Clobazam | 10 |
| Ethosuximide | 250 |
| Felbamate | 300 |
| Lamotrigine | 100 |
| Phenobarbitone | 30 |
| Phenytoin | 100 |
| Primidone | 125 |
| Valproate | 500 |
| Vigabatrin | 500 |

### 4.6.4 The adverse effects of continuing medication

Surprisingly, there is little information about the actual risks of continuing antiepileptic medication. A particular issue has concerned the cognitive and sedative actions of the drugs and their effects on learning, particularly in children (Ch. 9, 9.5). Although often stressed, recent studies have failed to show any great effects in this regard (Aldercamp et al 1993, Dodrill & Troupin 1991). The other chronic side-effects of the conventional AEDs are well documented (see above, 4.5) but in general in seizure-free patients on stable therapy these are often unimportant. Teratogenic effects need to be considered in females of childbearing potential (Ch. 6, 6.3.3).

### 4.6.5 Individual factors

It is important not to overlook these when deciding about withdrawal of therapy, and to include the attitude of the patient towards medication, the social and medical consequences of seizure recurrence, the side-effects of medication, the patient's employment and the requirement for a driving licence. The psychological effects of having to take therapy should not be underestimated. Taking medication is a confirmation of 'illness', it implies a state of dependence on others, it reduces self confidence and encourages a sickness role. In addition, the cost of medication, particularly with modern drugs, is a significant factor in some clinical settings.

### 4.6.6 Overall advice

It should be clear from the above that advice regarding the withdrawal of medication is difficult and must be individually based. Practice varies widely, but a few broad guidelines can be given.

1. It would be wise to refer all patients to a physician with experience in epilepsy to discuss the relevant issues.
2. As a rule of thumb, withdrawal of medication can be considered after 2 or more years of freedom from seizures. The longer the seizure-

free period the less likely is subsequent recurrence to occur, but if prognostic factors are unfavourable, the risks of recurrence even after longer periods are high. The application of the MRC prognostic model can be helpful (Table 4.7). If the period of active epilepsy prior to the remission is short, however, withdrawal of medication may be attempted earlier. After a single attack, for instance, 6 months may suffice.

3. Withdrawal should usually be carried out gradually and in stages, sometimes over a period of many months (Table 4.8). The patient should be carefully supervised over this period and if seizures recur, therapy should be recommenced.

4. The risks of recurrence should be very clearly explained to the patient, balanced against the risks of continuing therapy, and the advice recorded in the medical notes. The possible medical and social implications should be made explicit.

5. Only one drug at a time should be withdrawn or reduced.

## 4.7 NON-PHARMACOLOGICAL TREATMENTS OF EPILEPSY

Pharmacological treatments of epilepsy are not uniformly successful in patients. Even if good seizure control is obtained, many patients experience troublesome side-effects of treatments that must often be continued for many years. The need to take medication on a long-term basis has obvious implications for women wishing to become pregnant. In addition, many individuals describe feelings of oppression and an increased fear of being labelled as ill because of their need for regular drug-taking. Surgical treatment (Ch. 10) is an option only for a minority of patients and is also not without physical and psychological sequelae. It is therefore not surprising that alternative treatment approaches are sought by some patients (Table 4.9).

**Table 4.9** Non-medical treatments of epilepsy

*Psychological*
- Reward programmes
- General relaxation (? includes aromatherapy)
- Contingent relaxation
- Specific counter-measures
  Primary inhibition
  Secondary inhibition

*Biofeedback*
- Slow cortical potentials
- Non-specific EEG rhythms

*Vagal stimulation*

*Diet*
- Ketogenic
- Hypoallergenic
- Exclusion
- For inborn errors of metabolism

In mainstream clinical management it is easy to focus exclusively on seizure response and the latest change in AED therapy. An important aspect of many 'non-medical' treatments of epilepsy is that, while they are of intrinsically very limited efficacy, they encompass a more holistic approach to a patient's problems.

### 4.7.1 Psychological approaches (HA Ring, MR Trimble)

It has been suggested that many patients with epilepsy have a mental mechanism that they use to attempt to inhibit their seizures. In one study of 70 patients, 36% claimed that they could sometimes stop their seizures (Fenwick 1991). A behavioural approach to the treatment of epilepsy is based on these and other observations that epilepsy can be manipulated in a systematic way through environmental, psychological and physical changes. The initial stage in this approach is a behavioural analysis of the ways in which environmental and behavioural factors interact with seizure occurrence (Dahl et al 1987).

It has been demonstrated that significant reductions in seizure frequency may be achieved by teaching patients a specific contingent relaxation technique, which they must be able to employ rapidly when they identify a situation when they are at high risk of having a seizure (Dahl et al 1987). In a study of three children with intractable seizures it was found that contingent relaxation alone did not significantly reduce seizures but that such a reduction was obtained following the addition of specific counter-measures. The latter aimed at changing the arousal level relevant to and contingent on early seizure cues, for instance suddenly jerking the head to the right when it would habitually move to the left with a feeling of drowsiness at the onset of a seizure (Dahl et al 1988). Other specific approaches to seizure inhibition have been reviewed by several authors (Mostofsky & Balaschak 1977, Fenwick 1991).

Some patients suffer from reflex seizures and their seizures are reliably precipitated by external stimuli. A proportion of people can identify specific environmental or affective triggers and may be able to develop specific strategies to abort or delay a seizure. These methods may involve motor or sensory activity or they may be purely mental. However, in one study it was found that 50% of patients who inhibited their seizures found the procedures uncomfortable (Antebi & Bird 1992).

Primary seizure inhibition describes the direct inhibition of seizures by an act of will; for instance a man whose seizures were precipitated by a feeling of unsteadiness tackled this by keeping his gaze fixed on a point when walking down an incline (Fenwick 1991). The nature of the successful act varies from person to person and if this treatment approach is to be pursued then it must be individually tailored, based on an analysis of the patient's seizures and of any actions they may already have noticed which modifies them.

The term secondary inhibition is employed by Fenwick (1991) to describe behavioural techniques that are thought to act by changing cortical activity in neurones around a focus, without deliberately intending to do so. This reduces the risk both of partial and of a generalized seizure discharge, which may otherwise follow recruitment of surrounding normal brain by these neurones firing abnormally (Lockard 1980). An example of this is the act of maintaining alertness by a patient whose seizures appear in a state of drowsiness. Treatment in this case starts with trying to identify situations where the subject reliably tends to have seizures, or alternatively seems to be free of them.

As well as these seizure-related approaches, more general psychological strategies have also been investigated. Several anecdotal reports have been published demonstrating benefit from reward programmes that aim to reward seizure-free periods.

Based on the observation that some patients with olfactory auras can prevent progression of the seizure by applying a sudden, usually unpleasant olfactory counter-stimulus, Betts has explored the use of aromatherapy techniques in the control of epilepsy (Betts & Boden 1992). Currently it is not clear what are the relative contributions of specific olfactory stimuli and the general relaxation, that is a part of the treatment, to any clinical benefit that might be observed.

### 4.7.2 Biofeedback

(HA Ring, MR Trimble)

Specific biofeedback techniques have also been explored. Measurement of scalp electrical activity has demonstrated that there is an increase in surface-negative slow cortical potentials (SCPs) in the seconds before a seizure occurs. These SCPs represent the extent to which apical dendrites of cortical pyramidal cells are depolarized and hence indicate neuronal excitability (Rockstroh et al 1993). Studies using visual feedback of this effect have demonstrated that some patients are able to modulate cortical electrical activity with an associated decrease in seizure frequency (Birbaumer 1992). However it appears that patients with epilepsy are less able than normal controls to regulate their cortical excitability. This impairment can be minimized by extending the amount of training received by those with epilepsy. In a study that gave 28 1-h training sessions to 18 patients followed up for at least 1 year, six became seizure-free (Rockstroh et al 1993). However, not every patient who achieved reliable SCP control experienced a change in seizure frequency.

Non-specific EEG biofeedback has been used to modulate cerebral electrical rhythms; for instance to increase fast low-voltage activity and suppress slow wave activity surrounding the epileptic focus (Whyler et al 1976).

It has been pointed out that the teaching of any of these methods of self-control of seizures may increase morale, not only by reducing seizures but also by providing patients with a sense of control of their epilepsy.

### 4.7.3 Vagal stimulation

A quite different biological approach that has been explored in some centres is vagal stimulation using an implanted stimulator. This approach has the drawback that, while the nerve is being stimulated, usually for 30 s every 5–10 min, the voice changes. More intense stimulation may be associated with throat pain and coughing. In one series 39% of patients had at least a 50% reduction in seizures with high frequency stimulation, as did 19% receiving low frequency stimulation, and in some cases there was a worthwhile improvement in seizure severity (Ben-Menachem et al 1994).

The long-term place of this therapy is uncertain. At present its use is confined to patients with severe, refractory epilepsy who are not candidates for surgical treatment.

### 4.7.4 Diet

Rare patients with inborn errors of metabolism may require specific dietary manipulation, for example, protein restriction and arginine supplementation for urea cycle disorders; and restriction of protein and fat, with supplementation of essential amino acids and co-factors, for organic acidaemias (Leonard 1991).

A ketogenic diet is often tried by paediatricians after failure of AEDs adequately to control seizures. The diet is unpleasant, restricts carbohydrate and protein and supplies 80% of energy intake as fat. This diet is reported to be more effective in children with atypical absence, atonic and myoclonic seizures than other seizure types, particularly if they are under the age of 5 years. A ketogenic diet has no place in adult epilepsy.

Parents often report that diet, particularly food additives, may affect seizures, especially in children. In the setting of intractable epilepsy a trial of omission of certain foodstuffs seems reasonable, but it must be said that the reported association does not often stand up to critical assessment, with prospective recording of seizures and diet.

In other children, allergy to natural food constituents may be held responsible for some seizures and an oligoantigenic diet may be implemented. In such cases a good response is commonly found in atopic children, the atopy also responding to exclusion of certain foods. In addition, occasional patients report benefit from taking vegetarian or gluten-free diets.

REFERENCES

Albright P, Bruni J 1985 Reduction of polypharmacy in epileptic patients. Arch Neurol 42: 797–799

Aldercamp AP, Alpherts WCJ, Blennow G et al 1993 Withdrawal of antiepileptic medication in children – effects on cognitive function: the multicenter Holmfrid study. Neurology 43: 41–50

Annegers JF, Hauser WA, Elveback LR 1979 Remission of seizures and relapse in patients with epilepsy. Epilepsia 20: 729–734

Anonymous. 1989 Oxcarbazepine (editorial). Lancet 2: 196–198

Antebi D, Bird J 1992 The facilitation and evocation of seizures. Br J Psychiat 160: 154–164

Appleton RE, Montiel-Viesca F 1993 Vigabatrin in infantile spasms – why add on? Lancet 341: 962

Appleton R, Panayiotopoulos CP, Acomb AB et al 1993 Eyelid myoclonia with absences: an epilepsy syndrome. J Neurol Neurosurg Psychiat 56: 1312–1316

Ben-Menachem E, Mañon-Espaillat R, Ristanovic R et al 1994 Vagus nerve stimulation for treatment of partial seizures: 1. A controlled study of effect on seizures. Epilepsia 35: 616–626

Berg AT, Shinnar S 1994 Relapse following discontinuation of antiepileptic drugs: a meta-analysis. Neurology 44: 601–608

Betts T, Boden S 1992 Use of olfactory stimuli (aromatherapy). Seizure 1(suppl A): Abstract S25/3

Betts T, Thomas L 1990 Vigabatrin and behaviour disturbances. Lancet 335: 1279

Binnie CD, Debets RMC, Engelsman M et al 1989 Double blind crossover trial of lamotrigine as add-on therapy in intractable epilepsy. Epilepsy Res 4: 222–229

Birbaumer N 1992 Application of learnt cortical control to seizure behavior. Seizure 1(suppl A): S25/4

Bourgeois BFD 1995 Valproate; clinical use. In: Levy RH, Mattson RH, Meldrum BS (eds) Antiepileptic drugs, 4th edn. Raven Press, New York, p 633-639
Bourgeois BFD, Wad N 1988 Combined administration of carbamazepine and phenobarbital: effects on anticonvulsant activity and neurotoxicity Epilepsia 29: 482–487
Bourgeois B, Leppik IE, Sackellares JC et al 1993 Felbamate: a double-blind controlled trial in patients undergoing presurgical evaluation of partial seizures. Neurology 43: 693–696
Brodie MJ 1992 Drug interactions in epilepsy. Epilepsia 33(suppl 1): S13–S22
Brodie MJ 1993 Felbamate. Lancet 341: 1445–1446
Brown P, Steiger MJ, Thompson PD et al 1993 The effectiveness of piracetam in cortical myoclonus. Movement Disorders 8: 62–68
Browne TR 1978 Clonazepam. N Engl J Med 299: 812–816
Bruni J, Sanders M, Anhut H, Sauermann N 1991 Efficacy and safety of gabapentin (neurontin): a multicenter, placebo-controlled, double-blind study. Neurology 41(suppl 1): 330–331
Butler WH, Ford GP, Newberne JWA 1987 Study of the effects of vigabatrin on the central nervous system and retina of Sprague Dawley and Lister-hooded rats. Toxicol Pathol 15: 143–148
Callaghan N, O'Dwyer R, Keating J 1984 Unnecessary polypharmacy in patients with frequent seizures. Acta Neurol Scand 69: 15–19
Callaghan N, Kenny RA, O'Neill B, Crowley M, Goggin T 1985 A prospective study between carbamazepine, phenytoin and sodium valproate as monotherapy in previously untreated and recently diagnosed patients with epilepsy. J Neurol Neurosurg Psychiat 48: 639–644
Cannon DJ, Butler WH, Mumford JP, Lewis PJ 1991 Neuropathologic findings in patients receiving long-term vigabatrin therapy for chronic intractable epilepsy. J Child Neurol 6(suppl 1): 2S17–24
Chadwick DW 1994 The withdrawal of antiepileptic drugs. In: Hopkins A, Shorvon SD, Cascino G (eds) Epilepsy. Chapman & Hall, London p 215-220
Chadwick DW 1995 Gabapentin and felbamate. In: Duncan JS, Panayiotopoulos CP (eds) Typical absences and related epileptic syndromes. Churchill Livingstone, Edinburgh, p 376–380
Chataway J, Fowler A, Thompson PJ, Duncan JS 1993 Discontinuation of clonazepam in patients with active epilepsy. Seizure 2: 295–300
Chiron C, Dulac O, Beaumont D et al 1990 Vigabatrin in infantile spasms. Lancet 335: 363–364
Chugani HT, Shields WD, Shewmon DA, Olson DM, Phelps ME, Peacock WJ 1990 Infantile spasms: 1. PET identifies focal cortical dysgenesis in cryptogenic cases for surgical treatment. Ann Neurol 27: 406–413
Commission on Classification and Terminology of the International League against Epilepsy 1981 Proposal for revised clinical and electroencephalographic classification of epileptic seizures. Epilepsia 22: 489–501
Commission on Classification and Terminology of the International League against Epilepsy 1989 Proposal for revised classification of epilepsies and epileptic syndromes. Epilepsia 30: 389–399
Copani A, Genazzani AA, Aleppo G et al 1992 Nootropic drugs positively modulate α-amino-3-hydroxy-5-methyl-4-isoxazolepropionic acid sensitive glutamate receptors in neuronal cultures. J Neurochem 58: 1199–1204
Coulter DL 1991 Carnitine, valproate and toxicity. J Child Neurol 6: 7–14
Coulter DA, Huguenard JR, Prince DA 1989 Characterization of ethosuximide reduction of low-threshold calcium currents in thalamic neurons. Ann Neurol 25: 582–593
Cramer JA 1991 Overview of methods to measure and enhance patient compliance. In: Cramer JA, Spilker B (eds) Patient compliance in medical practice and clinical trials. Raven Press, New York, p 3–10
Cramer JA, Mattson RH 1991 Monitoring compliance with antiepileptic drug therapy. In: Cramer JA, Spilker B (eds) Patient compliance in medical practice and clinical trials. Raven Press, New York, p 123–137
Cramer JA, Mattson RH 1995 Phenobarbital; toxicity. In: Levy RH, Mattson RH, Meldrum BS (eds) Antiepileptic drugs, 4th edn. Raven Press, New York, p 409-420
Crawford P, Ghadiali E, Lane R, Blumhardt L, Chadwick D 1987 Gabapentin as an antiepileptic drug in man. J Neurol Neurosurg Psychiat 50: 682–686
Dahl J, Melin L, Lund L 1987 Effects of a contingent relaxation program on adults with refactory epileptic seizures. Epilepsia 28: 125–132
Dahl A, Melin L, Leissner P 1988 Effects of a behavioral intervention on epileptic seizure behavior and paroxysmal activity: A systematic replication of three cases of children with intractable epilepsy. Epilepsia 29: 172–183

Dam M 1990 Vigabatrin and behaviour disturbances. Lancet 335: 605
Dam M, Ostergaard LH 1995 Oxcarbazepine. In: Levy RH, Mattson RH, Meldrum BS (eds) Antiepileptic drugs, 4th edn. Raven Press, New York, p 987-995
Dodrill CB, Temkin NR 1989 Motor speed is a contaminating factor in evaluating the 'cognitive' effects of phenytoin. Epilepsia 30: 453–457
Dodrill CB, Troupin AS 1991 Neuropsychological effects of carbamazepine and phenytoin: a reanalysis. Neurology 41: 141–143
Dreifuss FE, Langer DH, Moline KA, Maxwell JE 1989 Valproic acid hepatic fatalities. II: US experience since 1984. Epilepsia 39: 201–207
Duncan JS 1988 Neuropsychiatric aspects of sedative drug withdrawal. Human Psychopharmacology 3: 171–180
Duncan JS 1990 Prescribing anticonvulsant drugs: 5. Primidone and phenobarbitone. Prescribers J 30: 131–137
Duncan JS 1991 Modern treatment strategies for patients with epilepsy: a review. J Roy Soc Med 84: 159–62
Duncan JS 1993 Conventional and clinimetric approaches to individualization of antiepileptic drug therapy. In: Meinardi H, Cramer JA, Baker G, da Silva M (eds) Quantitative assessment in epilepsy care. Plenum Press, New York, p 137–143
Duncan JS 1995 Treatment strategies for typical absences and related epileptic syndromes. In: Duncan JS, Panayiotopoulos CP (eds) Typical absences and related epileptic syndromes. Churchill Livingstone, Edinburgh, p 354–360
Duncan JS, Shorvon SD, Trimble MR 1988 Withdrawal symptoms from phenytoin, carbamazepine and sodium valproate. J Neurol Neurosurg Psychiat 51: 924–928
Duncan JS, Shorvon SD, Trimble MR 1990a Discontinuation of phenytoin, carbamazepine and sodium valproate in patients with active epilepsy. Epilepsia 31: 324–333
Duncan JS, Shorvon SD, Trimble MR 1990b The effects of removal of phenytoin, carbamazepine and sodium valproate on cognitive function. Epilepsia 31: 584–591
Duncan JS, Patsalos PN, Shorvon SD 1991 Effects of discontinuation of phenytoin, carbamazepine and valproate on concomitant antiepileptic medication. Epilepsia 32: 101–116
Faught E, Sachdeo RC, Remler MP et al 1993 Felbamate monotherapy for partial onset seizures: an active-control trial. Neurology 43: 688–692
Felbamate Study Group in Lennox–Gastaut Syndrome 1993 Efficacy of felbamate in childhood epileptic encephalopathy (Lennox–Gastaut syndrome). N Engl J Med 328: 29–33
Fenwick P 1991 Evocation and inhibition of seizures: behavioral treatment. In: Smith D, Treiman D, Trimble M (eds) Neurobehavioral problems in epilepsy. Advances in neurology 55. Raven Press, New York, p 163–183
Fish DR, Quirk JE, Smith SJM, Sander JWAS, Shorvon SD 1994 Videogames and epilepsy. Final Report. HMSO, London
Foy PM, Chadwick DW, Rajgopalan N, Johnson AL, Shaw MDM 1992 Do prophylactic anticonvulsant drugs alter the pattern of seizures after craniotomy. J Neurol Neurosurg Psychiat 55: 753–757
Gibson JP, Yarrington JT, Loudy DE, Gerbig CG, Hurst GH, Newberne JW 1990 Chronic toxicity studies with vigabatrin, a GABA-transaminase inhibitor. Toxicol Pathol 18: 225–238
Gillham RA, Blacklaw J, McKee PJW, Brodie MJ 1993 Effect of vigabatrin on sedation and cognitive function in patients with refractory epilepsy. J Neurol Neurosurg Psychiat: 56: 1271–1275
Goodridge DMG, Shorvon SD 1983a Epileptic seizures in a population of 6000. 1: Demography, diagnosis and classification, and the role of the hospital services. Br Med J 287: 641–644
Goodridge DMG, Shorvon SD 1983b Epileptic seizures in a population of 6000. 2: Treatment and prognosis. Br Med J 287: 645–647
Gram L 1995 Acetazolamide, lamotrigine and benzodiazepines. In: Duncan JS, Panayiotopoulos CP (eds) Typical absences and related epileptic syndromes. Churchill Livingstone, Edinburgh, p 368–375
Gram L, Klosterkov P, Dam M 1985 Gamma-vinyl GABA: a double-blind placebo-controlled trial in partial epilepsy. Ann Neurol 17: 262–266
Grunewald RA, Chroni E, Panayiotopoulos CP 1992 Delayed diagnosis of juvenile myoclonic epilepsy. J Neurol Neurosurg Psychiat 55: 497–499
Grunewald RA, Thompson PJ, Corcoran RS, Corden Z, Jackson GD, Duncan JS 1994 Effects of vigabatrin on partial seizures and cognitive function. J Neurol Neurosurg Psychiat 57: 1057–1063
Hammond EJ, Wilder BJ 1985 Effect of gamma-vinyl GABA on human pattern evoked visual potentials. Neurology 35: 1801–1803

Hart YM 1992 The early prognosis and care of people with epilepsy. University of London, MD thesis

Hart YM, Sander JWAS, Johnson AL, Shorvon SD 1990 The National General Practice Study of Epilepsy: recurrence after a first seizure. Lancet 336: 1271–1274

Hauser WA, Kurland LT 1975 The epidemiology of epilepsy in Rochester Minnesota 1935 through 1967. Epilepsia 16: 1–66

Heller AJ, Chesterman P, Elwes RDC et al 1995 Phenobarbitone, phenytoin, carbamazepine, or sodium valproate for newly diagnosed adult epilepsy: a randomised, comparative monotherapy trial. J Neurol Neurosurg Psychiat 58: 44–50

Henry TR, Leppik IE, Gumnit RJ et al 1988 Progressive myoclonus epilepsy treated with zonisamide. Neurology 38: 928–931

Jackson GD, Grunewald RA, Connelly A, Duncan JS 1994 Quantitative MR Relaxometry study of effects of Vigabatrin on the brains of patients with epilepsy. Epilepsy Res 18: 127–137

Janz D 1974 Epilepsy and the sleeping waking cycle. In: Magnus O, Lorentz de Haas AM (eds) The epilepsies. Handbook of clinical neurology, vol 15. Amsterdam, North Holland, p 457–490

Jawad S, Richens A, Goodwin G, Yuen WC 1989 Controlled trial of lamotrigine for refractory partial seizures. Epilepsia 30: 356–363

Johnsen SD, Tarby TJ, Sidell AD 1984 Carbamazepine-induced seizures. Ann Neurol 16: 392–393

Kellaway P, Frost JD, Hrachovy RA 1983 Infantile spasms. In: Morselli P, Pippenger CE, Penry JK (eds) Antiepileptic drug therapy in pediatrics. Raven Press, New York, p 115–136

Ketter TA, Malow B, White SR, Post RM, Theodore WH 1992 Anticonvulsant withdrawal-emergent psychopathology. Neurology 42(suppl 3): 450

Knott C 1983 Measurement of saliva drug concentrations in the control of antiepileptic medication. In: Pedley TA, Meldrum BS (eds) Recent advances in epilepsy 1. Churchill Livingstone, Edinburgh, p 57–73

Kramer G, Besser R, Katzmann K, Theisohn M 1985 Slow-release carbamazepine in the treatment of epilepsy. Acta Neurol 12: 70–74

Larkin JG, Herrick AL, McGuire GM, Percy-Robb I, Brodie MJ 1990 Anticonvulsant monitoring at the epilepsy clinic: a prospective evaluation. Epilepsia 32: 89–95

Lees G, Leach MJ 1993 Studies on the mechanism of action of the novel anticonvulsant lamotrigine (Lamictal) using primary neuroglial cultures from rat cortex. Brain Res 612: 190–199

Leonard J V 1991 Inherited metabolic disease: urea cycle disorders, organic acidaemias and non-ketotic hyperglycinaemia. In: Brett E M (ed) Paediatric neurology. Churchill Livingstone, Edinburgh, p 209–222

Leppik IE, Dreifuss FE, Pledger GW 1991 Felbamate for partial seizures: results of a controlled clinical trial. Neurology 41: 1785–1789

Leppik IE, Willmore LJ, Homan RW et al 1993 Efficacy and safety of zonisamide: results of a multicenter study. Epilepsy Res 14: 165–173

Lerman P, Lerman-Sagie T, Kivity S 1991 Effect of early corticosteroid therapy for Landau–Kleffner syndrome. Develop Med Child Neurol 33: 257–266

Levy RH, Mattson RH, Meldrum BS 1995 Antiepileptic drugs, 4th edn. Raven Press, New York

Lockard J S 1980 A primate model of clinical epilepsy: mechanisms of action through quantification of therapeutic effects. In: Lockard J S, Ward A A (eds) Epilepsy: a window to brain mechanisms. Raven Press, New York, p 11–49

Loiseau P, Hardenberg JP, Pestre M et al 1986 Double-blind placebo-controlled study of vigabatrin (gamma-vinyl GABA) in drug-resistant epilepsy. Epilepsia 27: 115–120

Loiseau P, Yuen AW, Duche B, Menager T, Arne-Bes MC 1990 A randomised, double-blind, placebo-controlled, add-on trial of lamotrigine in patients with treatment-resistant partial seizures. Epilepsy Res 7: 136–145

McGuire AM, Duncan JS, Trimble MR 1992 Effects of vigabatrin on cognitive function and mood, when used as add-on therapy in patients with intractable epilepsy. Epilepsia 33: 128–134

McKee PJW, Blacklaw J, Butler E, Gillham RA, Brodie MJ 1991 Monotherapy with conventional and controlled release carbamazepine: a double-blind, double-dummy comparison in epileptic patients. Br J Clin Pharmacol 32: 99–104

McKee PJW, Blacklaw J, Friel E, Thompson GG, Gillham RA, Brodie MJ 1993 Adjuvant vigabatrin in refractory epilepsy: a ceiling to effective dosage in individual patients? Epilepsia 34: 937–943

McKinlay I, Newton R 1989 Intention to treat febrile convulsions with rectal diazepam, valproate or phenobarbitone. Develop Med Child Neurol 31: 617–625

Matsuo F, Bergen D, Faught E et al 1993 Placebo-controlled study of the efficacy and safety of lamotrigine in patients with partial seizures. Neurology 43: 2284–2291

Mattson RH, Cramer JA, Collins JF et al 1985 Comparison of carbamazepine, phenobarbital, phenytoin and primidone in partial and secondarily generalized tonic-clonic seizures. N Engl J Med 313: 145–152

Mattson RH, Cramer JA, Collins JF et al 1992 A comparison of valproate and carbamazepine for the treatment of complex partial seizures and secondarily generalized tonic-clonic seizures in adults. N Engl J Med 327: 765–771

Meador KJ, Loring DW, Huh K, Gallagher BB, King DW 1990 Comparative cognitive effects of anticonvulsants. Neurology 40: 391–394

Messenheimer J, Ramsay RE, Willmore LJ et al 1994 Lamotrigine therapy for partial seizures: a multicenter, placebo-controlled, double-blind, cross-over trial. Epilepsia 35: 113–121

Mireles R, Leppik IL 1985 Valproate and clonazepam comedication in patients with intractable epilepsy. Epilepsia 26: 122–126

Mostofsky D, Balaschak B A 1977 Psychobiological control of seizures. Psychol Bull 84: 723–750

MRC Antiepileptic Drug Withdrawal Study Group 1991 Randomised study of antiepileptic drug withdrawal in patients in remission. Lancet 337: 1175–1180

MRC Antiepileptic Drug Withdrawal Study Group 1993 Prognostic index for recurrence of seizures after remission of epilepsy. Br Med J 306: 1374–1378

Mumford JP, Dam M 1989 Meta-analysis of placebo controlled studies of vigabatrin in drug resistant epilepsy. Br J Clin Pharmacol 27(suppl 1): 101S–108S

Mumford JP, Beaumont D, Gisselbrecht D 1990 Cognitive function, mood and behaviour in vigabatrin treated patients. Acta Neurol Scand 82(suppl 133): 15

Musicco M, Beghi E, Solari A et al 1994 Effect of antiepileptic treatment initiated after the first unprovoked seizure on the long-term prognosis of epilepsy. Neurology 44(suppl 2): A337–A338

Obeso JA, Artieda J, Quinn N et al 1988 Piracetam in the treatment of different types of myoclonus. Clin Neuropharmacol 11: 529–536

Oller LFV, Russi A, Oller Daurella L 1991 Lamotrigine in the Lennox–Gastaut syndrome. Epilepsia 32(suppl. 1): 58

Oommen K, Penry JK, Riela A et al 1993 Gabapentin as add-on therapy in refractory partial epilepsy: a double-blind, placebo-controlled, parallel-group study. Neurology 43: 2292–2298

Painter MJ, Gaus LM 1995 Phenobarbital; clinical use. In: Levy RH, Mattson RH, Meldrum BS (eds) Antiepileptic drugs, 4th edn. Raven Press, New York, p 401-407

Panayiotopoulos CP, Ferrie CD, Knott C, Robinson RO 1993 Interaction of lamotrigine with sodium valproate. Lancet 341: 445

Patsalos PN, Duncan JS 1993 Antiepileptic drugs: a review of clinically significant drug interactions. Drug safety 9: 156–184

Patsalos PN, Duncan JS 1994 New antiepileptic drugs: mechanisms of action, pharmacokinetics and therapeutic efficacy. CNS Drugs 2: 40–77

Patsalos PN, Sander JWAS, Oxley JR, Lascelles PT 1987 Immediate anticonvulsant drug monitoring in the management of epilepsy. Lancet 2: 39

Pedley TA 1988 Discontinuing antiepileptic drugs. N Engl J Med 318: 982–984

Post RM 1982 Use of the anticonvulsant carbamazepine in primary and secondary affective illness: clinical and theoretical implications. Psychol Med 12: 701–704

Preece NA, Jackson GD, Houseman JA, Duncan JS, Williams SR 1994 NMR detection of elevated cortical GABA in the vigabatrin-treated rat in vivo. Epilepsia 35: 431–436

Ramsay RE, Wilder BJ, Berger JR, Bruni J 1983 A double-blind study comparing carbamazepine with phenytoin as initial seizure therapy in adults. Neurology 33: 904–910

Remy C, Favel P, Tell G et al 1986 Etude en double aveugle contre placebo en permutations croisées du vigabatrin dans l'epilepsie de l'adulte résistant à la thérapeutique. Boll Lega Ital Epil 54/55: 241–243

Resor SR, Resor LD 1990 Chronic acetazolamide monotherapy in the treatment of juvenile myoclonic epilepsy. Neurology 40: 1677–1681

Resor SR, Resor LD, Woodbury DM, Kemp JW 1995 Acetazolamide. In: Levy RH, Mattson RH, Meldrum BS (eds) Antiepileptic drugs, 4th edn. Raven Press, New York, p 969-985

Reynolds EH, Shorvon SD 1981 Monotherapy or polytherapy for epilepsy? Epilepsia 22: 1–10

Reynolds EH, Ring HA, Farr IN et al 1991 Open, double-blind and long-term study of vigabatrin in chronic epilepsy. Epilepsia 32: 530–538

Rho JM, Donevan SD, Rogawski MA 1994 Mechanism of action of the anticonvulsant felbamate: opposing effects on *N*-methyl-D-aspartate and $\gamma$–amino butyric acid A receptors. Ann Neurol 1994; 35: 229–234

Richens A, Davidson DLW, Cartlidge NEF et al 1994 A multicentre comparative trial of sodium valproate and carbamazepine in adult onset epilepsy. J Neurol Neurosurg Psychiat 57: 682–687

Richens A, Chadwick DW, Duncan JS et al 1995 Adjunctive treatment of partial seizures with tiagabine: a placebo-controlled trial. Epilepsy Res: 21: 37-42

Rimmer EM, Richens A 1984 Double-blind study of gamma-vinyl GABA in patients with refractory epilepsy. Lancet 2: 189–190

Ring HA, Heller AJ, Farr IN, Reynolds EH 1990 Vigabatrin: rational treatment for chronic epilepsy. J Neurol Neurosurg Psychiat 53: 1051–1053

Ring HA, Crellin R, Kirker S, Reynolds EH 1993 Vigabatrin and depression. J Neurol Neurosurg Psychiat 56: 925–928

Rockstroh B, Elbert T, Birbaumer N et al 1993 Cortical self-regulation in patients with epilepsies. Epilepsy Res 14: 63–72

Rothman DL, Petroff OAC, Behar KL, Mattson RH 1993 Localized $^{1}$H NMR measurements of $\gamma$-aminobutyric acid in human brain *in vivo*. Proc Natl Acad Sci USA 90: 5662–5666

Rowan AJ, Meijer JW, de Beer-Pawlikowski N, van der Geest P, Meinardi H 1983 Valproate-ethosuximide combination therapy for refractory absence seizures. Arch Neurol 40: 797–802

Rowan J, Ahmann P, Wannamaker B et al 1993 Safety and efficacy of three doses of tiagabine HCl versus placebo as adjunctive treatment for complex partial seizures. Epilepsia 34(suppl 2): 157

Sachdeo R, Kramer LD, Rosenberg A, Sachdeo S 1992 Felbamate monotherapy: Controlled trial in patients with partial onset seizures. Ann Neurol 32: 386–392

Sander JWAS 1993 Some aspects of prognosis in the epilepsies: a review. Epilepsia 34: 1007–1016

Sander JWAS, Hart YM, Johnson AL, Shorvon SD 1990a The National General Practice Study of Epilepsy: newly diagnosed epileptic seizures in a general population. Lancet 336: 1276–1271

Sander JWAS, Patsalos PN, Oxley JR, Hamilton MJ, Yuen WC 1990b A randomised, double blind, placebo-controlled, add-on trial of lamotrigine in patients with severe epilepsy. Epilepsy Res 6: 221–226

Sander JWAS, Trevisol-Bittencourt PC, Hart YM, Patsalos PN, Shorvon SD 1990c The efficacy and long-term tolerability of lamotrigine in the treatment of severe epilepsy. Epilepsy Res 7: 226–227

Sander JWAS, Trevisol-Bittencourt PC, Hart YM, Shorvon SD 1990d Evaluation of the efficacy of vigabatrin as an add-on drug in the management of severe epilepsy. J Neurol Neurosurg Psychiat 53: 1008–1010

Sander JWAS, Hart YM, Patsalos PN, Duncan JS, Shorvon SD 1991a Lamotrigine and generalized seizures. Epilepsia 32(suppl 1): 59

Sander JWAS, Hart YM, Trimble MR, Shorvon SD 1991b Vigabatrin and psychosis. J Neurol Neurosurg Psychiatry 54: 435–439

Sato S, Malow BA 1995 Benzodiazepines: clonazepam. In: Levy RH, Mattson RH, Meldrum BS (eds) Antiepileptic drugs, 4th edn. Raven Press, New York, p725-734

Sato S, White BG, Penry JK, Dreifuss FE, Sackellares JC, Kupferberg HJ 1982 Valproic acid versus ethosuximide in the treatment of absence seizures. Neurology 32: 157–163

Schapel GJ, Beran RG, Vajdor FJE et al 1993 Double-blind, placebo-controlled, crossover study of lamotrigine in treatment resistant partial seizures. J Neurol Neurosurg Psychiat 56: 448–453

Schmidt D 1982 Two antiepileptic drugs for intractable epilepsy with complex partial seizures. J Neurol Neurosurg Psychiat 45: 1119–1124

Schmidt D 1983 How to use benzodiazepines. In: Morselli P, Pippenger CE, Penry JK (eds) Antiepileptic drug therapy in pediatrics. Raven Press, New York, p 271–278

Schmidt D, Jacob R, Loiseau P et al 1993 Zonisamide for add-on treatment of refractory partial epilepsy: a European double-blind trial. Epilepsy Res 15: 67–73

Sherwin AL 1995 Ethosuximide: clinical use. In: Levy RH, Mattson RH, Meldrum BS (eds) Antiepileptic drugs, 4th edn. Raven Press, New York, p667-673

Shields WD, Saslow E 1983 Myoclonic atonic and absence seizures following institution of carbamazepine therapy in children. Neurology 33: 1487–1489

Shinnar S, Berg AT, Moshe SL et al 1994 Discontinuing antiepileptic drugs in children with epilepsy: a prospective study. Ann Neurol 35: 534–545

Shorvon SD 1982 The drug treatment of epilepsy. University of Cambridge, MD thesis

Shorvon SD 1984 The temporal aspects of prognosis in epilepsy. J Neurol Neurosurg Psychiatry 47: 1157–1165

Shorvon SD. 1991 Medical assessment and treatment of chronic epilepsy. Br Med J 302: 363–366

Shorvon SD 1995 Clobazam. In: Levy RH, Mattson RH, Meldrum BS (eds) Antiepileptic drugs, 4th edn. Raven Press, New York, p 763-777

Shorvon SD, Reynolds EH 1977 Unnecessary polypharmacy for epilepsy. Br Med J 1: 1635–1637

Shorvon SD, Reynolds EH 1979 Reduction in polypharmacy for epilepsy. Br Med J 2: 1023–1025

Shorvon SD, Reynolds EH 1982 Early prognosis of epilepsy. Br Med J 285: 1699–1701

Sivenius J, Ylinen A, Murros K, Mumford JP, Riekkinen PJ 1991 Vigabatrin in drug resistant partial epilepsy: a 5 year follow-up study. Neurology 41: 562–565

Snead OC III 1990 Treatment of infantile spasms. Pediat Neurol 6: 147–150

Snead OC, Hosey LC 1985 Exacerbation of seizures in children with carbamazepine. N Engl J Med 313: 916–921

Sveinbjornsdóttir S, Sander JWAS, Upton D et al 1993 The excitatory aminoacid antagonist, D-CPP-ene (SDZ EAA-494) in patients with epilepsy. Epilepsy Res 16: 165–174

Tartara A, Manni R, Galimberti CA et al 1986 Vigabatrin in the treatment of epilepsy: a double-blind placebo-controlled study. Epilepsia 27: 717–723

Tartara A, Manni R, Galimberti CA, Mumford JP, Iudice A, Perucca E 1989 Vigabatrin in the treatment of epilepsy: a long-term follow-up study. J Neurol Neurosurg Psychiat 52: 467–471

Tassinari CA, Michelucci R, Ambrosetto G, Salvi F 1987 Double-blind study of vigabatrin in the treatment of drug-resistant epilepsy. Arch Neurol 44: 907–910

Temkin NR, Dikmen SS, Wilensky AJ, Reihm J, Chabal S, Winn HR 1990 A randomized, double-blind study of phenytoin for the prevention of posttraumatic seizures. N Engl J Med 323: 497–502

Theodore WH, Porter RJ 1983 Removal of sedative-hypnotic antiepileptics from the regimens of patients with intractable epilepsy. Ann Neurol 13: 320–324

Theodore WH, Raubertas RF, Porter RJ et al 1991 Felbamate: a clinical trial for complex partial seizures. Epilepsia 32: 392–397

Thompson PJ, Trimble MR 1982 Anticonvulsant drugs and cognitive functions. Epilepsia 23: 531–544

Thurston JH, Thurston DL, Hixon BB, Keller AJ 1982 Prognosis in childhood epilepsy: additional follow-up of 148 children 15–23 years after withdrawal of anticonvulsant therapy. N Engl J Med 306: 831–836

Timmings PL, Richens A 1992 Lamotrigine in primary generalized epilepsy. Lancet 339: 1300

Todt H 1984 The late prognosis of epilepsy of childhood: results of a prospective follow-up study. Epilepsia 25: 137–144

Triggs WJ, Bohan TP, Lin SN, Willmore J 1990 Valproate-induced coma with ketosis and carnitine insufficiency. Arch Neurol 47: 1131–1133

Troupin A, Ojemann LM, Halpern L, Dodrill C, Wilkus R, Friel P 1977 Carbamazepine – a double blind comparison with phenytoin. Neurology 27: 511–519

Troupin AS, Mendius JR, Cheng F, Risinger MW 1986 MK-801. In: Meldrum B, Porter R, eds. New anticonvulsant drugs. John Libbey, London, p 191–201

Turnbull DM, Rawlins MD, Weightman D, Chadwick DW 1982 A comparison of phenytoin and valproate in previously untreated adult epileptic patients. J Neurol Neurosurg Psychiat 45: 55–59

UK Gabapentin Study Group 1990 Gabapentin in partial epilepsy. Lancet 335: 1114–1117

Velez A, Dulac O, Plouin P 1990 Prognosis for seizure control in infantile spasms preceded by other seizures. Brain Develop 12: 306–309

Verity CM, Hosking G, Easter DJ 1995 A multicentre comparative trial of sodium valproate and carbamazepine in paediatric epilepsy. The Paediatric ERITEG Collaborative Group Develop Med Child Neuro: 37: 97-108

Vial H, Claustre Y, Pacheco H 1974 Effets de substances stimulantes, sedatives et hypnotiques sur le taux d'amino-acides cérébrales libres chez le rat. J Pharmacol 5: 461–478

Warner T, Patsalos PN, Prevett MC, Elyas AA, Duncan JS 1992 Pharmacokinetic interaction between lamotrigine and carbamazepine-epoxide. Epilepsy Res 11: 147–150

Whyler A R, Lockard J S, Ward A A, Finch C A 1976 Condition EEG desynchronisation and seizure occurrence in patients. Electroencephalog Clin Neurophysiol 41: 501–512

Wolf SM, Forsythe A 1978 Behaviour disturbance, phenobarbitone and febrile seizures. Paediatrics 61: 728

Yasuhara A, Yoshida H, Hatanaka T, Sugimoto T, Kobayashi Y, Dyken E 1991 Epilepsy with continuous spike-waves during slow sleep and its treatment. Epilepsia 32: 59–62

Ylinen A, Sivenius J, Pitkanen A et al 1992 γ-vinyl GABA (vigabatrin) in epilepsy: clinical, neurochemical, and neurophysiologic monitoring in epileptic patients. Epilepsia 35: 917–922

# 5 Emergency treatment: acute management of seizures, serial seizures and status epilepticus

The principles of emergency short-term treatment of seizures are very different from those of long-term therapy (Ch. 4). In this chapter the acute management of the single self-limiting seizure and serial seizures, and of status epilepticus, will be considered. The EEG aspects of status epilepticus are described in Chapter 3, 3.2.7.

## 5.1 ACUTE MANAGEMENT OF SEIZURES AND SERIAL SEIZURES

### 5.1.1 The acute management of a seizure

If the seizure is likely to occur in any particular situation (for instance at school, work etc) it is best to warn those in contact (e.g. fellow students, workmates, associates, supervisors etc), as the impact of a sudden epileptic seizure is all the greater if unexpected. Major attacks are frightening to onlookers, and the commotion caused is lessened with prior warning. Convulsive seizures are almost always short-lived and do not require immediate medical treatment. Nothing can be done to influence the course of the seizure. The sufferer should be made as comfortable as possible, preferably lying down (or eased to the floor if seated), the head should be protected and tight clothing or neckwear released. During the attack, measures should be taken to avoid injury (e.g. from hot radiators, top of stairs, hot water, road traffic, etc). No attempt should be made to open the mouth or force anything between the teeth. After the convulsive movements have subsided, roll the person into the recovery position, check that the airway is unobstructed and that there are no injuries requiring medical attention. When fully recovered, the patient should be comforted and reassured. An ambulance or emergency treatment is required only if:

- There is serious injury
- The convulsive movements continue for longer than 10 min, or longer than is customary for the individual patient
- The patient does not recover consciousness rapidly
- The seizures recur

Non-convulsive seizures are often less dramatic but can still be frightening to onlookers. Again, little can be done to hasten the resolution of the attacks, which will resolve spontaneously. If consciousness is not lost, the patient should be treated sympathetically and with the minimum of fuss.

Confusion is usual after a convulsive attack, and during and after non-convulsive attacks. During these periods of confusion, it is necessary to prevent injury or danger (for instance from wandering), at the same time minimizing restraint, which often exacerbates the confusion and causes agitation or occasionally violence.

Emergency antiepileptic drug (AED) therapy is needed in convulsive attacks only if the convulsions persist for longer than is customary for the individual patient, or when this is unknown, for more than 10 min. A fast-acting benzodiazepine drug is commonly given. The usual choice is diazepam, administered either intravenously or rectally. Intravenous diazepam is given in its undiluted form at a rate not exceeding 2–5 mg/min, using the Diazemuls® formulation. Rectal administration is given either as the intravenous preparation infused from a syringe via a plastic catheter, or as the ready made proprietary rectal tube preparation Stesolid®, the latter is a convenient and easy method. Diazepam suppositories should not be used, as absorption is too slow. The adult bolus intravenous or rectal dose in status is 10–20 mg, and in children the equivalent bolus dose is 0.2–0.3 mg/kg. The solution should be freshly prepared, and drugs should not be mixed. Alternatively, midazolam, loraze-pam or paraldehyde can be given (details of administration are given below).

## 5.1.2 Serial seizures and clusters of seizures

Serial seizures are those that recur at frequent intervals, with full recovery between attacks. In some patients, such seizure clusters occur on a regular basis (for instance around menstruation). In certain individuals, seizures occur only in clusters. The management of individual seizures in a small cluster is no different from that of an individual attack. If seizures recur at frequent intervals or at an accelerating rate, however, emergency therapy should be initiated, as for the premonitory stage of status epilepticus (see below).

In any individual, if seizure clusters are common, acute therapy after the first seizure can be given in an attempt to prevent subsequent attacks. Clobazam (10–20 mg) is a common choice, given orally, and this will take effect within 1 h. If seizures (either single or clusters) occur at predictable times, prophylactic treatment can be given for a few days, with intermittent oral clobazam 10–20 mg/d or acetazolamide 250–500 mg/d. Oral clobazam can similarly also be given on an occasional basis prophylactically in situations in which seizures would be particularly troublesome (e.g. when travelling, before a wedding, during exams, etc), or after a first seizure if a cluster is the usual pattern, in the hope of terminating the series of seizures.

A worsening of seizure control, with a cluster that may develop into status epilepticus, sometimes occurs as a result of withdrawal of an AED either because of an ill-advised drug change or poor compliance by the patient. The crucial therapy in this situation is to reintroduce the AED that has been withdrawn.

## 5.2 STATUS EPILEPTICUS

Status epilepticus is a condition in which epileptic activity persists for 30 min or more, causing a wide spectrum of clinical symptoms and with a highly variable pathophysiological, anatomical and aetiological basis (Shorvon 1994). It is not simply a rapid repetition of seizures, but a condition that has distinctive pathophysiological features. There are various types of status epilepticus and classification is controversial. The patterns of status are dependent on age, seizure type, underlying aetiology and underlying pathophysiology and a classification should reflect this (Table 5.1). Included in the classification are 'boundary syndromes', which are prolonged states in which the symptoms may be due to ongoing underlying epileptic activity. These include some cases of post-ictal confusion, peri-ictal psychosis and behavioural disorders, and states in which there is evidence of electrographic status without overt seizure activity.

**Table 5.1** Classification of status epilepticus (Shorvon 1994)

*Status epilepticus confined to the neonatal period*

- Neonatal status
- Status in neonatal epilepsy syndromes

*Status epilepticus confined to infancy and childhood*

- Infantile spasm (West's syndrome)
- Febrile status epilepticus
- Status in childhood myoclonic syndromes
- Status in benign childhood partial epilepsy syndromes
- Electrical status during slow wave sleep (ESES)
- Syndrome of acquired epileptic aphasia

*Status epilepticus occurring in childhood and adult life*

- Tonic-clonic status
- Absence status
- Epilepsia partialis continua (EPC)
- Myoclonic status in coma
- Specific forms of status in mental retardation
- Myoclonic status in other epilepsy syndromes
- Non-convulsive simple partial non-convulsive status
- Complex partial status
- Boundary syndromes

*Status epilepticus confined to adult life*

- De novo absence status of late onset

### 5.2.1 Tonic-clonic status epilepticus

Tonic-clonic status epilepticus is defined as a condition in which prolonged or recurrent tonic-clonic seizures persist for 30 min or more. The annual incidence of tonic-clonic status is approximately 18–28 cases per 100 000 persons (9000–14 000 new cases each year in the UK, and 45 000–70 000 cases in the US) (Shorvon 1994). It occurs most commonly in children, the mentally handicapped, and in those with structural cerebral pathology, especially in the frontal lobes. In established epilepsy, status may be precipitated by drug withdrawal, intercurrent illness or metabolic disturbance, or the progression of the underlying disease, and is commoner in symptomatic than in idiopathic epilepsy. About 5% of all adult patients attending an epilepsy clinic will have at least one episode of status in the course of their epilepsy, and in children the proportion is higher (10–25%). Most episodes of status, however, develop de novo and in such cases are almost always due to acute cerebral disturbances; common causes are cerebral infection, trauma, cerebrovascular disease, cerebral tumour, acute toxic or metabolic disturbances and childhood febrile illness. Alper's disease is an uncommon cause of acute status that may be exacerbated by valproate therapy.

There is often a premonitory stage of several hours, during which epileptic activity increases in frequency or severity from its habitual level (Clark & Prout 1903/4). This clinical deterioration is a warning of impending status, and urgent therapy at this stage can prevent full-blown status. At the onset of status, the attacks typically take the form of discrete tonic-clonic seizures; the motor activity then becomes continuous; then the jerking becomes less pronounced, and finally ceases altogether (Roger et al 1974). This is the stage of 'subtle status epilepticus', by which time the patient will be deeply unconscious. There is also sometimes a progressive change in the EEG (Treiman et al 1990). Autonomic changes in status include hyperpyrexia, tachycardia, cardiac arrhythmia, blood pressure changes, apnoea, sweating, hypersecretion and massive noradrenaline and adrenaline release.

The physiological changes in status can be divided into two phases, the transition from phase 1 to phase 2 occurring after about 30–60 min of continuous seizures (Meldrum 1983, Simon 1985, Lothman 1990):

*Phase 1*: At the onset of status, cerebral metabolism is markedly increased. Generally speaking, though, physiological mechanisms are initially sufficient to compensate for these changes. There is a massive increase in cerebral blood flow and the delivery of glucose to the active cerebral tissue is maintained. Systemic and cerebral lactate levels rise and a profound lactic acidosis may develop. Endocrine changes result in initial hyperglycaemia. Blood pressure rises, as does cardiac output and rate. Massive autonomic activity results in sweating, hyperpyrexia, bronchial secretion, salivation and vomiting, and adrenaline and noradrenaline release.

*Phase 2*: Compensatory physiological mechanisms begin to fail as seizure activity continues. Cerebral autoregulation breaks down progressively, and thus cerebral blood flow becomes increasingly dependent on systemic blood pressure. Hypotension develops as a result of seizure-related autonomic and cardiorespiratory changes and drug treatment, and in terminal stages may be severe. The falling blood pressure results in falling cerebral blood flow and cerebral metabolism. The high metabolic demands of the epileptic cerebral tissue cannot be met and this results in ischaemic or metabolic damage (Meldrum 1983). The hypotension can be greatly exacerbated by intravenous antiepileptic drug therapy, especially if infusion rates are too fast.

Other common problems in status are hypoxia and cardiac arrythmias, both of which may require urgent therapy. Intracranial pressure can rise dramatically in late status, and the combined effects of systemic hypotension and intracranial hypertension can result in a compromised cerebral circulation and cerebral oedema, particularly in children. Pulmonary hypertension and oedema occur, and pulmonary artery pressures can exceed the osmotic pressure of blood, causing oedema and stretch injuries to lung capillaries. Cardiac output can fall because of decreasing left ventricular contractility and stroke volume, and cardiac failure can ensue. Profound hyperpyrexia is also a risk in tonic-clonic status.

There are many metabolic and endocrine disturbances in status, the commonest and most important are acidosis, hypoglycaemia, hypo/hyperkalaemia and hyponatraemia. Lactic acidosis is almost invariable in tonic-clonic status epilepticus from its onset (Aminoff & Simon 1980). Other potentially fatal metabolic complications include acute tubular necrosis, renal failure, hepatic failure and disseminated intravascular coagulation. Rhabdomyolysis, resulting from persistent convulsive movements, can precipitate renal failure if severe. This can be prevented by artificial ventilation and muscle paralysis.

The mortality of tonic-clonic status is about 5–10%, most patients dying of the underlying condition rather than the status itself or its treatment. Permanent neurological and mental deterioration may result from status, particularly in young children, the risks of morbidity being greatly increased the longer the duration of the status episode; for this reason urgent effective therapy is vital (Ch. 8, 8.3.2). See Chapter 3, 3.2.7 for EEG investigation of status epilepticus.

## 5.2.2 Epilepsia partialis continua (EPC)

This form of status epilepticus is defined as 'spontaneous regular or irregular clonic twitching of cerebral cortical origin, sometimes aggravated by action or sensory stimuli, confined to one part of the body, and continuing for hours, days or weeks (Obeso et al 1985).

The first cases were reported by Kojewnikoff (1895), who described 'a particular type of cortical epilepsy' in four patients, which he named *epilepsia corticalis sive partialis continua*. The seizure disorder consisted of frequent jerks continuing for years in the same part of the body, uninfluenced by treatment. This condition was due to focal encephalitis with the Russian Spring–Summer tick-borne virus. The jerks typically affect agonist and antagonist muscles, with a rhythmic quality, in short bursts of 1–2 s duration alternating with quiescent phases of 2–4 s persisting in sleep and worsened by action or stress. Jacksonian or generalized epileptic seizures are almost invariable and sometimes frequent accompaniments, although with a strong tendency to improve with time. Sensory symptoms occur in about one-fifth of cases, and 80% of cases have a persisting hemiparesis. A similar clinical picture was described in three patients with a chronic focal encephalitis (Rasmussen et al 1958), a condition henceforward known as Rasmussen's chronic encephalitis. The onset is usually in childhood (mean age 6.8 years, and 85% before the age of 10 years), in about 50% there is a history of preceding infections and all present with epilepsy, usually but not always focal. About half exhibit episodes of epilepsia partialis continua (EPC) (usually within 2 years of the onset of epilepsy). These episodes last hours in some patients and years in others, and are often discontinuous. The condition is progressive and, after a highly variable period, fixed focal deficits develop, notably hemiplegia, hemianopia or aphasia. Other forms of epilepsy occur, and EPC may be a relatively minor feature. Pathological examination reveals changes suggestive of chronic encephalitis confined to the cerebral cortex of one hemisphere (Oguni et al 1991). Cytomegalovirus infection has been implicated but no infective agent has been definitively identified. Since the early 1970s, EPC has come to be seen simply as a form of simple partial motor status epilepticus. Viewed in this light, cases with widely varying aetiologies can be included (Thomas et al 1977, Shorvon 1994).

The clonic jerks in EPC can affect any muscle group. In some individuals, the jerks are confined to a single muscle or muscle group, but in others the distribution is more widespread, and the distribution of the jerks can vary over time. Agonists and antagonists are affected together, and distal muscles are more commonly involved than proximal musculature. When widespread, the jerking is usually synchronous, and palatal myoclonus is occasionally seen. The jerks are spontaneous and often exacerbated on action, startle or sensory stimuli. They can be single or cluster and may have a rhythmic quality and a wide range of frequencies and amplitudes. Some jerks recur only every few minutes and others are more frequent. In chronic cases the myoclonus may have continued relentlessly for months or years. In some individuals with long-lasting myoclonus, periods of freedom from jerking are experienced, without obvious cause.

The presence of other neurological signs, other seizure types depend on the underlying pathology, as do the EEG findings which are often relatively non-specific, showing simply focal ictal and interictal epileptic features often in with a wider distribution than the clinical picture would lead one to expect.

The Russian and Canadian cases of EPC are due to encephalitic conditions. Pathological examination of tissue from other patients with EPC who do not conform to the picture of a chronic encephalitis may show degenerative or inflammatory changes which are not easily characterized. Other reported aetiologies include cerebral infarction or haemorrhage, cerebral tumour, metabolic encephalopathy, mitochondrial disease, subacute measles encephalopathy in immunosuppressed children, non-ketotic hyperglycinaemia and Alper's disease.

### 5.2.3 Complex partial status epilepticus

This form of non-convulsive status can be defined as a prolonged epileptic episode in which fluctuating or frequently recurring focal electrographic epileptic discharges result in a confusional state. There are highly variable clinical symptoms and the focal epileptic discharges may arise in temporal or extratemporal cortical regions.

Periods of complex partial status can last for days or even weeks, although typically an episode will persist for several hours. It is commonest in adults, usually developing in patients with long histories of complex partial epilepsy. Precipitating factors include menstruation, alcohol and drug withdrawal (but not usually photic stimulation or overbreathing as in typical absence status). The onset and offset are usually less well defined than in absence status and the response to intravenous therapy more gradual. Complex partial status may typically follow a secondary generalized tonic-clonic seizure (or cluster of seizures), but is rarely terminated by a generalized convulsion, in contrast to the case in typical absence status. Episodes of complex partial status are usually recurrent, and occasionally there is a remarkable periodicity (Cockerell et al 1994).

Confusion is the leading clinical feature of complex partial status. This can fluctuate or be fairly continuous. The severity of the confusion can varying from profound stupor with little response to external stimuli in some cases to others in whom subtle abnormalities on cognitive testing are the only sign. Amnesia is usual but not invariable.

Associated with the confusion are other symptoms (Williamson et al 1985, Tomson et al 1986, Dunne et al 1987, Rohr-Le Floch et al 1988, Shorvon 1994), including:

*Behavioural features*: These are vary variable, ranging from agitation, even occasionally mania, to severe psychomotor retardation or stupor. Occasionally, behaviour may appear almost normal. Commonly, the patient appears alert but rather sluggish, behaves in a restless and apparently questing fashion and may seem facile or silly. Reactions are usually slow. Aggressive, hostile or anxious behaviour can occur. Psychotic symptoms are often prominent, including delusions, catatonia, visual or auditory hallucinations, ideas of reference, paranoia, illogical responses and often a curious perseverative obsessive insistence on oppositions, such as black/white, good/bad, left/right. Severe schizophrenic or autistic features can be present and a misdiagnosis of a psychiatric condition is common.

*Speech and language disturbance*: Speech patterns are often abnormal, with aphasia, perseveration, confabulation, echolalia and stereotyped repetitive utterances. Language is usually sparse and responses to questions, although eventually appropriate, may show a marked delay.

*Motor features*: Posturing, clonic jerks, tonic spasm, adversion of the head and eyes and motor automatisms occur. Lip-smacking, orofacial automatism, posturing and gestural automatisms are common but not usually as marked as in isolated complex partial seizures.

*Other clinical features*: Autonomic disturbances, including belching, flatulence, change in colour, pupillary dilatation or fever, and sensory symptoms or signs may occur.

*Fluctuation and cycling of signs*: In some cases, the confusional state is continuous or virtually continuous over long periods of time and in others, fluctuations or cycling of signs are a prominent feature. Sometimes, rapidly repeated discrete complex partial seizures can be identified within the confusional state. In some cases, individual seizures are subtle in form and difficult to detect, manifest only by brief motor automatisms, colour changes, dilatation of the pupil, or sometimes nothing more than a blank spell.

The scalp EEG findings may be slight although seldom normal. A whole range of EEG patterns are seen including continuous or frequent spike or spikes/slow wave, or spike/wave paroxysms that are sometimes widespread or focal, and also episodes of desynchronization. The longer the status proceeds, the less likely is discrete ictal activity to be noticeable. The focal abnormalities can be maximal in temporal or extratemporal sites. Intracranial EEG has been much more informative than scalp EEG and discrete and continuous focal ictal activity is usually seen. This is often from frontal rather than temporal cortex, and an extratemporal origin for the status is common (Williamson et al 1985).

Complex partial status can arise in focal epilepsies of widely varying aetiologies and carries no aetiological specificity. Neuroimaging will often show an underlying structural lesion, but transient focal abnormalities suggestive of vasogenic cerebral oedema are occasionally seen on X-ray CT or MRI scans, which disappear when the seizures resolve.

The prognosis of complex partial status is good. It is not usually life-threatening and resolves with oral or intravenous therapy. There is a strong tendency for recurrence however. Permanent neurological or psychological sequelae are rare, in contrast to the poor prognosis of tonic-clonic status.

## 5.2.4 Absence status

Absence status can be best subdivided into at least two separate syndromes, with overlapping clinical and EEG features.

*Typical absence status*: Non-convulsive status occurring in the syndrome of idiopathic generalized epilepsy.

*Atypical absence status*: Status that occurs largely in secondarily generalized epilepsy of the Lennox–Gastaut type, and also in other patients with compromised cerebral function and transitional cases. These two conditions should be distinguished from *complex partial status*, which is non-convulsive focal status and which may have a very similar clinical and electrographic form (see above, 5.2.3).

### *Typical absence status*

This occurs only in patients with idiopathic generalized epilepsy and thus in a context very different from that of either atypical absence status or complex partial status (Roger et al 1974, Rohr-Le Floch et al 1988, Shorvon 1995). A history of absence status occurs in about 3–9% of patients with a history of typical absences. The attacks can recur and can last for hours or occasionally days. Precipitating features are common and include menstruation, withdrawal of medication, hypoglycaemia, hyperventilation, flashing or bright lights, sleep deprivation, fatigue, stress and grief.

The principal clinical feature of typical absence status is clouding of consciousness. This can vary from slight clouding to profound stupor. At one extreme, patients have nothing more than slowed ideation and expression and deficits in activities requiring sustained attention, sequential organization or spatial structuring. Amnesia may be slight or even absent. At the other extreme, there may be immobility, mutism, simple voluntary actions performed only after repeated requests, long delays in verbal responses and monosyllabic and hesitant speech. Typically the patient is in an expressionless, trance-like state with slow responses and a stumbling gait.

Motor features occur in about 50% of cases, including myoclonus, atonia, rhythmic eyelid blinking, quivering of the lips, facial grimacing and smiling. Facial, especially eyelid, myoclonus is common in absence status but rare in complex partial status. Episodes of absence status are often terminated by a tonic-clonic seizure.

The diagnostic electrographic pattern is continuous or almost continuous bilaterally synchronous and symmetrical spike/wave activity, with little or no reactivity to sensory stimuli. The classical EEG appearance with 3 Hz spike/wave is usually seen in the setting of idiopathic generalized epilepsy, and the closer the EEG is to this classic pattern the more typical the clinical features. Other heterogeneous forms have been described, including irregular and slow spike/wave (1.5–4 Hz), prolonged bursts of spike activity, generalized periodic triphasic sharp waves and polyspike and wave at frequencies from 2–6 Hz. Whether to include such cases within the rubric of absence status and quite where to draw the nosological line is uncertain. The cycling of EEG changes seen in complex partial status is not usual in typical absence status, but does occur, and in some patients the spike/wave is not continuous but rather broken into frequent bursts.

*Atypical absence status*

This form of status is common in patients with diffuse cerebral damage and is typically seen as part of the Lennox–Gastaut syndrome (Ch. 2, 2.6.8) (Dravet et al 1985, Beaumanoir et al 1988, Shorvon 1994). The clinical phenomenology of typical and atypical absence status overlap greatly, although there are important differences. The clinical context is very different: typical absence status occurs in patients without intellectual deterioration, very unlike the clinical picture of the Lennox–Gastaut syndrome. The temporal course of the status differs, with episodes of atypical absence status usually being longer and more frequent, with a gradual onset and offset. Atypical absence status is often preceded by changes in motor activity, mood or intellectual ability for hours or days before the overt seizures develop. This prodromal stage might be due to subclinical status. Once atypical absence status has developed, it tends to fluctuate and minor motor, myoclonic or more typically tonic seizures interrupt but do not terminate an episode. In some patients, the mental state fluctuates gradually in and out of this ill defined epileptic state over long periods of time (some attacks last weeks or even months), with little distinction possible between ictal and interictal phases. Unlike typical absence status, tonic-clonic seizures seldom occur at the beginning or end of the status episode, and atypical absence status often responds poorly to injection of a benzodiazepine. Indeed antiepileptic drug therapy can have little effect and the condition fluctuates apparently uninfluenced by external factors. Atypical absence status is more likely to occur if the patient is drowsy or understimulated and it is thus important not to overmedicate these patients.

The EEG during atypical absence status may show continuous irregular slow (2 Hz) spike/wave, or hypsarrhythmia, or more discrete ictal patterns. 3 Hz spike-wave can be seen in some patients and is difficult to differentiate from that of typical absence status (Ch. 3, 3.2.7).

## 5.3 THE EMERGENCY TREATMENT OF TONIC-CLONIC STATUS EPILEPTICUS

The principles of treatment of status are very different from those of chronic epilepsy (Shorvon 1994). The priorities are to halt seizure activity as rapidly as possible, prevent injury, maintain cardiorespiratory function and avoid secondary medical complications. The potential long-term side-effects of medication and pharmacokinetics of chronic therapy are of no importance. Treatment consists of (1) general measures and (2) antiepileptic drug therapy.

### 5.3.1 General measures

The treatment of tonic-clonic status epilepticus is best considered in successive stages (Table 5.2).

*1st stage (0–10 min)*

In all patients presenting in status, the protection of cardiorespiratory function takes first priority. Cardiorespiratory function should be assessed, the airway secured and resuscitation carried out if necessary. Hypoxia is usually much worse than appreciated and oxygen should always be administered.

*2nd stage (1–60 min)*

*a. Monitoring* should be instituted, including: neurological observations, measurements of pulse, blood pressure, ECG and temperature. Regular measurements should be made of: blood urea, electrolytes, liver function, sugar, calcium and phosphorus; blood gases and pH; haematological and clotting parameters.

*b. Emergency anticonvulsant therapy* should be started (see below).

*c. Intravenous lines* should be set up. Drugs should not be mixed and if two antiepileptic drugs are needed (e.g. phenytoin and diazepam) two intravenous lines are required. Many antiepileptic drugs cause severe phlebitis and thrombosis at the site of infusion, and the lines should beplaced in large veins. Arterial lines must *never* be used for drug administration as arterial spasm, necrosis, thrombosis and embolism can result.

*d. Emergency investigations*: Emergency measurement should be made of: blood gases; sugar; renal and liver function, calcium and magnesium levels; haematological and blood clotting measures (including platelets); and serum antiepileptic drug concentrations. 20 ml of serum should also be saved for future analysis if the cause of the status is unknown.

*e. Intravenous glucose and thiamine*: Hypoglycaemia may cause status and 50 ml of a 50% glucose solution should be given immediately intravenously if this is suspected. 250 mg of thiamine should also be given with glucose if there is a history of alcoholism or other compromised nutritional state, as glucose without thiamine can precipitate Wernicke's encephalopathy in susceptible patients. Routine glucose administration in non-hypoglycaemic patients should be avoided because of this and also because of evidence that hyperglycaemia can itself aggravate neuronal damage. A suitable preparation of thiamine is the high-potency intravenous formulation Parenterovite (10 ml of which contains 250 mg). The intravenous injection should be given slowly (e.g. 10 ml over 10 min), with facilities for treating anaphylaxis, to minimize the dangers of an allergic reaction.

*f. Acidosis*: The rapid control of respiration and abolition of motor seizure activity will usually reverse the acidosis which is common in status. Additional bicarbonate infusion is seldom necessary, but can be given in severe acidosis to lessen the chance of cardiorespiratory shock.

**Table 5.2** General measures in the treatment of tonic-clonic status epilepticus

*1st (0–10 min)*

- Assess cardiorespiratory function
- Secure airway and resuscitate
- Administer oxygen

*2nd (0–60 min)*

- Institute regular monitoring (see text)
- Emergency antiepileptic drug therapy (see text)
- Set up intravenous lines
- Emergency investigations (see text)
- Administer glucose (50 ml of 50% solution) and/or thiamine (250 mg as HPIV parenterovite) where appropriate
- Treat acidosis if severe

*3rd (0–60/90 min)*

- Establish aetiology
- Identify and treat medical complications
- Pressor therapy

*4th (30–90 min)*

- Transfer to intensive care
- Establish intensive care and EEG monitoring (see text)
- Initiate seizure and EEG monitoring
- Initiate intracranial pressure monitoring
- Initiate long-term maintenance antiepileptic therapy

These four stages should be followed chronologically; stages 1 and 2 within 10 min and stage 4 (transfer to ITU) in most settings within 60-90 min of presentation

*3rd Stage (1–60/90 min)*

*a. Establish aetiology*: Investigations depend on clinical circumstances and causes differ in patients with or without histories of existing epilepsy and in different age groups. A CT brain scan and CSF examination are often required, the latter being carried out only where facilities for resuscitation are available, as intracranial pressure is often elevated in status.

*b. Physiological changes and medical complications*: Treatment is often necessary to counter such complications as hypoxia, hypotension, raised intracranial pressure, pulmonary oedema and hypertension, cardiac arrhythmias, cardiac failure, lactic acidosis, hyperpyrexia, hypoglycaemia, electrolyte disturbance, acute hepatic or renal failure, rhabdomyolysis and disseminated intravascular coagulation.

*c. Pressor therapy*: Pressor therapy is required by many patients in prolonged status, especially if intravenous sedative drugs have been given. Dopamine is the most commonly used agent, given by continuous intravenous infusion. The dose should be titrated to attain the desired haemodynamic and renal responses (usually initially between 2–5 μg/kg/min, but this can be increased to over 20 μg/kg/min in severe hypotension), and ECG monitoring to detect effects on conduction is required, especially in the presence of cardiac failure. Dopamine should be given into a large vein as extravasation causes tissue necrosis. Dobutamine at a rate of 2.5 μg/kg/min is an alternative.

*4th stage (30–90 min)*

*a. Intensive care:* If seizures are continuing in spite of the measures taken above, the patient must be transferred to an intensive care setting.

*b. Intensive care monitoring*: In prolonged status, intensive monitoring is desirable, including intra-arterial blood pressure, capnography, oximetry, central venous pressure and Swan–Ganz monitoring.

*c. Seizure and EEG monitoring*: Motor activity in status diminishes over time and may become barely apparent, especially in comatose or ventilated patients. Electrographic activity and burst suppression can be detected by using either a full EEG or a cerebral function monitor (CFM) (Altafullah et al 1991). The CFM has to be calibrated for each individual patient but then has the advantage over EEG of simplicity of use. Burst suppression provides an arbitrary physiological target for the titration of barbiturate or anaesthetic therapy, with drug dosing commonly set at a level that aims to produce burst suppression with interburst intervals of between 2–30 s (Ch. 3, 3.2.6).

*d. Intracranial pressure (ICP) monitoring and cerebral oedema*: If there is evidence of persisting, severe or progressively elevated intracranial pressure, ICP monitoring is advisable. The need for this is usually determined by the underlying cause rather than the status. If ICP is critically raised, intermittent positive pressure ventilation, high-dose corticosteroid therapy (4 mg dexamethasone every 6 h) or mannitol infusion can be used to lower the pressure, and neurosurgical decompression is occasionally required.

*e. Long-term antiepileptic drug therapy*: Maintenance antiepileptic therapy must be initiated as soon as possible, along with emergency treatment. The choice of drug depends on previous therapy, the type of epilepsy and the clinical setting. Both phenytoin or phenobarbitone can be used as emergency and maintenance therapy and can be continued orally (through a nasogastric tube) after intravenous loading. Other maintenance AEDs can also be given via oral loading doses, and blood level estimations can help define the optimal dosage.

### 5.3.2 Emergency antiepileptic drug treatment

The emergency drug treatment of tonic-clonic status epilepticus can be usefully divided into four stages. There are several options for drug treatment in each stage, and choice is to an extent arbitrary. The authors' preferred regimen for the typical case of newly developing status presenting to a casualty department is shown in Table 5.3. In cases of status epilepticus precipitated by AED withdrawal or non-compliance, the immediate restitution of the withdrawn drug will usually avert or rapidly terminate the status.

**Table 5.3** Emergency antiepileptic drug regimen for tonic-clonic status epilepticus in newly presenting adult patients

*Premonitory stage*

- Diazepam 10 mg given i.v. or rectally, repeated once 15 min later if status continues to threaten, at a rate not exceeding 2–5 mg/min

— If seizures continue, treat as below

*Early status*

- Lorazepam (i.v.) 4 mg bolus, repeated after 10 min (rate not critical)

— If seizures continue 30 min after first injection, treat as below

*Established status*

- Phenobarbitone bolus of 10 mg/kg at a rate of 100 mg/min (e.g. about 700 mg over 7 min in an adult)

*and/or*

- Phenytoin infusion at a dose of 18 mg/kg at a rate of 50 mg/min (e.g. 1000 mg in 20 min) with 10 mg diazepam if not already given

— If seizures continue for 30/60 min or longer, treat as below

*Refractory status*

- General anaesthesia, with either propofol or thiopentone
- Anaesthetic continued for 12–24 h after the last clinical or electrographic seizure, then dose tapered

In the above scheme, the refractory stage (general anaesthesia) is reached 60–90 min after the initial therapy. This scheme is suitable for usual clinical hospital settings. In some situations, general anaesthesia should be initiated earlier, and occasionally it should be delayed.

*In all stages*

- Ensure that the patient's regular AEDs are administered, including any AED that has recently been withdrawn or omitted. If the patient was not on maintenance therapy before the status, this should be initiated

*Premonitory stage*

Parenteral drug treatment in this phase will often prevent the development of full-blown status. One of three drugs is used, and each is highly effective: diazepam, midazolam or paraldehyde. The earlier treatment is given the more successful it is. If the patient is at home, antiepileptic drugs should be administered before transfer to hospital, or in the casualty department before transfer to the ward. Acute parenteral therapy will cause drowsiness or sleep, and occasionally cardiorespiratory collapse, and should therefore be carefully supervised.

*Stage of early status epilepticus (0–30 min)*

Once status epilepticus has developed, treatment should be carried out in hospital, under close supervision. It is usual to initiate treatment with a fast-acting benzodiazepine drug. Intravenous lorazepam or diazepam (but not both together) is the usual drug of choice. Rectal or intramuscular paraldehyde is a useful alternative where facilities for intravenous injection or for resuscitation are not freely available (for instance in nursing homes, where it can be administered by nursing staff). Intravenous lignocaine may be preferable in patients with respiratory disease. In most episodes of status, initial treatment will be highly effective. Even if seizures cease, 24-h in-patient observation should follow. In persons without a previous history of epilepsy, chronic AED treatment should be introduced, and in those already on maintenance antiepileptic therapy this should be reviewed.

*Stage of established status epilepticus (30–60-90 min)*

If status continues for 30 min despite early-stage treatment, intensive care facilities are mandatory. There are three alternative first-line treatment options, but each has drawbacks and status at this stage carries an appreciable morbidity. These are subanaesthetic doses of phenobarbitone, or phenytoin, both given by intravenous loading followed by repeated oral or intravenous supplementation, or chlormethiazole given by intravenous bolus and continuous infusion. Diazepam is often given with phenytoin (either at this or the early stage of status), combining the fast-acting but short-lasting effect of diazepam with the slow-onset but long-lasting effect of phenytoin. Second-line treatment options include continuous intravenous infusions of clonazepam, diazepam, paraldehyde, or midazolam, at various dosages. However, continuous benzodiazepine infusions carry a significant risk of cardiorespiratory collapse and should not be undertaken without ITU support. Lorazepam and lignocaine are essentially short-term therapies and so should not be employed at this stage.

*Stage of refractory status epilepticus (after 60-90 min)*

In most patients, if seizures continue for 60–90 min after the initiation of therapy, full anaesthesia is required. In some emergency situations (e.g. postoperative status, severe or complicated convulsive status, patients already in ITU), anaesthesia can and should be introduced earlier. The prognosis is now much poorer and there is a high risk of mortality and morbidity.

The principles of therapy are similar for all anaesthetics, and presumably a wide range of barbiturate and non-barbiturate anaesthetic agents could be used. Thiopentone and pentobarbitone are the usual barbiturate drugs used in status. They have strong antiepileptic action but problematic pharmacokinetic properties. The non-barbiturate drugs used in status are isoflurane, etomidate and propofol. These have convenient pharmacokinetics, in particular short half-life, lack of accumulation, non-saturable kinetics, lack of autoinduction and tolerance, and are also much less toxic, without the cardiorespiratory risks of barbiturate therapy. Experience with these agents in status is, however, meagre and furthermore, although all are powerful anaesthetics, they do not generally have anti-epileptic properties; indeed, some exhibit proconvulsant properties at subanaesthetic doses. Whether such non-anticonvulsant anaesthesia is as effective in status as anticonvulsant anaesthesia is quite unclear. All the drugs are given in doses sufficient to induce deep unconsciousness; therefore assisted respiration, intensive cardiovascular monitoring and the full panoply of intensive care are essential. The depth of anaesthesia should be sufficient to abolish all clinical and EEG epileptic activity (often requiring sedation to the point of burst suppression on the EEG), and cerebral electrical activity must by necessity be visualized, either with a formal EEG or a cerebral function monitor (Ch. 3, 3.2.6).

*Failure to respond to treatment*

In the great majority of cases, the above measures will control the seizures and the status will resolve. If drug treatment fails, there are often complicating factors. Common reasons for the failure to control seizures in status epilepticus are:

- *Inadequate drug treatment*
  - Insufficient emergency antiepileptic drug therapy. A particular problem is the administration of intravenous drugs at too low a dosage (for instance with phenobarbitone or phenytoin)
  - Failure to initiate or continue maintenance antiepileptic drug therapy in parallel with the acute emergency therapy. This will result in recrudescence of seizures once the effects of the emergency drug treatment has worn off
- *Additional medical factors*
  - Medical complications can exacerbate seizures (Table 5.4)
  - A failure to treat (or identify) the underlying cause can result in intractable status. This is particularly the case in acute progressive cerebral disorders and cerebral infections
- *Misdiagnosis*
  - A common problem is to fail to diagnose pseudostatus (see below, 5.5) which, in specialist practice, is commoner than true epileptic status

### 5.3.3 Complications of status epilepticus

Tonic-clonic status is a serious condition, with appreciable morbidity and mortality (Table 5.4). Focal neurological deficit may follow status, especially in children and after prolonged status. Mental and personality changes are not infrequent in the wake of a severe episode, and chronic epilepsy may also be a sequel. Status has been shown to result in neuronal loss and gliosis in hippocampus, cerebral cortex and other regions in experimental models. The neuropathological damage may be due directly to excitotoxin release, and occur in the presence of adequate oxygenation, cerebral glucose levels and circulatory function. The relevance of this work to human status is not clear.

Status epilepticus can result in death, mortality rates in different series falling between 3–60%. The most important factor influencing mortality in tonic-clonic status is the underlying cause. The mortality rate of idiopathic status is low (1–5%) compared with rates as high as 50% recorded in symptomatic status. Up to 90% of deaths in status are directly attributable to the underlying cerebral or metabolic disorder. The duration of status is also a factor determining outcome, with morbidity and mortality rising sharply in cases that persist for 24 h or more. The highest mortality rates are experienced in neonatal status, in infancy and in the elderly.

**Table 5.4** Medical complications of tonic-clonic status epilepticus

*Cerebral*

- Hypoxic/metabolic cerebral damage
- Seizure-induced cerebral damage
- Cerebral oedema and raised intracranial pressure
- Cerebral venous thrombosis
- Cerebral haemorrhage and infarction

*Cardiovascular, respiratory and autonomic*

- Hypotension
- Hypertension
- Cardiac failure, tachy- and bradyarrhythmia, arrest
- Cardiogenic shock
- Respiratory failure
- Disturbances of respiratory rate and rhythm, apnoea
- Pulmonary oedema, hypertension, embolism
- Pneumonia, aspiration
- Hyperpyrexia
- Sweating, hypersecretion, tracheo-broncheal obstruction
- Peripheral ischaemia

*Metabolic*

- Dehydration
- Electrolyte disturbance (especially hyponatraemia, hyperkalaemia, hypoglycaemia)
- Acute renal failure (especially acute tubular necrosis)
- Acute hepatic failure
- Acute pancreatitis

*Other*

- Disseminated intravascular coagulopathy/multiorgan failure
- Rhabdomyolysis
- Fractures
- Infections (especially pulmonary, skin, urinary)
- Thrombophlebitis, dermal injury

## 5.3.4 Drugs used in status epilepticus

*Diazepam*

Diazepam (Delgado-Escueta & Enrile-Bacsal 1983, Rémy et al 1992, Schmidt 1995) is useful in the premonitory or early stages of status. There is extensive clinical experience in adults, children and the newborn; the drug has well-proved efficacy in many types of status, a rapid onset of action and well-studied pharmacology and pharmacokinetics. Diazepam has a number of important disadvantages, however, which limit its usefulness in status. Although it has a rapid onset of action, it is highly lipid-soluble and thus has a short duration of action after a single injection, with a strong tendency for seizures to relapse after initial control. Furthermore, diazepam accumulates on repeated injections or after continuous infusion, with a high risk of sudden respiratory depression, sedation and hypotension. Other disadvantages are its dependency on hepatic metabolism and its metabolism to an active metabolite, which can complicate prolonged therapy. A combination of diazepam and phenytoin is popular, combining the rapid onset but short-lived action of diazepam with the slow onset but long-lasting effects of phenytoin. Diazepam has a tendency to precipitate from concentrated solutions and to interact with other drugs, and is absorbed on to plastic on prolonged contact.

*Usual preparations:* i.v. formulation – diazepam emulsion, 1 ml ampoule containing 5 mg/ml or i.v. solution 2 ml ampoules containing 5 mg/ml. Rectal formulation – 2.5 ml rectal tube containing 2 mg/ml or, using the i.v. solution, 2 ml ampoule containing 5 mg/ml.

*Usual dosage:* i.v. bolus (undiluted) – 10–20 mg (adults); 0.25–0.5 mg/kg (children), at a rate not exceeding 2–5 mg/min. The bolus dosing can be repeated. Rectal administration – 10–30 mg (adults); 0.5–0.75 mg/kg (children); and this can be repeated.

*Midazolam*

Midazolam (Dundee et al 1984, Galvin & Jellinek 1987) is another benzodiazepine, an alternative to diazepam, which can be used in the premonitory or early stages of status. It has one major advantage over diazepam, that it is rapidly absorbed by intramuscular (i.m.) injection. It is therefore useful in situations in which i.v. administration is difficult or ill advised. It has a rapid onset of action after i.m. administration (Jawad et al 1986) and, although there is a danger of accumulation on prolonged or repeated therapy, this tendency is less than with diazepam. There is, however, only limited published experience in adults with status, and none in children. Occasionally, severe cardiorespiratory depression occurs after i.m. administration, and other adverse effects include hypotension, apnoea, sedation and thrombophlebitis. Like diazepam, the drug is short-acting, and there is a strong tendency for seizures to relapse after initial control; as with diazepam, its metabolism is altered by hepatic disease.

*Usual preparation*: 5 ml ampoule containing 2 mg/ml midazolam hydrochloride.

*Usual dosage*: i.m. or rectally – 5–10 mg (adults); 0.15–0.3 mg/kg (children). This can be repeated once after 15 min. i.v. bolus of 0.1–0.3 mg/kg, at a rate not to exceed 4 mg/min, which can be repeated once after 15 min. An i.v. infusion can be given at a rate of 0.05–0.4 mg/kg/h.

*Paraldehyde*

Paraldehyde (Koren et al 1986, Browne 1983, Lockman 1995) still has a useful place in premonitory and early status, as an alternative to diazepam, especially in situations where facilities for resuscitation are not available. Paraldehyde is rapidly and completely absorbed after i.m. injection or rectally. The risks of drug accumulation are low. The risks of hypotension and cardiorespiratory arrest are small, and seizures do not often recur after control has been obtained. Paraldehyde has been used for many years in status, and although there is wide experience in patients of all ages, no modern pharmacokinetic or clinical studies have been carried out. Toxicity is unusual provided the solution is freshly made, used immediately and correctly diluted. The use of decomposed or inadequately diluted i.v. solutions is dangerous, causing precipitation, microembolism, thrombosis and cardiorespiratory collapse. The i.m. injection of paraldehyde is painful and can cause sterile abscess and sciatic nerve damage if wrongly placed. Other side-effects include cardiorespiratory depression, sedation and metabolic or lactic acidosis. The drug rapidly binds to plastic, and glass tubing and syringes are advisable unless injected immediately upon drawing the solution up. The drug should not be exposed to light. The half-life of paraldehyde is markedly increased by hepatic disease.

*Usual preparation:* Ampoule containing 5 ml paraldehyde (equivalent to approximately 5 g; in darkened glass).

*Usual dosage:* Paraldehyde can be given rectally (or i.m.) 5–10 ml, diluted by the same volume of water for injection (adults), or 0.07–0.35 ml/kg (children). This dose can be repeated after 15–30 min.

*Chlormethiazole*

Chlormethiazole (Harvey et al 1975, Miller & Kovar 1983, Lingam et al 1980, Laxenaire et al 1966) is a valuable drug in established status epilepticus. It is given by i.v. bolus followed by a continuous infusion. The drug is rapidly distributed and has a very rapid and short-lived initial action. Dosage can be initially titrated against response, on a moment-by-moment basis, without inducing respiratory arrest or anaesthesia, a unique property among drugs used in status. The danger of chlormethiazole is that it accumulates on prolonged use, with the risk of sudden cardiorespiratory collapse, hypotension and sedation. There is also a danger of respiratory arrest and hypotension if the maximum rate of injection is exceeded. Other side-effects include cardiac rhythm disturbances, vomiting and thrombophlebitis, and there is a tendency for seizure recurrence on discontinuing therapy. Prolonged therapy carries the risk of fluid overload and electrolyte disturbance. There is limited published experience in status, particularly in children, and insufficient published data for neonatal use. Hepatic disease reduces the metabolism and elimination of the drug. Chlormethiazole is slowly absorbed by plastic.

*Usual preparation*: 0.8% solution of chlormethiazole edisylate in 500 ml in 4% dextrose (8 mg/ml).

*Usual dosage*: i.v. infusion of 40–100 ml (320–800 mg), at rate of 5–15 ml/min, followed by a continuous infusion, with dosage titrated according to response (usually 1–4 ml/min, range 0.5 ml–20 ml/min) (adults); initially 0.1 ml/kg/min (0.08 mg/kg/min) increasing progressively every 2–4 h as required (children).

*Clonazepam*

The main indication of clonazepam in status is as an alternative to diazepam in early status, and there is little to choose between the two drugs (Gastaut et al 1971, Gimenez-Roldán et al 1972, Congdon & Forsythe 1980). It has a similar onset of action, a longer duration of action and a lower incidence of late relapse. There is wide experience with the drug in adults and children, although not in neonates, and the drug has proven efficacy in tonic-clonic, partial and absence status. Clonazepam accumulates on prolonged infusion, with the resulting risk of respiratory arrest, hypotension and sedation – a side-effect profile similar to that of diazepam. There is also a danger of sudden collapse if the recommended rate of injection is exceeded. A continuous infusion of clonazepam may be used, but only in ITU settings because of the risks of sudden cardiorespiratory collapse.

*Usual preparation:* 1 ml ampoule containing 1 mg of clonazepam.

*Usual dosage*: 1–2 mg bolus injection over 30 s (adults). 250–500 μg (children), which can be repeated up to four times. The 1 ml ampoule of clonazepam is mixed with 1 ml of water for injection (provided as diluent) *immediately* before administration. The rate of injection should not exceed 1 mg in 30 s. The drug can also be given more slowly in a dextrose (5%) or 0.9% sodium chloride solution (1–2 mg in 250 ml). A continuous infusion in 0.9% sodium chloride or dextrose (5%) at a dose of 10 mg/24 h (3 mg in 250 ml) can be given if the patient is in an intensive care unit.

*Lignocaine*

Lignocaine (Pascual et al 1992, De Giorgio et al 1991) is given in early status only, as a bolus injection or short i.v. infusion. The clinical effects and pharmacokinetics have been extensively studied in patients of all ages, and the drug is highly effective. The main disadvantage of lignocaine is that its antiepileptic effects are short-lived and seizures are controlled for a matter of hours only; the drug is thus useful only while more definitive antiepileptic drug treatment is administered. The risk of drug accumulation is low, and the incidence of respiratory or cerebral depression and hypotension is lower than with other antiepileptics. The drug may be particularly valuable in patients with respiratory disease. The risk of drug accumulation is low. Other disadvantages include: a possible pro-convulsant effect at high levels; an active metabolite that may accumulate on prolonged therapy; the need for cardiac monitoring as cardiac rhythm disturbances are common; and the dependency of the clearance of lignocaine on hepatic blood flow.

*Usual preparations*: 5 ml ready-prepared syringe containing lignocaine 20 mg/ml (2%) *or* 10 ml ready-prepared syringe containing lignocaine 10 mg/ml (1%) (i.e. both syringes containing 100 mg). Lignocaine is also available as a 5 ml vial containing 20 mg/ml (i.e. 100 mg) of lignocaine (2%) or a 5 ml vial containing 200 mg/ml (i.e. 1000 mg) of lignocaine (20%), and as ready-made 0.1% (1 mg/ml) and 0.2% (2 mg/ml) infusions (in 500 ml containers in 5% dextrose).

*Usual dosage*: Intravenous bolus injections of 1.5–2.0 mg/kg (usually 100 mg in adults), at a rate of injection not exceeding 50 mg/min. The bolus injection can be repeated once if necessary. A continuous infusion can be given at a rate of 3–4 mg/kg/h (usually of 0.2% solution in 5% dextrose, for no more than 12 h); 3–6 mg/kg/h (neonates).

*Lorazepam*

Lorazepam is a drug of choice in the early stage of status, given by i.v. bolus injection (Leppik et al 1983a, Crawford et al 1987, Mitchell & Crawford 1990, Maytal et al 1991). A single injection is highly effective and the drug has a longer initial duration of action and a smaller risk of cardiorespiratory depression than diazepam. There is little risk of drug accumulation and also a lower risk of hypotension. The main disadvantage of lorazepam is a stronger tendency for tolerance to develop, the drug being usually effective for about 12 h only. It is thus usable only as initial therapy, and longer-term maintenance antiepileptic drugs must be given in addition. There is a large clinical experience in adults, children and the newborn, with well-proven efficacy in tonic-clonic and partial status, and the pharmacology and pharmacokinetics of the drug are well characterized. Lorazepam is a stable compound, which is not likely to precipitate in solution, and is relatively unaffected by hepatic or renal disease.

*Usual preparation:* 1 ml ampoule containing 4 mg/ml for i.v. injection

*Usual dosage*: i.v. bolus of 0.07 mg/kg (usually 4 mg), repeated after 10 min if necessary (adults); bolus of 0.1 mg/kg (children). The rate of injection is not crucial.

*Phenytoin*

Phenytoin is a highly effective medication for the established stage of status (Wallis et al 1968, Leppik et al 1983b, Cranford et al 1978, Shaner et al 1988). Extensive clinical experience has been gained in adults, children and neonates, and phenytoin has proven efficacy in tonic-clonic and partial status. The drug has a prolonged action, with a relatively small risk of respiratory or cerebral depression and no tendency for tachyphylaxis. Its main disadvantage is the time necessary to infuse the drug and its delayed onset of action; it is for this reason that it is often given with diazepam, the combination theoretically providing a rapid-onset and long-lasting antiepileptic effect. The pharmacokinetics of phenytoin are problematic, with zero-order kinetics at conventional dosages and wide variation between individuals. Toxic side-effects include cardiac rhythm disturbances, thrombophlebitis and hypotension. The risk of cardiac side-effects is greatly increased if the recommended rate of injection is exceeded, and cardiac monitoring is advisable during phenytoin infusion. There is a risk of precipitation if phenytoin is diluted in other solutions than 0.9% saline or if mixed with other drugs.

*Usual preparations*: 5 ml ampoule containing 250 mg stabilized in propylene glycol, ethanol and water (alternatives exist, e.g. phenytoin in Tris buffer or in infusion bottles of 750 mg in 500 ml of osmotic saline).

*Usual dosage*: In adults, an 15–18 mg/kg i.v. infusion. This can be given via the side arm of a drip or preferably directly via an infusion pump. The rate of infusion should not exceed 50 mg/min (20 mg/min in the elderly). In children a 20 mg/kg i.v. infusion is usually given, at a rate not exceeding 25 mg/min. The drug should never be given by i.m. injection.

*Phenobarbitone*

Phenobarbitone is used at the stage of established status, as a first-line alternative to phenytoin (Lockman et al 1979, Gal et al 1982, Crawford et al 1988, Shaner et al 1988). It is a highly effective antiepileptic drug, with well proven effectiveness in tonic-clonic and partial status, and there is extensive clinical experience in adults, children and neonates. Phenobarbitone has a stronger anticonvulsant action than other barbiturates and an additional potential cerebral protective action. It has a rapid-onset and long-lasting action and can be administered much faster than can phenytoin. Its safety at high doses has been established and the drug can be continued as chronic therapy. The disadvantages of the drug relate to prolonged use, when, because of the long elimination half life, there is a risk of drug accumulation and inevitable sedation, respiratory depression and hypotension. Marked autoinduction may also occur.

*Usual preparation*: 1 ml ampoule, containing phenobarbitone sodium 200 mg/ml in propylene glycol 90% and water for injection 10%.

*Usual dosage*: i.v. loading dose of 10 mg/kg at rate of 100 mg/min (usual adult dose 600–800 mg), followed by maintenance dose of 1–4 mg/kg (adults); i.v. loading dose of 15–20 mg/kg, followed by maintenance dose of 3–4 mg/kg (children and neonates). Higher doses can be given, with monitoring of blood concentrations (Crawford et al 1988).

*Thiopentone*

Thiopentone is the usual choice for barbiturate anaesthesia. It is a highly effective antiepileptic drug, with additional potential cerebral protective action (Partinen et al 1981, Young et al 1980, Orlowski et al 1984, Lowenstein et al 1988). It reduces intracranial pressure and cerebral blood flow, and has a very rapid onset of action, and there is wide experience of its use. The drug has a number of pharmacokinetic disadvantages including saturable kinetics, a strong tendency to accumulate and a prolonged recovery time after anaesthesia is withdrawn. Blood level monitoring of the parent drug and its active metabolite (pentobarbitone) is advisable on prolonged therapy. There is often some tachyphylaxis to its sedative and to a lesser extent its anticonvulsant properties. Respiratory depression and sedation is inevitable, and hypotension is common. Other less common side-effects include pancreatitis, hepatic dysfunction and spasm at the injection site. Full intensive care facilities with artificial ventilatory support and intensive EEG and cardiovascular monitoring are needed. It can react with co-medication, and with plastic giving sets, and is unstable when exposed to air. Autoinduction occurs, and hepatic disease prolongs the elimination of thiopentone.

*Usual preparations*: Injection of thiopentone sodium 2.5 g with 100 ml and 5 g with 200 ml diluent (to make 100 ml and 200 ml of a 2.5% solution). It is also available as 500 mg and 1 g vials to make 2.5% solutions.

*Usual dosage*: 100 mg–250 mg i.v. bolus given over 20 s, with further 50 mg boluses every 2–3 min until seizures are controlled, followed by a continuous i.v. infusion to maintain a burst suppression pattern on the EEG (usually 3–5 mg/kg/h). The dose should be lowered if systolic blood pressure falls below 90 mmHg despite cardiovascular support. Thiopentone should be slowly withdrawn 12 h after the last seizure.

*Pentobarbitone*

Pentobarbitone is an alternative to thiopentone (although not available in the UK) (Rashkin et al 1987, Lowenstein et al 1988, Yaffe & Lowenstein 1992). It has certain advantages, which include a shorter elimination half-life than thiopentone, non-saturable kinetics, no active metabolites and a longer duration of action. It is a stable compound and is unreactive with plastic. There is however much more limited clinical experience, and published trials have shown a uniformly poor outcome. Respiratory depression and sedation are invariable, and hypotension and cardio-respiratory dysfunction are common. Decerebrate posturing and flaccid paralysis occur during induction of anaesthesia, and a flaccid weakness can persist for weeks in survivors. There is a tendency for seizures to recur when the drug withdrawn. It requires intensive care, artificial ventilatory support, EEG and cardiovascular monitoring. Blood level monitoring is usually advised, although there is in fact only an inconsistent relationship between serum level and seizure control.

*Usual preparation*: 100 mg in a 2 ml injection vial, formulated in propylene glycol 40% and ethyl alcohol 10%.

*Usual dosage*: i.v. loading dose of 10–20 mg/kg, at a rate not exceeding 25 mg/min, followed by a continuous infusion of 0.5–1.0 mg/kg/h, increasing if necessary to 1–3 mg/kg/h. Additional 5–20 mg/kg boluses can be given if breakthrough seizures occur. The dose should be tapered 12 h after the last seizure by 0.5–1 mg/kg/h every 4–6 h (depending on blood level).

*Isoflurane*

Isoflurane is the drug of choice for inhalational anaesthesia in status (Ropper et al 1986, Kofke et al 1989, Hilz et al 1992) and has significant advantages over other inhalational anaesthetics such as halothane or enflurane – lower solubility, less hepatotoxicity or nephrotoxicity, less effect on cardiac output, fewer cardiac arrhythmias, less hypotension, less effect on cerebral blood flow and autoregulation, less increase in intracranial pressure, less convulsant effect and linear kinetics. It has a very rapid onset of action and recovery, and no tendency to accumulate.

Although hypotension is common it is generally mild. There is no hepatic metabolism and the drug is unaffected by hepatic or renal disease. There is, however, little published experience in status or of long-term use, and the major disadvantage is logistical, as isoflurane requires the use of an anaesthetic system with a scavenging apparatus, which is inconvenient in most ITU situations. The other facilities required are the usual ones of assisted ventilation, intensive care and cardiorespiratory monitoring.

*Usual preparation*: Nearly pure (99.9%) liquid, for use in a correctly calibrated vaporizer via an anaesthetic system.

*Usual dosage*: Inhalation of isoflurane at dosages producing end tidal concentrations of 0.8–2%, with the dose titrated to maintain a burst suppression pattern on the EEG.

*Propofol*

Propofol is a good anaesthetic, with excellent pharmacokinetic properties (Wood et al 1988, MacKenzie et al 1990, De Maria et al 1991). In status it has a very rapid onset of action and rapid recovery. There are few haemodynamic side-effects and the drug has been used at all ages. There is however little published experience of its use in status, or indeed of prolonged infusions. Unlike isoflurane, it is metabolized in the liver and affected by severe hepatic disease. As with all anaesthetics, its use requires assisted ventilation, intensive care and intensive care monitoring. It causes lipaemia and acidosis, which may complicate its use, especially on long-term therapy and in infants. Involuntary movements (without EEG change) can occur, and should not be confused with seizure activity.

*Usual preparation*: 20 ml ampoule containing 10 mg/ml (i.e. 200 mg) as an emulsion.

*Usual dosage*; 2 mg/kg bolus, repeated if necessary, and then followed by a continuous infusion of 5–10 mg/kg/h initially, reducing to 1–3 mg/kg/h. When seizures have been controlled for 12 h, the drug dosages should be slowly tapered over 12 h.

*Etomidate*

Etomidate is an alternative to propofol as a non-barbiturate infusional anaesthetic in status (Yeoman et al 1989). It is a highly effective anaesthetic with low risk of cardiorespiratory toxicity, and is particularly safe in patients with cardiovascular disease, although mild hypotension is common. Corticosteroid co-medication (hydrocortisone 100 mg 6-hourly) is obligatory, as etomidate interferes with adrenocortical function. Seizures tend to recur if the drug is weaned too fast. It reduces cerebral blood flow and metabolism, which is of uncertain benefit in status. There is very little experience of prolonged etomidate usage and very few reports of its use in status. It may have antiepileptic properties, which would be an advantage over other non-barbiturate anaesthetics, but drug-induced myoclonus, muscular twitching and other involuntary movements can occur during etomidate anaesthesia. As is the case with all anaesthetics, assisted ventilation, intensive care and cardiorespiratory monitoring are required.

*Usual preparation*: Etomidate is dissolved in 35% propylene glycol (which can be allergenic) and is presented as a solution containing 20 mg in a 10 ml ampoule (2 mg/ml). A more concentrated solution of 125 mg/ml in 1 ml ampoules is also available for dilution as a continuous infusion.

*Usual dosage*: i.v. bolus of 0.3 mg/kg, repeated if necessary, followed by a continuous infusion at an initial rate of about 20 μg/kg/min (5 mg/ml of etomidate in 5% dextrose), titrated up or down to maintain burst suppression. After 24 h the drug is slowly tapered, and the infusion reinstituted if seizures recur, for a further 24 h. Corticosteroid co-medication must be given in a dose of 100 mg every 6 h and continued for 72 h after cessation of the etomidate infusion.

## 5.4 TREATMENT OF OTHER FORMS OF STATUS EPILEPTICUS

Urgent therapy is necessary in tonic-clonic status, to avoid or reverse the pathophysiological changes induced by status. In general, the homoeostatic perturbations are less severe in other forms of status and the same degree of urgency is not required. For most non-convulsive forms, oral therapy is sufficient, and treatment should follow the normal principles of antiepileptic drug usage (Shorvon 1994) (see Ch. 4, 4.4.3 for the treatment of the Landau–Kleffner syndrome and electrical status in slow wave sleep).

*Typical absence status*

Typical absence status (petit mal status) can usually be terminated by intravenous benzodiazepine therapy: diazepam 0.2–0.3 mg/kg, clonazepam 1 mg (0.25–0.5 mg in children) or lorazepam 0.07 mg/kg (0.1 mg/kg in children), repeated if required. If this is ineffective, intravenous chlormethiazole, phenytoin or valproate may be needed, although absence status is seldom life-threatening and aggressive intravenous therapy is therefore seldom required. Atypical absence status (for instance, in the Lennox–Gastaut syndrome) is treated in the same way, although therapy is often less effective. Oral therapy with valproate, lamotrigine or felbamate is sometimes useful in typical or atypical absence status.

*Complex partial status*

Complex partial status can be treated by intravenous therapy in the same way as generalized absence status, although the effect of i.v. benzodiazepines is often less rapid or complete (Tomson et al 1986, Dunne et al 1987). Some cases are refractory to initial i.v. therapy and in this situation oral therapy with carbamazepine, phenytoin or phenobarbitone is advisable. It is seldom necessary to use more aggressive i.v. therapy but if this is required the principles of treatment are the same as for tonic-clonic status.

*Epilepsia partialis continua*

The seizures generally remit spontaneously in acute cases. In a well-established case, however, epilepsia partialis continua (EPC) can be particularly resistant to therapy, and i.v. therapy even to the point of anaesthesia can produce only temporary respite. Phenytoin, carbamazepine or phenobarbitone are probably the drugs of first choice, and oral corticosteroids are sometimes helpful. The long-term outcome depends on the underlying cause, but in many cases the clonic movements continue in spite of medical therapy. Resective neurosurgical treatment can be considered in refractory cases (Olivier 1991).

Steroids and intravenous immunoglobulin (Hart et al 1994) and zidovudine (DeToledo & Smith 1994) have been tried in Rasmussen's chronic encephalitis, but definitive evidence of long-term efficacy is lacking and controlled studies are necessary.

## 5.5 PSEUDOSTATUS EPILEPTICUS

Pseudostatus epilepticus is a condition in which repeated or continuous seizures occur, which are psychogenic in origin and which resemble (at least superficially) convulsive status epilepticus (Toone & Roberts 1979, Howell et al 1989) (see also Ch. 9, 9.1). In contemporary specialist practice, pseudostatus is as common as true status epilepticus. To the experienced observer, the differentiation from true status epilepticus is usually easy. The motor movements do not have the classic features of convulsive seizures but fluctuate in intensity, frequency or distribution as the status proceeds, often influenced by emotional external factors. Vocalization is common, as is bizarre behaviour, explosive emotional expression and resistance to examination. Preservation of consciousness can often be deduced in spite of the continuing convulsions. Incontinence, tongue-biting and cyanosis do occur but are less common than in true status. Opisthotonus was first depicted by Charcot and is a dramatic motor manifestation, sometimes accompanying flapping and twisting of the limbs (Bateman 1989). There is often a long history of psychiatric or personality disorder, often with hysterical features, and previous episodes of pseudostatus or other non-organic illnesses. The epilepsy history is usually atypical, showing an odd pattern of seizures over time, an inconsistent response to treatment and repeatedly normal interictal EEG. An EEG during the episode will definitively confirm or refute the diagnosis, if there is clinical doubt (Ch. 3, 3.2.6).

If mistaken for true status epilepticus, a disastrous therapeutic cycle is all too commonly embarked upon. Intravenous anticonvulsants are given. Seizures persist and more drugs are administered, to the point of unconsciousness. These have a temporary effect but, as consciousness is regained, seizures recur and more intravenous anticonvulsants are given, often including i.v. anaesthetics. Sedation occurs, and full ITU care then is necessary, often with assisted ventilation. Seizures recur whenever the patient recovers consciousness, and further treatment is given. The cycle can persist even to the stage of tracheostomy.

This is unfortunate for, once the true diagnosis is made, treatment is straightforward. All anticonvulsant and sedative therapy should be immediately withdrawn, and sympathetic but firm verbal encouragement given. This will rapidly terminate the episode. A few patients exhibit both true epilepsy and non-epileptic seizures, and occasionally an episode of pseudostatus will follow a true tonic-clonic seizure.

Most patients have no formal psychiatric diagnosis, but in others there is evidence of malingering, psychopathic disorder, a history of sexual abuse or neurotic personality disorder. In some the seizures seem to occur simply in the context of unhappiness or loneliness. Long-term treatment should attempt to prevent repeated episodes of this hazardous behaviour. Recidivism is more common if there is a lack of family support, in chronic cases and in the absence of a clear psychogenic mechanism (Meierkord et al 1991, Pakalnis et al 1991).

## REFERENCES

Altafullah I, Asaikar S, Torres F 1991 Status epilepticus: clinical experience with two special devices for continuous cerebral monitoring. Acta Neurol Scand 84: 374–381.

Aminoff MJ, Simon RP 1980 Status epilepticus: causes, clinical features and consequences in 98 patients. Am J Med 69: 657–666.

Bateman DE 1989 Pseudostatus epilepticus. Lancet 2: 1278–1279.

Beaumanoir A, Foletti G, Magistris M, Volanschi D 1988 Status epilepticus in the Lennox–Gastaut Syndrome. In: Niedermeyer E, Degen R (eds) The Lennox–Gastaut syndrome. Neurology and Neurobiology 45. Alan R Liss, New York, p 283–300.

Browne TR 1983 Paraldehyde, chlormethiazole, and lidocaine for treatment of status epilepticus. In: Delgado Escueta AV, Wasterlain CG, Treiman DM, Porter RJ (eds) Advances in neurology 34. Status epilepticus: mechanisms of brain damage and treatment. Raven Press, New York, p 509–517.

Clark LP, Prout TP 1903/4 Status epilepticus: a clinical and pathological study in epilepsy (an article in 3 parts). Am J Insanity 60: 291–306; 60: 645–675; 61: 81–108.

Cockerell OC, Walker CM, Sander JWAS, Shorvon SD 1994 Complex partial status epilepticus: a recurrent problem. J Neurol Psychiat Neurosurg 57: 835–837

Congdon PJ, Forsythe WI 1980 Intravenous clonazepam in the treatment of status epilepticus in children. Epilepsia 21: 97–102.

Cranford RE, Leppik IE, Patrick B, Anderson CB, Kostick B 1978 Intravenous phenytoin: clinical and pharmacokinetic aspects. Neurology 28: 874–880.

Crawford TO, Mitchell WG, Snodgrass SR 1987 Lorazepam in childhood status epilepticus and serial seizures: effectiveness and tachyphylaxis. Neurology 37: 190–195.

Crawford TO, Mitchell WG, Fishman LS, Snodgrass R 1988 Very-high-dose phenobarbital for refractory status epilepticus in children. Neurology 38: 1035–1040.

De Giorgio CM, Rabinowicz AL, Bird EH, Altman K 1991 Lidocaine in refractory nonconvulsive status epilepticus: confirmation of efficacy with continuous EEG monitoring. Epilepsia 32(suppl. 1): 77.

Delgado-Escueta AV, Enrile-Bacsal F 1983 Combination therapy for status epilepticus: intravenous diazepam and phenytoin. In: Delgado Escueta AV, Wasterlain CG, Treiman DM, Porter RJ (eds) Advances in neurology 34. Status epilepticus: mechanisms of brain damage and treatment. Raven Press, New York, p 477–485.

De Maria G, Guarneri D, Pasolini MP, Antonini L 1991 Stato di male versivo trattato con propofol. Boll Lega Ital Contro L'Epilessia 74: 191–192.

DeToledo JC, Smith DB 1994 Partially successful treatment of Rasmussen's encephalitis with zidovudine: symptomatic improvement followed by involvement of the contralateral hemisphere. Epilepsia 35: 352–355.

Dravet C, Natale O, Magaudda A et al 1985 Les etats de mal dans le syndrome de Lennox–Gastaut. Rev d'Electroencephalog Neurophysiol Clin 15: 361–368.

Dundee JW, Halliday NJ, Harper KW, Brogden RN 1984 Midazolam: a review of its pharmacological properties and therapeutic uses. Drugs 28: 519–543.

Dunne JW, Summers QA, Stewart-Wynne EG 1987 Non-convulsive status epilepticus: a prospective study in an adult general hospital. Q J Med 62: 117–126.

Gal P, Toback J, Boer HR, Erkan NV, Wells TJ 1982 Efficacy of phenobarbital monotherapy in treatment of neonatal seizures – relationship to blood levels. Neurology 32: 1401–1404.

Galvin GM, Jellinek GA 1987 Midazolam: an effective intravenous agent for seizure control. Arch Emerg Med 4: 169–172.

Gastaut J, Courjon J, Poiré R, Weber M 1971 Treatment of status epilepticus with a new benzodiazepine more active than diazepam. Epilepsia 12: 197–214.

Gimenez-Roldán S, Lopéz Agreda JM, Martin FJ 1972 Un nuevo medicamento eficaz en el tratamiento del status epilepticus – Ro 5-4023. Med Clin 58: 133.

Harvey PKP, Higenbottam TW, Loh L 1975 Chlormethiazole in treatment of status epilepticus. Brit Med J 2: 603–605.

Hart YM, Cortez M, Andermann F et al 1994 Medical treatment of Rasmussen's syndrome (chronic encephalitis and epilepsy): effect of high-dose steroids or immunoglobulins in 19 patients. Neurology 44: 1030–1036

Hilz MJ, Bauer J, Claus D, Stefan H, Neundörfer B 1992 Isoflurane anaesthesia in the treatment of convulsive status epilepticus. J Neurol 239: 135–137.

Howell SJL, Owen L, Chadwick DW 1989 Pseudostatus epilepticus. Q J Med 71: 507–519.

Jawad S, Oxley J, Wilson J, Richens A 1986 A pharmacodynamic evaluation of midazolam as an antiepileptic compound. J Neurol Neurosurg Psychiat 49: 1050–1054.

Kofke WA, Young RSK, Davis P et al 1989 Isoflurane for refractory status epilepticus: a clinical series. Anesthesiology 71: 653–659.

Kojewnikoff AY 1895 Eine besondere Form von corticaler Epilepsie. Neurol Zentralblatt 14: 47–48.

Koren G, Butt W, Rajchgot P et al 1986 Intravenous paraldehyde for seizure control in newborn infants. Neurology 36: 108–111.

Laxenaire M, Tridon P, Poiré P 1966 Effect of chlormethiazole in treatment of delirium tremens and status epilepticus. Acta Psychiat Scand 42(suppl 192): 87–102.

Leppik IE, Derivan AT, Homan RW, Walker J, Ramsay RE, Patrick BK 1983a Double-blind study of lorazepam and diazepam in status epilepticus. JAMA 249: 1452–1454.

Leppik IE, Patrick BK, Cranford RE 1983b Treatment of acute seizures and status epilepticus with intravenous phenytoin. In: Delgado Escueta AV, Wasterlain CG, Treiman DM, Porter RJ (eds) Advances in neurology 34. Status epilepticus: mechanisms of brain damage and treatment. Raven Press, New York, p 447–452.

Lingam S, Bertwistle H, Elliston H, Wilson J 1980 Problems with intravenous chlormethiazole (Heminevrin) in status epilepticus. Brit Med J i: 155–156.

Lockman LA 1995 Paraldehyde. In: Levy RH, Mattson RH, Meldrum BS (eds) Antiepileptic drugs, 4th edn. Raven Press, New York, p 963-967.

Lockman LA, Kriel R, Zaske D, Thompson T, Virnig N 1979 Phenobarbital dosage for control of neonatal seizures. Neurology 29: 1445–1449.

Lothman E 1990 The biochemical basis and pathophysiology of status epilepticus. Neurology 40(suppl 2): 13–22

Lowenstein DH, Aminoff MJ, Simon RP 1988 Barbiturate anesthesia in the treatment of status epilepticus: clinical experience of 14 patients. Neurology 38: 395–400.

MacKenzie SJ, Kapadia F, Grant IS 1990 Propofol infusion for control of status epilepticus. Anaesthesia 45: 1043–1045.

Maytal J, Novak GP, King KC 1991 Lorazepam in the treatment of refractory neonatal seizures. J Child Neurol 6: 319–323.

Meierkord H, Will RG, Fish D, Shorvon S 1991 The clinical features and prognosis of pseudoseizures diagnosed using video-EEG telemetry. Neurology 41: 1643–1646.

Meldrum BS 1983 Metabolic factors during prolonged seizures and their relation to cell death. In: Delgado Escueta AV, Wasterlain CG, Treiman DM, Porter RJ (eds) Advances in neurology 34. Status epilepticus: mechanisms of brain damage and treatment. Raven Press, New York, p 261–275

Miller P, Kovar I 1983 Chlormethiazole in the treatment of neonatal status epilepticus. Postgrad Med J 59: 801–802

Mitchell WG, Crawford TO 1990 Lorazepam is the treatment of choice for status epilepticus. J Epilepsy 3: 7–10.

Obeso JA, Rothwell JC, Marsden CD 1985 The spectrum of cortical myoclonus. Brain 108: 193–224.

Oguni H, Andermann F, Rasmussen TB 1991 The natural history of chronic encephalitis and epilepsy: a study of the MNI series of forty-eight cases. In: Andermann F (ed) Chronic encephalitis and epilepsy: Rasmussen's syndrome. Butterworth-Heinemann, London, p 7–36.

Olivier A 1991 Corticectomy for the treatment of seizures due to chronic encephalitis. In: Andermann F (ed) Chronic encephalitis and epilepsy: Rasmussen's syndrome. Butterworth-Heinemann, London, p 205–212.

Orlowski JP, Erenberg G, Lüders H, Cruse RP 1984 Hypothermia and barbiturate coma for refractory status epilepticus. Crit Care Med 12: 367–372.

Pakalnis A, Drake ME, Phillips B 1991 Neuropsychiatric aspects of psychogenic status epilepticus. Neurology 41: 1104–1106.

Partinen M, Kovanen J, Nilsson E 1981 Status epilepticus treated with barbiturate anaesthesia with continuous monitoring of cerebral function. Brit Med J 282: 520–521

Pascual J, Ciudad J, Berciano J 1992 Role of lidocaine (lignocaine) in managing status epilepticus. J Neurol Neurosurg Psychiat 55: 49–51.

Rashkin MC, Youngs C, Penovich P 1987 Pentobarbital treatment of refractory status epilepticus. Neurology 37: 500–503.

Rasmussen T, Olszweski J, Lloyd-Smith DL 1958 Focal seizures due to chronic localized encephalitis. Neurology 8: 435–445.

Rémy C, Jourdil N, Villemain D, Favel P, Genton P 1992 Intrarectal diazepam in epileptic adults. Epilepsia 33: 353–358.

Roger J, Lob H, Tassinari CA 1974 Status epilepticus. In: Magnus O, Lorentz de Haas AM (eds) The epilepsies. Handbook of clinical neurology, vol. 15. North-Holland, Amsterdam, p 145–188.

Rohr-Le Floch J, Gauthier G, Beaumanoir A 1988 Etats confusionnels d'origine épileptique interêt de l'EEG fait en urgence. Rev Neurol 144: 6–7, 425–436.

Ropper AH, Kofke WA, Bromfield EB, Kennedy SK 1986 Comparison of isoflurane, halothane, and nitrous oxide in status epilepticus. Ann Neurol 19: 98–99.

Schmidt D 1995 Diazepam. In: Levy R, Mattson R, Meldrum B (eds) Antiepileptic drugs, 4th edn. Raven Press, New York, p 705-724.

Shaner DM, McCurdy SA, Herring MO, Gabor AJ 1988 Treatment of status epilepticus: a prospective comparison of diazepam and phenytoin versus phenobarbital and optional phenytoin. Neurology 38: 202–207.

Shorvon SD 1994 Status epilepticus: its clinical features and treatment in children and adults. Cambridge University Press, Cambridge.

Shorvon SD 1995 Absence status epilepticus. In: Duncan JS, Panayiotopoulos CP (eds) Typical absences and related epileptic syndromes. Churchill Livingstone, Edinburgh, p 263–274.

Simon RP 1985 Physiological consequences of status epilepticus. Epilepsia 26(suppl 1): S58–S66

Thomas JE, Reagan TJ, Klass DW 1977 Epilepsia partialis continua: a review of 32 cases. Arch Neurol 34: 266–275.

Tomson T, Svanborg E, Wedlund J-E 1986 Nonconvulsive status epilepticus: high incidence of complex partial status. Epilepsia 27: 276–285.

Toone BK, Roberts J 1979 Status epilepticus: an uncommon hysterical conversion syndrome. J Nerv Ment Dis 167: 548–552.

Treiman DM, Walton NY, Kendrick C 1990 A progressive sequaence of electroencephalographic changes during generalized convulsive status epilepticus. Epilepsy Res 5: 49–60

Wallis W, Kutt H, McDowell F 1968 i.v. diphenylhydantoin treatment of acute repetitive seizures. Neurology 18: 513–525.

Williamson PD, Spencer DD, Spencer SS, Novelly RA, Mattson RH 1985 Complex partial status epilepticus: a depth-electrode study. Ann Neurol 18: 647–654.

Wood PR, Browne GPR, Pugh S 1988 Propofol infusion for the treatment of status epilepticus. Lancet 1: 480–481

Yaffe K, Lowenstein DH 1992 Pentobarbital coma for refractory status epilepticus: prognostic factors in the outcome of 17 patients. Neurology 42(suppl 3): 263.

Yeoman P, Hutchinson A, Byrne A, Smith J, Durham S 1989 Etomidate infusions for the control of refractory status epilepticus. Int Care Med 15: 255–259.

Young GB, Blume WT, Bolton CF, Warren KG 1980 Anesthetic barbiturates in refractory status epilepticus. Can J Neurol Sci 7: 291–292.

# 6 Epilepsy and reproduction

## 6.1 EPILEPSY AND MENSTRUATION

### 6.1.1 Catamenial epilepsy

Although many women link occurrence of epileptic seizures to their menstrual period, when data is collected prospectively a positive association is unusual; being present in 10 of 226 women in one series (Rosciszewska 1987) and in five of 40 women in another (Duncan et al 1993). In some the period was associated with a fall in plasma phenytoin concentrations. Changes in hormone concentrations, with oestrogen being proconvulsant and progesterone anticonvulsant, have been considered as contributory factors. An increase in seizures has also been reported during the follicular phase, when oestrogen concentrations are high; and a decrease has been noted in the mid-luteal phase, at which time progesterone levels are high. Premenstrual tension and fluid retention have also been proposed as contributory factors to catamenial exacerbation of seizures, but are of uncertain significance (Crawford 1991).

There have been various approaches to the treatment of catamenial seizures. Trials of administered progesterone or norethisterone have been open and add-on and have shown only equivocal benefit, although there have been anecdotal reports of marked benefit. Acetazolamide taken over the menstrual period has been advocated in view of its antiepileptic and diuretic effects, but is not very effective. Intermittent clobazam has been reported to be useful in 78% of women, and given in this way avoids the development of benzodiazepine tolerance (Feely et al 1982). Practical limitations, however, to the effective use of intermittent medication are that the patient must have a regular cycle and remember the dosing instructions, and the fact that a catamenial exacerbation is often not reliably linked to any particular day in the cycle.

### 6.1.2 Fertility

The fertility of men and women with epilepsy has been estimated to be 85% and 80% of the expected levels, respectively (Weber et al 1986). Menstrual disorders are common in women with epilepsy, particularly polycystic ovarian syndrome and hypogonadotrophic hypogonadism (Herzog et al 1986, Bilo et al 1988). The incidence of spontaneous abortions in these groups appeared not to differ from the general population (Annegers et al 1988). Choice not to raise children, reduced sexual appetite and associated abnormalities of endocrine function are likely to be contributory factors. Phenytoin has been reported to be associated with reduced sperm production and motility. The effects of individual AEDs on male and female fertility, however, are not clear.

## 6.2 HORMONAL CONTRACEPTION

Antiepileptic drugs that induce the activity of hepatic microsomal enzymes (barbiturates, phenytoin, carbamazepine) increase the rate at which the steroid hormones present in the oral contraceptive pill are metabolized. Vigabatrin, valproate, benzodiazepines and gabapentin do not induce hepatic enzymes. Oxcarbazepine and lamotrigine appear to have weak enzyme-inducing effects. A consequence of increased metabolism of oestrogen in women taking enzyme-inducing drugs is reduced contraceptive efficacy and breakthrough bleeding during a cycle of pill administration. In a prospective study, 8.5% of pregnant women with epilepsy reported failure of oral contraceptives (Koch et al 1983).

Women taking enzyme-inducing AEDs who wish to rely on an oral contraceptive pill should be prescribed a preparation containing 50 μg oestradiol. Breakthrough bleeding is a clear sign of inadequate oestrogen levels and in some women 80 or even 100 μg of ethinyloestradiol per day may be needed. Giving 80 μg of ethinyloestradiol per day, however, carries a risk of causing nausea. An alternative strategy is to 'tricycle' a 50 μg-oestradiol-containing preparation. This entails taking three packets of pills without a break, followed by an interval of only 4 days, rather than the usual seven. If need be, 60 μg of ethinyloestradiol per day can be given by prescribing a double dose of a 30 μg-containing preparation. Serial ultrasound scans may be used to ensure that ovarian follicular activity has ceased.

These larger doses of oestrogen, being given solely to keep pace with more rapid metabolism, carry no higher risk of complications. Women need to be counselled, however, that, even with the precaution of taking higher doses of oestrogen that prevent breakthrough bleeding, there is an elevated risk of contraceptive failure, increasing from 0.3 to about 3/100 woman years. This risk is comparable to that associated with barrier methods of contraception.

While oestrogen is proconvulsant and progesterone is anticonvulsant, there is no clear evidence that taking the oral contraceptive pill adversely affects seizure control (Dana-Haeri & Richens 1983).

*Injectable contraceptives*

Injectable long-term contraceptives such as Depo-Provera are a useful alternative to oral contraception, particularly if the patient has difficulty with taking oral medication regularly, and there have been anecdotal reports of significant improvements in seizure control. A dose of 150 mg Depo-Provera every 12 weeks gives excellent contraceptive efficacy, with a failure rate of 0.5/100 woman years. As the rate-limiting step of elimination is hepatic blood flow and not hepatic enzyme activity, this is not affected by enzyme-inducing AEDs. Unless there are concomitant risk factors for vascular disease, long-term therapy with Depo-Provera is reasonable.

## 6.3 PREGNANCY IN WOMEN WITH EPILEPSY

### 6.3.1 Effect of pregnancy on epilepsy

Most women with epilepsy do not have an increase in seizures while pregnant. Between 17% and 37% of women have an increase in seizures during pregnancy; in many of these cases the increase can be attributed to factors such as poor compliance with prescribed AEDs, sometimes compounded by vomiting, inappropriate reduction of AED therapy, pregnancy-related fall in plasma drug concentrations and sleep deprivation. Increased seizure frequency is more likely in women with a high pregravid seizure frequency or multiple seizure types. An episode of status epilepticus occurs in less than 1% of pregnancies. The risk of seizures is greatest in the delivery period and tonic-clonic seizures complicate labour in 1–2% of cases. Up to 50% of women report that their epilepsy is better controlled during preg-nancy, for reasons that include avoidance of excessive fatigue, better compliance and hormonal changes (Schmidt et al 1983, Delgado-Escueta & Janz 1992).

### 6.3.2 Effect of epilepsy on pregnancy

Some series have not indicated any increased risk of obstetric complications in women with epilepsy, but others have found an approximately 1.5–3 times increase in the risk of common complications such as toxaemia, pre-eclampsia, placental bleeding and premature labour and a 1.2–2 times increase in perinatal mortality. Many studies, however, have been retrospective or based on registries and are likely to be complicated by ascertainment bias (Delgado-Escueta & Janz 1992).

There is no evidence that simple partial, complex partial, absence and myoclonic seizures adversely effect a pregnancy or developing fetus, other than by the effects of trauma. Tonic-clonic seizures can also lead to injury and carry additional potential risk by virtue of impaired oxygenation. There are anecdotal reports of miscarriage following a single tonic-clonic seizure (Beaussant-Defaye et al 1985) and of fetal bradycardia following generalized tonic-clonic seizures during labour; but there is a lack of definitive data and other factors such as administered sedation may be complicating factors (Yerby 1987).

### 6.3.3 Teratogenic risks from AEDs

Although a major concern of women with epilepsy who are contemplating pregnancy is the teratogenic potential of AEDs, it is important to put these risks in perspective. The background risk of fetal malformation is approximately 3% in developed countries and the consensus from many studies is that this increases to 7% if one AED is taken and to 15% if two or more are taken (Annegers et al 1978, Nakane et al 1980, Koch et al 1992). There is also circumstantial evidence that larger doses of AEDs are associated with an increase in risk. Some combinations of drugs appear to carry a particularly high risk, e.g. valproate + carbamazepine + phenytoin or phenobarbitone has been associated with a 50% malformation rate (Lindhout et al 1984). The mechanisms whereby AEDs are teratogenic have not been definitely established. Possibilities include the formation of epoxide and arene oxide metabolites and of cytotoxic free radicals.

*Is there any difference between the major antiepileptic drugs?*

There is no conclusive evidence for a differential overall risk of teratogenicity from phenytoin, valproate, carbamazepine or phenobarbitone. There have been suggestions that valproate is more teratogenic than the others (Lindhout et al 1984, Koch et al 1992). In a recent prospective study of 159 women who took AEDs during pregnancy, abnormal outcomes occurred in 10.7%, compared with 3.4% in the control group. Phenobarbitone was associated with the highest relative risk, followed by phenytoin and then carbamazepine. There were insufficient numbers of women treated with valproate to assess the risk associated with this drug (Waters et al 1994). Different studies have drawn different inferences and interpretation of the findings is confounded by patients taking different doses and combinations of drugs, and there have been insufficient studies of monotherapy to draw definitive conclusions. One AED, trimethadione, stands out as having a particularly high teratogenic risk and is contraindicated in pregnancy (Zackai et al 1975).

*Phenytoin*

Although doubt has been cast on the existence of a true 'fetal hydantoin syndrome' (see below), phenytoin is particularly associated with an increased risk of cleft lip and palate and, less commonly, with cardiac defects.

*Valproate*

The use of valproate in pregnancy has generally been associated with a 1–2% risk of neural tube defects, particularly an open lumbosacral myelocele, against a background risk of 0.2–0.5%; and with an increased incidence of cardiovascular and urogenital malformations. Higher daily doses of valproate, e.g. more than 1000 mg/d, probably carry greater risk than lower doses (Lindhout et al 1992). It has been suggested on the basis of studies in rodents that high peak concentrations of valproate increase the risk and that this may be reduced by dividing the daily dose into three or four fractions. Although conclusive evidence is lacking, this strategy appears reasonable providing that compliance is not compromised. An alternative, which has not been evaluated, would be to prescribe the slow release formulation of valproate.

*Carbamazepine*

Carbamazepine has enjoyed a reputation as the AED associated with the least teratogenic risk. One recent study, however, reported a 0.9% risk of neural tube defects in offspring of mothers who took carbamazepine through pregnancy (Rosa 1991). There have also been reports of reduced head circumference at birth, although not at 5 years, and of developmental delay in 20% of infants (Jones et al 1989). These studies have been of small numbers and of uncontrolled data; and need to be replicated before being regarded as definitive.

*Other drugs*

There is very little human data on the teratogenic risk associated with the new AEDs, vigabatrin and lamotrigine. However, exposure of pregnant rabbits to vigabatrin has been associated with an increased incidence of fetal cleft palate. The birth of 16 normal infants to women taking vigabatrin has been reported, as have three spontaneous abortions in the first trimester and one stillbirth with congenital absence of the diaphragm.

12 normal births to women taking lamotrigine have been reported, with one miscarriage and one elective termination after the prenatal diagnosis of a neural tube defect. There are very few data on the use of gabapentin in pregnant women.

*Dysmorphic features*

Dysmorphic features such as epicanthal folds, long philtrum, flat nasal bridge, digital hypoplasia and hypertelorism are commonly associated with minor abnormalities that cause disability but do not result in serious impairment or death. Such abnormalities have, in the past, been ascribed to syndromes related to specific AEDs, such as the 'fetal hydantoin syndrome' (Hanson & Buehler 1982). A subsequent view has been to recognize a 'fetal AED syndrome'. More recently still the extent of the causal relationship with AEDs has been questioned and evidence has been put forward for maternal genetic factors influencing the development of epicanthus and digital hypoplasia (Gaily et al 1988). Larger prospective studies of women treated with monotherapy are necessary to resolve these issues.

Dysmorphic features may require the attentions of a plastic surgeon, although a recent study has indicated that digital and craniofacial hypoplasia tend to resolve over the first few years of life (Koch et al 1992). Some investigations have reported that babies exposed to AEDs in utero tend to be small for dates and to have slow postnatal growth and cognitive development. There is a lack of controlled data and most studies have suggested a very low risk of children exposed to AEDs prenatally being of low intelligence. A recent controlled prospective study found only a 1.4% increased risk of mental retardation in children exposed to AEDs (Granstrom & Gaily 1992). Furthermore, many other factors also come into play, including maternal and paternal genetic and psychosocial influences.

## 6.3.4 The role of folic acid

Serum folic acid concentrations less than 4 mg/ml have been associated with an increased risk of anomalies and spontaneous abortion. A UK Medical Research Council study found that 4 mg/d of folic acid given from preconception to women who had previously given birth to an infant with a neural tube defect was associated with a 72% protective effect (Medical Research Council Vitamin Study Research Group 1991). Folic acid supplementation has also been shown to have a protective role in the primary prevention of neural-tube defects (Czeizel & Dudas 1992, Rosenberg 1992). Although there has been no specific study of the effect of folic acid supplementation on the risk of neural-tube defects and other congenital malformations in women taking valproate or other AEDs it seems reasonable to extrapolate from the published studies and to recommend folic acid supplements (4 mg/d) during pregnancy for all women taking AEDs, starting before conception.

4 mg of folic acid per day is most probably more than is needed to achieve a maximal reduction of risk and this dose does not appear to cause adverse effects. It is also uncertain whether the measurement of red blood cell folate concentrations, so that supplementation may be adjusted

to result in high normal levels, is a useful exercise. In practical terms, if a supramaximal dose of folic acid results in an optimal risk reduction in all patients, without adverse effects and obviates the need for blood test monitoring, this is a reasonable policy to continue.

### 6.3.5 Preconception review of AED treatment

The importance of reviewing antiepileptic medication before conception should be emphasized to all female patients with epilepsy who are of reproductive potential. All too often women with epilepsy are referred for review of their treatment when they are 10–14 weeks pregnant, by which time the most critical period with regard to malformations has probably passed. The withdrawal of AEDs should be considered and discussed with the patient if she has been seizure-free for more than 2–3 years. She will need to know the risks of teratogenic effects from her medication and the risks of seizure recurrence should AEDs be tapered. The consequences of a recurrence of seizures, such as loss of driving licence and earning potential also need consideration (see Ch. 4, 4.6 for further details on these issues).

For most women with active epilepsy, the appropriate course is to establish them on the minimally effective dose of the single AED that gives the best control of their seizures, before they conceive. There have not, however, been good studies to establish that higher doses of a single AED carry a greater risk of teratogenesis than do lower doses.

It is useful to measure the serum drug concentration(s) that give the optimal control of the epilepsy before conception. These values can form a useful baseline against which to judge subsequent alterations.

We would not generally advocate changing from a particular AED, such as valproate, if that drug gave optimal seizure control, for example in a patient with juvenile myoclonic epilepsy, for whom the alternative may be a combination of carbamazepine and clonazepam.

In addition to advice about AEDs and the importance of regular medication-taking, patients should be reminded to avoid alcohol, smoking and other drugs and to ensure good nutrition throughout pregnancy, as failure to attend to these factors may have a deleterious effect on fetal development.

### 6.3.6 Management of epilepsy through pregnancy

Having established the patient on optimal monotherapy and determined the serum drug concentration prior to conception, subsequent management of AED doses through pregnancy is generally straightforward, but requires careful attention (Table 6.1). Serum AED concentrations often fall during pregnancy, particularly in the first and third trimesters. Many factors may be contributory, including increased hepatic clearance, increased renal clearance, increased plasma volume and reduced plasma albumin concentration. Reduced bioavailability, as a result of impaired absorption from the gastrointestinal tract, has also previously been regarded as an important factor, but recently its relevance has been cast in doubt. It is generally appropriate to measure serum concentrations of phenytoin, carbamazepine and phenobarbitone every

**Table 6.1** Important practice points: pregnancy and epilepsy

- Preconception counselling of patient about risks of teratogenesis and possible adverse effects of uncontrolled seizures to maternal health and pregnancy
- Preconception review of antiepileptic drugs; aim for minimal effective monotherapy if active epilepsy; consider drug withdrawal if seizure-free
- Commence folic acid supplements preconception
- Screen for malformations
- Monitor condition and antiepileptic drug concentrations through pregnancy
- Vitamin $K_1$ in last month of pregnancy, or for neonate
- Reassure patient that > 90% pregnancies proceed with no problem in women with epilepsy

2–3 months through gestation. Decreased drug concentrations do not necessarily require an increase in dose if there has not been any deterioration of seizure control. The advantage, however, of measuring concentrations at regular intervals is that it is then possible to advise an appropriate dose increment without delay, to return the concentrations to the levels that gave optimum seizure control preconception, should there be an increase in seizures. In some patients taking phenytoin measurement of free phenytoin may be more useful than the total concentrations, if seizure control is finely balanced with toxicity, and if hypoalbuminaemia develops. It pays dividends if time is taken to ensure that patients understand and agree with their prescription and the strategy of dose changes. Similarly, it is important to know exactly what medication the patient is actually taking if rational decisions about dosing are going to be made.

### 6.3.7 Prenatal diagnosis of malformations

Before conception, the patient and her partner need to be counselled about the fetal abnormalities that may be detected, and those that may be missed, by prenatal testing; and need to consider how they would react to the finding of an abnormal fetus and their views on a possible termination of the pregnancy.

At 16 weeks of gestation, alphafetoprotein concentration may be usefully measured in maternal blood. Maternal levels are elevated in 80% of pregnancies with fetal neural-tube defects. Estimation of alphafetoprotein concentration in amniotic fluid is much more sensitive but carries a 1% risk of causing an abortion; a risk that is of the same order as the 1–2% risk of neural-tube defect in women taking valproate. High-resolution fetal ultrasonography by an experienced operator at 16–18 weeks of pregnancy detects over 94% of neural-tube defects. In consequence, it may reasonably be argued that amniocentesis, for the purposes of alphafetoprotein determination, should be reserved for patients who have raised alphafetoprotein concentrations in maternal blood or in whom an ultrasound scan does not reliably exclude a neural-tube defect (Nadel et al 1990, Hobbins 1991).

Careful ultrasound studies at 20–24 weeks may also identify major cardiac, facial and limb anomalies. Patients and families need to be advised, however, that even the most sophisticated scans cannot detect 100% of abnormalities.

### 6.3.8 Management of labour

1–2% of women with active epilepsy will have a tonic-clonic seizure during labour, and further 1–2% will have such a seizure in the following 24 h. Generalized tonic-clonic seizures are likely to result in more profound hypoxia than in the non-gravid state, because of increased maternal oxygen requirements, and this may have deleterious effects on the fetus. Facilities for cardiopulmonary resuscitation should be immediately available.

The patient's regular AEDs should be continued through labour. All drugs may be given by nasogastric tube and phenytoin, valproate, phenobarbitone and some benzodiazepines may be given intravenously. It is useful to check serum drug concentrations if there is concern about inadequate dosing.

Most women with epilepsy have normal vaginal deliveries. Overbreathing, sleep deprivation, pain and emotional stress increase the risk of seizures during labour and it is appropriate to consider epidural anaesthesia early on, to minimize these factors. An elective caesarean section may be appropriate if the patient is having frequent tonic-clonic or prolonged complex partial seizures in the last weeks of pregnancy. A caesarean section would become indicated if frequent tonic-clonic, or complex partial seizures occurred during labour. Intravenous lorazepam has been advocated as the best acute treatment for serial seizures during labour (Yerby 1987). Intravenous phenytoin carries the theoretical concern that it inhibits myometrial contraction and so may prolong labour. In practical terms, however, a patient needing aggressive acute treatment for seizures is likely to be being prepared for caesarean section.

### 6.3.9 Vitamin K deficiency bleeding in infants

This is not a rare complication, carries a mortality rate in excess of 30%, is due to deficiency of factors II, VII, IX and X and is more likely to occur in women who have taken hepatic enzyme-inducing drugs through pregnancy. It is widely, but not universally, agreed that 20 mg/d of vitamin $K_1$ orally in the last month of pregnancy protects against this complication. There is a consensus that infants born of women with epilepsy should also receive 1 mg of vitamin $K_1$ intramuscularly at birth. Recently, concerns have been raised that the latter treatment is associated with an increased risk of childhood neoplasia (Golding et al 1992). The evidence is far from conclusive, however, and further studies are required before recommendations are made to alter an effective prophylactic therapy. Infants should receive intravenous fresh frozen plasma if there is evidence of bleeding or if the concentrations of two or more of factors II, VII, IX and X fall to less than 25% of normal.

### 6.3.10 Breast feeding and the puerperium

If the dose of AEDs has been increased during pregnancy, this should be reduced to preconception levels over the few weeks following delivery or toxicity will result.

Breast feeding is to be generally encouraged. When there is a risk of dropping the baby the mother should be advised to sit on floor cushions during feeding and to wash and change the baby on a plastic floor mat, rather than in a bath or on a raised surface. Bottle feeding, which the partner may share, may be appropriate if maternal fatigue is a factor that results in increased seizures. The amount of AEDs that enter breast milk depends on the free plasma concentration and lipophilicity of the drug. The breast milk/maternal plasma fraction of phenytoin is 10%, 5% for valproate, 45% for carbamazepine and 40% for pheno-barbitone. Barbiturates and benzodiazepines can result in the baby being drowsy, irritable and feeding poorly. The half-life of pheno-barbitone in the neonate is 40–300 h and the free fraction may exceed 90%, increasing the effect of the drug (Delgado-Escueta & Janz 1992). If the infant becomes sedated or irritable, the mother should be advised to reduce breast feeds and supplement with bottle feeds. Abrupt withdrawal of sedative medication from an infant, for example if s/he is fed entirely by bottle, may result in a withdrawal syndrome with agitation and tremor.

### 6.3.11 Development of seizures in pregnancy

The annual incidence of new cases of epilepsy in the reproductive years from the teens to 40 years is 20–30/100 000/year. In consequence, the development of epilepsy during pregnancy is not that unusual and, overall, the incidence is not increased. There are however a few specific aetiologies that may be encountered, such as an enlarging meningioma or arteriovenous malformation and vascular disease. The risk of ischaemic stroke is increased by a factor of 10 in the last 6 months of pregnancy, 50% of these strokes being attributable to specific causes, such as a coagulopathy, arteritis or cardiomyopathy. Approximately 4% of cerebral infarctions may be expected to result in seizures. Other specific vascular disorders which may occur in pregnancy and be complicated by seizures include cerebral venous thrombosis, subarachnoid haemorrhage and eclamptic hypertensive encephalopathy. In these conditions seizures will generally be just one manifestation of an acute neurological catastrophe, which requires urgent evaluation and treatment.

Investigation of seizures that develop in pregnancy should follow the same principles as for a non-gravid patient (Ch. 3). MRI is generally favoured over X-ray CT scanning in view of the superior resolution and the lack of ionizing radiation. It must be said, however, that the potential effects of a strong magnetic field on a developing fetus are not entirely clear, and that with the use of lead shielding the uterus may be largely protected from exposure during an X-ray CT scan.

The principles of initiating AED treatment in pregnancy are generally the same as for the non-pregnant patient. Concern about the teratogenic potential of AEDs will often raise the threshold for initiating therapy. Specific underlying causes such as stroke and eclamptic hypertensive encephalopathy will require their own treatment.

Status epilepticus arising as a consequence to eclampsia should be treated initially with phenytoin and a benzodiazepine such as lorazepam, in concert with the management of the eclampsia itself. Magnesium sulphate has found favour with obstetricians but is a poor AED and an inhibitor of uterine activity, and may have adverse effects on the baby.

## 6.4 THE GENETICS OF EPILEPSY

The study of the genetics of epilepsy is complex. A few uncommon conditions are inherited as single-gene or chromosomal disorders, with epilepsy as part of the phenotype. More frequent are the syndromes of idiopathic generalized epilepsy, which have a strong genetic contribution, the basis of which in most cases is not fully understood. Most cryptogenic epilepsies, however, fall into neither of these categories, with many factors contributing to the production of epilepsy, some genetic and some acquired. In such patients, the genetic contribution may be difficult to identify or quantify. Even in patients with a clearly defined acquired cerebral abnormality (for instance in head injury, stroke, cerebral tumour), epilepsy is a more common sequel in those with a positive family history than in those without – testament to a genetic predisposition to epilepsy even in predominantly acquired conditions. An inherited predisposition to epilepsy is presumably mediated through genetically determined alterations of cerebral structure or biochemistry, but little is currently known about the mechanisms of such effects (Anderson et al 1991).

### 6.4.1 Single gene and chromosomal disorders

Epilepsy is a major feature of over 160 single-gene disorders, in two-thirds of which mental retardation is also present (McKusick 1983). These conditions, however, contribute only about 1% of all cases of epilepsy. The most common examples of such genetically inherited epilepsies are as follows.

*Benign familial neonatal convulsions*

This is a rare condition, inherited as an autosomal dominant, with a penetrance of about 85% (Plouin 1992). The male and female incidence is equal. Convulsions develop in the first week of life in 80% of cases, with peak incidence of onset on the third day. Seizures remit within a few months in about one-third of cases, and in the first year in 70%. Seizures continue beyond the age of 5 in only about 10% of patients. There are no specific EEG changes. In some but not all affected families, the gene has been mapped to the long arm of chromosome 20 by linkage analysis (Leppert et al 1989, Ryan et al 1991). In a more recent unlinked family, a marker on chromosome 8q has been determined (Lewis et al 1993). Genetic counselling should advise that there is a 40–45% risk of an affected infant, although the relatively benign course of the condition should also be stressed.

*Tuberous sclerosis*

Tuberous sclerosis (synonyms: tuberose sclerosis, epiloia, Bourneville's disease) is the commonest of the mendelian-inherited epileptic conditions causing epilepsy (Ch. 2, 2.5.10). It is present in about 1/10 000 live births and is inherited in an autosomal dominant pattern. Recent linkage studies have suggested loci on chromosome 9q and 16 and the gene on chromosome 16 has recently been cloned (European Chromosome 16 Tuberous Sclerosis Consortium 1993).

*Other neurocutaneous syndromes*

Epilepsy is a common feature of other neurocutaneous syndromes (Smith 1982). Those that are autosomally dominantly inherited include neurofibromatosis and hypomelanosis of Ito. Autosomal recessive conditions include xeroderma pigmentosa and neuroichthyosis. Incontinentia pigmentosa has X-linked inheritance. Congenital non-genetic neurocutaneous syndromes with epilepsy include Sturge–Weber syndrome, neurocutaneous melanosis, and linear sebaceous naevus. Epilepsy is also an uncommon feature in other neurocutaneous syndromes including Chediak–Higashi syndrome, von Hippel–Lindau disease and Klippel–Trenaunay syndrome.

*Progressive myoclonus epilepsy syndromes*

These disorders have highly characteristic manifestations, with well-defined clinical features and prognosis (Chs 2, 2.8 and 3, 3.6.5) (Berkovic et al 1986, 1989, So et al 1989). Genetic counselling is required in most cases, fundamental to which is the identification of the underlying aetiology. Autosomal recessive inheritance occurs in Unverricht–Lundborg disease and sialidosis (types I and II), sphingolipidosis (Gaucher's disease, $GM_2$ gangliosidosis) and most forms of ceroid lipofuscinosis, although some cases of Kuf's disease may be autosomal dominant.

The gene for Unverricht–Lundborg disease (Baltic myoclonus) has recently been located on the long arm of chromosome 21 (Lehesjoki et al 1992, Malafosse et al 1992). Lafora body disease is autosomal recessive, although the location of the gene and the gene products have not been identified. Mitochondrial encephalopathy (MERRF) is transmitted by mitochondrial inheritance, the most common identified mutation being in the mitochondrial-coded lysine t-RNA (Hammans et al 1991, Berkovic et al 1991). Dentato-rubro-pallido-luysian atrophy (DRPLA) is inherited as an autosomal dominant condition with variable penetrance, and recently the genetic mechanism has been determined (Koide et al 1994).

*Other single-gene disorders causing epilepsy*

Many of the inborn errors of metabolism of the nervous system include epilepsy among their clinical features. Most are recessively inherited, and the epilepsy is only part of much more widespread abnormalities: the more common examples of the metabolic encephalopathies causing epilepsy are phenylketonuria, organic acidaemias, hyper-ammonaemia, disorders of purine metabolism (including Lesch–Nyhan disease), porphyrias, Wilson's disease, and peroxisomal disorders (including Zellweger's syndrome and the adrenoleuco-dystrophies). The metabolic storage disorders also commonly cause epilepsy, including some types of neuronal ceroid lipofuscinoses, mucopolysaccharidoses and sphingolipidoses. Menkes disease is inherited in an X-linked fashion; seizures may be the presenting feature and usually occur early in its course. Other genetic conditions of uncertain basis with epilepsy include Alper's disease, in which seizures (often status) and myoclonus are a common manifestation. Seizures may also occur in the hereditary ataxias, although they are seldom a predominant symptom. Benign familial myoclonus and benign familial neonatal seizures are epileptic syndromes inherited by an autosomal dominant mechanism, and some of the syndromes of benign partial epilepsy have putative autosomal dominant or multifactorial inheritance with age-specific penetrance (Heijbel et al 1975, Degen & Degen 1990).

*Chromosomal disorders causing epilepsy*

Chromosomal disorders can also cause epilepsy (Smith 1982). Seizures are frequent and severe in the rare syndromes of trisomy and deletion of 4p, trisomy of chromosome 13, and monosomy of 9p. In Down's syndrome, (chromosome 21 trisomy, mosaicism or translocation) epilepsy occurs in about 5–10% of cases, can take partial or generalized forms and may be very severe. In Klinefelter's syndrome (with XXY, XXXY or XXYY chromosomal patterns) epilepsy occurs in about 5%, usually associated with behavioural or cognitive disturbances. Not surprisingly, for a condition with such a heterogeneous aetiological, physiological and neurochemical substrate, no single chromosome or gene site has been found to be responsible for epilepsy.

### 6.4.2 Idiopathic generalized epilepsies

The clinical features of this range of conditions are described in Chapter 2, 2.7. These are the most common of the epilepsies with a strong genetic basis. The genetics of the idiopathic generalized epilepsies have been investigated in twin and family studies, with the clinical and EEG features considered separately, and more recently by molecular genetic methods (Duncan & Panayiotopoulos 1995). As yet, a clear understanding of the basic genetic mechanisms has not been reached.

The clinical studies are confounded by problems of definition and case ascertainment. Thus, both the occurrence of seizures and the EEG signature of idiopathic generalized epilepsy (the generalized spike wave discharge) have a highly age-dependent expression and, furthermore, EEG changes can be observed in persons without a history of seizures. Less specific EEG changes are found in an even higher proportion of relatives without a history of seizures. In the first comprehensive study of epilepsy with generalized spike wave discharges, Metrakos and Metrakos (1960, 1961) identified 211 patients with a centrencephalic EEG pattern and obtained a history of epilepsy from 13.5% of parents and 12.7% of 519 siblings. Centrencephalic EEG patterns were found in 7.7% of 195 parents, 36.7% of 223 siblings and 35% of 82 offspring. and less specific patterns in 9.2% of parents and 46.2% of siblings. In studies of absence seizures, Doose et al (1973) found a history of epilepsy (including febrile convulsions) in 7% of first-degree relatives and Tsuboi and Christian (1973) in 27%. A history of seizures was also found in 12.4% of offspring of 113 probands with awakening grand mal/absence/myoclonus and an abnormal EEG in 48%. Twin studies have also shown a concordance rate for idiopathic generalized epilepsy of the order of 80% in monozygotic and much lower rates in dizygotic twins.

A number of general conclusions can be drawn from these investigations.

- The idiopathic generalized epilepsies have a predominantly (perhaps exclusively) genetic basis. It is possible that there is an autosomal dominant mode of inheritance with variable penetrance, although a more complex multigenetic mechanism is more likely.
- The phenotypic expression of both the EEG and clinical manifestations of the condition is highly age-specific.
- For a child, the risks of inheritance are greatly increased by a positive family history. The risk runs from 80% for a person with an affected monozygotic twin, to over 25% if two first-degree relatives are affected, and between 5% and 20% if there is one affected first-degree relative. The risks of EEG abnormalities are greater.

The gene for juvenile myoclonic epilepsy (a subtype of idiopathic generalized epilepsy) was thought to be situated on the short arm of chromosome 6 (Greenberg et al 1988), but the validity of this localization has recently been questioned (Whitehouse et al 1993). Further clinical studies of this and other idiopathic generalized epilepsies are in progress. Alternative genetic approaches include analyses of animal models of generalized epilepsy and the search for candidate genes that determine proteins that are components of neuronal membrane ion channels and GABA and excitatory receptors (Noebels 1992, Gardiner 1995).

### 6.4.3 Genetic influences in other types of cryptogenic epilepsy

Hippocrates thought epilepsy to be a *familial condition*, and ever since an underlying genetic propensity in epilepsy has not been questioned. Indisputable, perhaps, but attempts to quantify this propensity in the generality of cases of epilepsy have been fraught with difficulty. Investigation has been greatly hampered in the past by the difficulty in establishing aetiology in the great majority of secondarily generalized and partial epilepsies. While it has been recognized that almost any cerebral disorder might result in epilepsy, in over two-thirds of cases none could be identified. The advances in neuroimaging of the past few years have revolutionized this situation, however, and a positive aetiological diagnosis of epilepsy is possible in over two-thirds of all cases. Many apparently cryptogenic cases are in fact due to congenital developmental disorders, some of which have a strong genetic basis. Until genetic studies have been carried out among these subcategories of cryptogenic epilepsy, there will be little progress in understanding the genetic basis of the condition. Similarly, advances in neurochemistry may reveal hitherto undetermined genetic syndromes, although this research is at an early stage.

Recently an autosomal dominant form of frontal lobe epilepsy, with a propensity to seizures occurring in sleep, has been described (Scheffer et al 1994) and it is likely that other inherited forms of partial seizure disorders will soon be identified.

Traditionally, an overall sibling risk of epilepsy in cryptogenic partial epilepsy has been said to be between 1% and 10%, with most studies citing figures between 2% and 5%. If EEG abnormalities are looked for, these are present in up to 20–30% of siblings, most of whom do not have a history of seizures. In one study of the effect of age of onset of seizures, the risk of seizures to siblings was 7.5% if the proband age of onset was 0–3 years and 4.3 if the proband age of onset was 4–15 years; the risk among controls without a sibling with epilepsy was 1.5% (Eisner et al 1959).

The overall cumulative incidence of unprovoked seizures among the offspring of patients with epilepsy is about 6%, and is twice as high amongst the offspring of female compared with male patients, and higher in those with an early onset of epilepsy. The risk of a patient with idiopathic generalized epilepsy having an affected child is about 9–12%, falling to 3% in the offspring of patients with cryptogenic partial epilepsy. The higher risk of transmission from affected female rather than male subjects raises the possibility at least that some of the genetic propensity to epilepsy may be passed on by mitochondrial inheritance. This information needs to be conveyed when counselling patients with epilepsy who are contemplating having children.

## REFERENCES

Anderson VE, Hauser WA, Leppik IE, Noebels JL, Rich SS 1991 Genetic strategies in epilepsy research. Epilepsy Res (suppl 4)

Annegers JF, Elveback LR, Hauser WA et al 1978 Congenital malformations and seizure disorders in the offspring of parents with epilepsy. Int J Epidemiol 7: 241–247

Annegers JF, Baumgartner KB, Hauser WA, Kurland LT 1988 Epilepsy, antiepileptic drugs, and the risk of spontaneous abortion. Epilepsia 29: 451–458

Beaussant-Defaye J, Basten N, Demarca C, Beaussart M 1985 Epilepsies and reproduction. Nord Epilepsy Research and Information Group, vol II. Grine, Lille

Berkovic SF, Andermann F, Carpenter S, Wolfe LS 1986 Progressive myoclonic epilepsies: specific causes and diagnosis. N Engl J Med 315: 296–305

Berkovic SF, Carpenter S, Evans A et al 1989 Myoclonus epilepsy and ragged-red fibres (MERRF): 1. A clinical, pathological, biochemical, magnetic resonance spectrographic and positron emission tomographic study. Brain 112: 1231–1260

Berkovic SF, Shoubridge EA, Andermann F, Andermann E, Carpenter S, Karpati G 1991 Clinical spectrum of mitochondrial DNA mutation at base pair 8344. Lancet 338: 457

Bilo L, Meo R, Nappi C et al 1988 Reproductive endocrine disorders in women with primary generalized epilepsy. Epilepsia 29: 612–619

Crawford P 1991 Catamenial seizures. In Trimble MR (ed) Women and epilepsy. John Wiley, Chichester, p 159–165

Czeizel AE, Dudas I 1992 Prevention of the first occurrence of neural-tube defects by periconceptional vitamin supplementation. N Engl J Med 327: 1832–1835

Dana-Haeri J, Richens A 1983 Effects of norethisterone on seizures associated with menstruation. Epilepsia 24: 377–381

Degen R, Degen HE 1990 Some genetic aspects of rolandic epilepsy: waking and sleep EEGs in siblings. Epilepsia 31: 795–801

Delgado-Escueta A V, Janz D 1992 Consensus guidelines: preconception counselling, management, and care of the pregnant woman with epilepsy. Neurology 42(suppl 5): 149–160

Doose H, Gerken H, Horstmann T, Volzke E 1973 Genetic factors in spike-wave absences. Epilepsia 14: 57–75

Duncan JS, Panayiotopoulos CP 1995 Typical absences and related epileptic syndromes. Churchill Livingstone, Edinburgh

Duncan S, Read CL, Brodie MJ 1993 How common is catamenial epilepsy? Epilepsia 34: 827–831

Eisner V, Pauli LL, Livingston S 1959 Hereditary aspects of epilepsy. Bull Johns Hopkins Hosp 105: 245–271

European Chromosome 16 Tuberous Sclerosis Consortium 1993 Identification and characterization of the tuberous sclerosis gene on chromosome 16. Cell 75: 1305–1315

Feely M, Calvert R, Gibson J 1982 Clobazam in catamenial epilepsy: a model for evaluating anticonvulsants. Lancet 2: 71–73

Gaily E, Granstrom M-L, Hiilesmaa V et al 1988 Minor abnormalities in children of mothers with epilepsy. J Pediatr 112: 520–529

Gardiner RM 1995 Genetics of human typical absence syndromes. In: Duncan JS, Panayiotopoulos CP (eds). Typical absences and related epileptic syndromes. Churchill Livingstone, Edinbugh, p 320–327

Golding J, Birmingham K, Greenwood R, Mott M 1992 Childhood cancer, intramuscular vitamin K, and pethidine given during labour. Br Med J 305: 341–346

Granstrom M-L, Gaily E 1992 Psychmotor development in children of mothers with epilepsy. Neurology 42(suppl 5): 144–148

Greenberg DA, Delgado-Escueta AV, Widlitz H, Sparkes RS, Treiman L, Maldonado HM 1988 Juvenile myoclonic epilepsy may be linked to the BF and HLA loci on human chromosome 6. Am J Med Genet 31: 185–192

Hammans SR, Sweeney MG, Brockington M, Morgan-Hughes JA, Harding AE 1991 Mitochondrial encephalopathies: molecular genetic diagnosis from blood samples. Lancet 337: 1311–1313

Hanson JW, Buehler BA 1982 Fetal hydantoin syndrome: current status. J Pediatr 101: 816–818

Heijbel J, Blom S, Rasmussen M 1975 Benign epilepsy of childhood with centrotemporal EEG foci: a genetic study. Epilepsia 16: 285–293

Herzog AG, Seibel MM, Schomer DL, Vaitukaitis JL, Geschwind N 1986 Reproductive endocrine disorders in women with partial seizures of temporal lobe origin. Arch Neurol 43: 341–346

Hobbins JC 1991 Diagnosis and management of neural-tube defects today. N Engl J Med 324: 690–691

Jones KL, Lacro RV, Johnson KA et al 1989 Pattern of malformations in the children of women treated with carbamazepine during pregnancy. N Engl J Med 320: 1661–1666

Koch S, Gopfert-Geyer J, Jager-Roman E et al 1983 Antiepileptika während der Schwangerschaft. Deutsche Med Wochenschr 108: 250–257

Koch S, Losche G, Jager-Roman E et al 1992 Major birth malformations and antiepileptic drugs. Neurology 42 (suppl 5): 83–88

Koide R, Ikeuchi T, Onodera O et al 1994 Unstable expansion of CAG repeat in hereditary dentatorubral-pallidoluysian atrophy (DRPLA). Nature Genet 6: 9–11

Lehesjoki AE, Koskiniemi M, Pandolfo M et al 1992 Linkage studies in progressive myoclonnus epilepsy: Unverricht–Lundborg and Lafora disease. Neurology 42: 1545–1550

Leppert MF, Anderson VE, Quattlebaum T et al 1989 Benign familial neonatal convulsions linked to genetic markers on chromosome 20. Nature 337: 647–648

Lewis TB, Leach RJ, Ward K, O'Connell P, Ryan SG 1993 Genetic heterogeneity in benign familial neonatal convulsions: identification of a new locus on chromosome 8q. Am J Hum Genet 53: 670–675

Lindhout D, Hoppener RJEA, Meinardi H 1984 Teratogenicity of antiepileptic drug combinations with special emphasis on epoxidation of carbamazepine. Epilepsia 25: 77–83

Lindhout D, Omtzigt JGC, Cornel MC 1992 Spectrum of neural-tube defects in 34 infants prenatally exposed to antiepileptic drugs Neurology 42(suppl 5): 111–118

McKusick VA 1983 Mendelian inheritance in man: catalogs of autosomal dominant, autosomal recessive and X-linked phenotypes, 6th edn. Johns Hopkins Press, Baltimore, MD

Malafosse A, Lehesjoki AE, Genton P et al 1992 Identical genetic locus for Baltic and Mediterranean myoclonus. Lancet 339: 1080–1081

Medical Research Council Vitamin Study Research Group 1991 Prevention of neural-tube defects: results of the Medical Research Council Vitamin Study. Lancet 338: 131–137

Metrakos JD, Metrakos K 1960 Genetics of convulsive disorders, part 1 (Introduction, problems, methods and base lines). Neurology 10: 228–240

Metrakos JD, Metrakos K 1961 Genetics of convulsive disorders, part 2 (genetics and electroencephalographic studies in centrencephalic epilepsy). Neurology 11: 474–483

Nadel AS, Green JK, Holmes LB, Frigoletto FD, Benacerraf BR 1990 Absence of need for amniocentesis in patients with elevated levels of maternal serum a fetoprotein and normal ultrasonographic examinations. N Engl J Med 323: 557–561

Nakane Y, Okuma T, Takahishi R et al 1980 Multi-institutional study on the teratogenicity and fetal toxicity of anticonvulsants: a report of a collaborative study group in Japan. Epilepsia 21: 663–680

Noebels JL 1992 Molecular genetics and epilepsy. In: Pedley TA, Meldrum BS (eds) Recent advances in epilepsy 5. Churchill Livingstone, Edinburgh, p 1–13

Plouin P 1992 Benign idiopathic neonatal convulsions (familial and non-familial). In: Roger J, Bureau M, Dravet C, Dreifuss FE, Perret A, Wolf P (eds) Epileptic syndromes in infancy, childhood and adolescence, 2nd edn. John Libbey, London, p 3–11

Rosa FW 1991 Spina bifida in infants of women treated with carbamazepine during pregnancy. N Engl J Med 324: 674–677

Rosciszewska D 1987 Epilepsy and menstruation. Epilepsia 12: 373–378

Rosenberg IH 1992 Folic acid and neural-tube defects – time for action? New Engl J Med 327: 1875–1876

Ryan SG, Wiznitzer M, Hollman C, Torres MC, Szekeresova M, Schneider S 1991 Benign familial neonatal c6+onvulsions: evidence for clinical and genetic heterogenity. Ann Neurol 29: 469–473

Scheffer IE, Bhatia KP, Lopes-Cendes I et al 1994 Autosomal dominant frontal epilepsy misdiagnosed as sleep disorder. Lancet 343: 515–517

Schmidt D, Canger R, Avanzini G et al 1983 Change of seizure frequency in pregnant epileptic women. J Neurol Neurosurg Psychiat 46: 751–755

Smith DW 1982 Recognisable patterns of human malformation. Major problems in clinical pediatrics, 3rd edn, vol VII. WB Saunders, Philadelphia, PA

So N, Berkovic S, Andermann F, Kuzniecky R, Gendron D, Quesney LF 1989 Myoclonus epilepsy and ragged-red fibres (MERRF): 2. electrophysiological studies and comparison with other progressive myoclonus epilepsies. Brain 112: 1261–1276

Tsuboi T, Christian W 1973 On the genetics of the primary generalised epilepsy with sporadic myoclonias of impulsive petit mal. Humangenetik 19: 155–182

Waters CH, Belai Y, Gott PS, Shen P, De Giorgio CM 1994 Outcomes of pregnancy associated with antiepileptic drugs. Arch Neurol 51: 250–253

Weber MP, Hauser WA, Ottman R, Annegers JF 1986 Fertility in persons with epilepsy. Epilepsia 27: 746–752

Whitehouse WP, Rees M, Curtis D et al 1993 Linkage analysis of idiopathic generalised epilepsy (IGE) and marker loci on chromosome 6p: no evidence for an epilepsy locus in the HLA region. Am J Hum Genet 53: 652–662

Yerby MS 1987 Problems in the management of pregnant women with epilepsy. Epilepsia 28(suppl 3): S29–S36

Zackai E, Mellman W, Neiderer B et al 1975 The fetal trimethadione syndrome. J Pediatr 87: 280–284

# 7 Managing the patient and their family

## 7.1 OVERALL MANAGEMENT OF THE PATIENT WITH EPILEPSY

### 7.1.1 Education and information giving

A satisfactory relationship between the patient and their physician is necessary for optimal management. This generally entails the patient and their family being actively involved in management decisions and not being dictated to. Education is very important. In general, patients need to have adequate information about how to deal with living with epilepsy, rather than detailed technical explanations about the pathophysiology of the condition. Some patients, however, seek and should be provided with more detailed medical information if they want it.

For education and counselling to be effective the provider needs to recognize the stress induced by a diagnosis of epilepsy and the fears patients have about the unpredictability of seizures. People with epilepsy can never be sure when, where or if a seizure will occur. Such a preoccupation may exist even if seizures have not occurred for years. People with epilepsy are often fearful of dying or endangering themselves or others during a seizure. Many types of seizures, particularly complex partial seizures, may involve bizarre behaviour that can give rise to personal embarrassment. In addition, there is a common fear that cumulative brain damage occurs with each seizure and that continued epilepsy inevitably results in dementia. Even when a child with epilepsy is very young some parents become preoccupied with whether their child can expect to lead a normal life in terms of school, work and marriage. Even quite young children with epilepsy express concerns such as: why do they have seizures? will they get worse? will seizures kill them? and might they go mad? Epilepsy may also have a detrimental effect on siblings, who may fear that they will 'catch the condition' or feel marginalized because parental attention is focused upon their brother or sister.

The primary care physician is in the best position to acknowledge such fears and explore them at the outset, before deep-seated worries become entrenched and have a deleterious effect upon emotional adjustment. Many misconceptions that exist regarding potential performance at school and work can be corrected. Unfortunately, clinic visits tend to focus on seizure counts and medication changes and side-effects, and psychosocial issues are seldom raised. Many patients with epilepsy and their families cope well, but benefit from this being acknowledged.

Information will often be conveyed in the course of an interactive discussion at the time of clinic appointments but, as only a small proportion of such data is generally retained, repetition is necessary. This can be usefully supplemented by written information sheets and videotape programmes that patients may study and discuss. Such written material is widely available, generally produced by voluntary agencies, such as the National Society for Epilepsy and the British Epilepsy Association in the UK and the Epilepsy Foundation of America in the United States.

In particular, patients and their relatives or carers need to be aware of: the nature of their seizures; precipitating factors that may be mitigated; activities and situations that should be avoided; reasonable risk taking; the prognosis of their epilepsy (Ch. 8.1); the role of medication, including its limitations and possible adverse effects, and the need for regular administration (Ch. 4). The nature and purpose of investigations need to be explained (Ch 3). Advice about first-aid and the acute management of seizures and indications for seeking emergency help should be given early on to patients and also to relatives, friends, colleagues and teachers (Ch. 5). Issues relating to contraception, pregnancy and heredity may need to be raised (Ch. 6). Social aspects also need to be discussed, including the implications for employment, driving, education and leisure activities (see below, 7.2).

The strategy and tactics of treatment and the organization of care, including the roles of the family doctor and primary care team and hospital-based specialists, need to be made clear and defined so that patients know how to work the system and who to approach for help with different problems. Advice needs to be individualized to a patient's particular circumstances. For example, avoidance of excessive fatigue in a student needs to centre on partygoing and timetables of studying that do not last all night. For the family taking young children with epilepsy on a long journey, adequate periods for rest and sleep need to be planned.

### 7.1.2 Adolescence

As with other conditions, such as diabetes, the management of epilepsy in adolescence can be particularly difficult and compounded by emotional upsets and rejection of parental authority. Epilepsy may become the focus of intrafamily conflict, being used both as a reason to restrict the adolescent's activities and as a rationale for under-achievement. Many adolescents with epilepsy feel great resentment and embarrassment, which adversely affect the development of social skills and may result in withdrawal and school avoidance.

Compliance with prescribed medications is often a major problem in this group and causes difficulties with making rational management decisions (Ch. 4, 4.2.5). For many, the antiepileptic medications are the visible evidence of epilepsy and are rejected along with the diagnosis. The establishment of a rapport with the treating physician, nurse practitioner or social worker is essential and there is a need for repeated non-confrontational counselling about the place, goals and limitations of drug therapy.

Other issues that are particularly likely to arise in this group are appropriate risk-taking and restriction of activities, the effects of alcohol and lack of sleep and the consequences of epilepsy for sexual functioning, relationships, reproduction, learning, scholastic performance and career choices.

### 7.1.3 Old age

The age-specific incidence of epilepsy rises after the age of 50 years, primarily on the basis of cerebrovascular disease. While the general principles of the diagnosis and treatment of epilepsy are the same as in the younger age-group, particular attention needs to be paid to the possible interactions with the other conditions and medications that an elderly patient may have. Further, the elderly patient is likely to metabolize AEDs more slowly and to be more susceptible to dose-related adverse effects. The possibility of impairment of memory needs serious consideration, and drug treatment regimens should be made as simple as possible and with appropriate reminders and cues.

### 7.1.4 Roles of voluntary agencies, self-help groups and professional counsellors

Voluntary agencies for people with epilepsy have been established in many countries. In the UK, for example, the National Society for Epilepsy produces written and videotape material for patients, relatives and professionals (including physicians, nurses, social workers and teachers). Frequent study days are organized and a network of community support groups provides self-help for patients and their families at a local level. Some patients derive considerable benefit from attending a self-help group, particularly from sharing problems and experiences with others. Some may find the multiplicity of voluntary organizations confusing. The British Epilepsy Association, for example, also produces educational material and sponsors local patient groups and there are separate regional societies in Wales, Scotland and Merseyside (Appendix). A similar situation pertains in many countries, with national, regional and local associations fulfilling different functions, but with some overlap.

Epilepsy nurse practitioners are becoming established, modelled on diabetes nurses, and have a very useful role at a primary care level, providing information and advice to patients and acting as a liaison with hospital-based clinics (Ch. 11, 11.3).

Counselling may be needed by some patients and their families who have difficulty coming to terms with epilepsy and its consequences and who as a result do not achieve their full potential in terms of occupation, living arrangements and behaviour. Non-specialist counselling may be provided by resources available in schools, colleges and community health centres. Counsellors with particular experience in epilepsy are generally only to be found in large epilepsy centres. Counselling has to be tailored to the individual's particular requirements and may be carried out in groups or singly and consist of practical discussions or more formal psychotherapy. In the case of children with epilepsy, family therapy may be needed to unravel and improve complicated family dynamics in order to optimize the quality of life not only of the patient with epilepsy but also of their siblings and parents. It is important that counselling is not viewed in isolation. Counselling needs to be integrated with social work, psychological and psychiatric input (Ch. 9). These may all have a significant role to play, for example in the patient with epilepsy, impaired language comprehension, depression and aggressive outbursts that threaten the break-up of the family unit.

## 7.2 SOCIAL CONSEQUENCES OF A DIAGNOSIS OF EPILEPSY

### 7.2.1 Driving in the UK and elsewhere

Research has repeatedly shown a substantially increased rate of road traffic accidents (and accidental deaths) in drivers suffering from epilepsy (Van der Lugt 1975, Taylor 1983, Parsonage 1986, Hansotia & Broste 1991, 1993), and for this reason the licensing for driving is subject to legislation in most countries of the world; indeed, this is one of the few areas where there is restrictive legislation concerned with epilepsy, in the developed world at least. Ideally, legislation should balance the excess risks of driving against the social and psychological disadvantage to individuals of prohibiting driving.

Driving regulations pertaining to epilepsy differ markedly from country to country. These range from a complete ban, as in Russia or Japan, to a 3-month seizure-free interval (Connecticut, USA). In some US States (e.g. California) the right to drive is left to the discretion of the patient's physician and the Driving Licence Board. There is a similar national variation as regards whether notification should come from the patient or their physician. The regulations in various countries have been summarized in a recent publication (Fisher et al 1994).

In the UK, documentation is produced by the licensing authority and a factsheet is provided by the National Society for Epilepsy (Espir & Godwin-Austin 1985, Driving and Vehicle Licensing Agency 1994, Shorvon 1994).

In the UK, the Driving and Vehicle Licensing Agency (DVLA) has a medical department which, on behalf of the Secretary of State, is empowered to consider the medical history of a licence applicant/holder and can (with an applicant's consent) obtain medical details from an applicant's personal doctors (hospital doctor or general practitioner). It is the DVLA, and not the sufferer's personal medical advisors, that makes the decision to allow/bar licensing. This arrangement (not shared by most other countries) has the important advantages that the medical aspects of the doctor–patient relationship are not overly compromised by questions of driving and that the personal doctors are not liable for the consequences.

The regulations are based on research into the risks of seizure recurrence in different clinical circumstances. The DVLA has an honorary medical advisory panel, which reviews individual cases in which doubt exists about eligibility for licensing and which reviews the regulations in the light of new findings. Stricter conditions are applied to group 2 licences because, in general, more time is spent driving, the consequences of accidents are often more serious and there is a greater risk of seizures occurring during driving.

Epilepsy is a 'prescribed disability', which means that a sufferer from epilepsy is barred in law from holding a licence unless the following criteria concerned with the control of seizures are met.

*Group 1 licences* (those for motorcars and motorcycles): An applicant for a licence suffering from epilepsy shall satisfy the following conditions:

a. He shall have been free of any epileptic attack during the period of

1 year immediately preceding the date when the licence is granted: or

b. In the case of an applicant who has epileptic attack(s) only while asleep, shall have demonstrated a sleep-only pattern for 3 years or more, without attacks while awake.
c. The driving of a vehicle is not likely to be a source of danger to the public.

The sleep regulations are designed so as not to prejudice the small subgroup of epilepsy sufferers whose attacks are confined to sleep and therefore will not constitute a danger to driving. The third condition is an important one, and is concerned with situations in which drug therapy, associated neurological or neuropsychiatric conditions may compromise road safety.

*Group 2 licences* (those for large goods vehicles (LGV) and public service vehicles (PSV) – i.e. vehicles over 7.5 tonnes, and nine seats or more, for hire or reward): An applicant for a licence shall satisfy the following conditions:

a. No epileptic attacks have occurred in the preceding 10 years and the sufferer has taken no antiepileptic drug treatment during this period.
b. There is no continuing liability to epileptic seizures.

The purpose of the second condition is to exclude persons from driving (whether or not epileptic seizures have actually occurred in the past) who have a potentially epileptogenic cerebral lesion or who have had a craniotomy or complicated head injury, for instance.

In relation to car driving, questions about the following circumstances commonly arise and may not be subject to the regulations:

*Single seizures*: These are not considered as 'epilepsy' by the DVLA unless a continuing liability can be demonstrated (usually by EEG or imaging). The licensing authority usually prohibits driving for a 12-month period after the attack.

*Provoked seizures*: If a seizure is considered to be 'provoked' by an exceptional condition that will not recur, epilepsy (defined as a condition exhibiting a continuing liability to seizures) is not deemed to be present. Driving is usually allowed once the provoking factor has been successfully or appropriately treated or removed, and provided that a 'continuing liability' to seizures is not also present. These cases are treated on an individual basis by the DVLA. A cautious attitude to 'provocation' is taken, however, and the provoking factor must be exceptional. Seizures related to alcohol or illicit drugs, for instance, are not considered 'provoked'.

*Mild seizures (e.g. myoclonic jerks)*: In the UK, the regulations apply regardless of the type of epileptic attacks. In Canada, in contrast, myoclonic jerks are not a bar to driving.

*Seizures without apparent alteration of consciousness (partial seizures, auras, etc)*: The regulations apply, because of the practical difficulty of being certain that consciousness is not altered during attacks. In many other countries, for examples the USA, simple partial seizures do not generally affect the holding of a driver's licence.

*Antiepileptic drug withdrawal*: The DVLA recommends that driving be suspended from the commencement of drug reduction and for 6 months after drug withdrawal. This is advisory and is not covered by legislation. The patient should be warned there is an increased risk of seizure recurrence, quoting an overall 40% risk in the first year of drug withdrawal, although this risk varies according to individual patient factors (Ch. 4, 4.6).

*Attacks occurring during changes in medication*: Any recurrence of attacks during drug changes (or withdrawal) in a person with epilepsy will result in the application of the epilepsy regulations and a licence will be barred. This is the case regardless of circumstance and whether or not the drug change was deliberate or accidental.

*Electroencephalographic changes*: Although an EEG can provide useful confirmation of epilepsy, the diagnosis of epilepsy is essentially clinical. Unequivocal episodes of 3 Hz spike/wave discharges in idiopathic generalized epilepsy are considered to be seizures, even if in the apparent absence of clinical accompaniment. This is because evidence shows that consciousness is invariably impaired during such electrographic bursts. This is the only situation in which the DVLA considers a clinically inapparent EEG change to be classifiable as a seizure.

*Neurosurgery*: If epilepsy occurs following neurosurgery, the epilepsy regulations must be applied. An exception can be made when seizures occur at the time of surgery. Following intracranial surgery, even if seizures have not occurred, driving is usually prohibited for a period that varies according to the type of underlying pathology and the nature and site of the neurosurgery (Table 7.1).

*Cerebral lesions*: When certain cerebral lesions are demonstrated, a single seizure is considered to be epilepsy (on the basis that a continuing liability to seizures is present). In the following conditions, even when epilepsy has not occurred, restrictions are still applied because of the known risk of epilepsy: malignant brain tumours, cerebrovascular disease, serious head injury, intracranial haemorrhage and cerebral infection. The duration of the period of restriction is based on research evidence of the risks of seizures (Table 7.1).

*Treatment status*: The epilepsy regulations apply whether or not the sufferer is receiving antiepileptic drug treatment and starting (or changing) antiepileptic drug treatment does not influence a decision about licensing.

The regulations have the virtue of simplicity but may be unfair to a small number of borderline cases (e.g. those whose seizures are mild, confined to a specific situations or in which awareness is fully maintained, those where accidental drug changes occurred), but legislation in these areas would be very difficult to draft or apply and there is a general perception that the current rules are both fair and sensible.

**Table 7.1** Cerebral lesions where driving is restricted because of the risk of epilepsy (when seizures have not yet occurred). This is a summary of the rules, which also depend on other clinical features (derived from DVLA 1994)

| Condition | | Duration of restriction on driving (Group 1 licences) |
|---|---|---|
| *Cerebral tumours* | | |
| ● Benign supratentorial tumour treated by craniotomy | | 12 months |
| ● Grade 1 malignant brain tumour | | 12 months |
| ● Grade 2/3 malignant brain tumour | | 24 months |
| ● Grade 4 malignant brain tumour | | 48 months |
| ● Pituitary tumour treated by craniotomy | | 6 months |
| *Cerebral vascular diseases* | | |
| ● Extradural haematoma treated by craniotomy | | |
| – without cerebral damage | | 6 months |
| – with cerebral damage | | 12 months |
| ● Acute subdural haematoma | | |
| – treated by burr holes | | 6 months |
| – treated by craniotomy | | 12 months |
| ● Acute intracerebral haematoma treated by surgery (burr holes or craniotomy) | | 6 months |
| ● Subarachnoid haemorrhage treated by surgery | | |
| – Ant./post. cerebral aneurysm with neurological deficit | | 6 months |
| – Middle cerebral aneurysm | without deficit | 6 months |
| | with deficit | 12 months |
| ● Subarachnoid haemorrhage due to aneurysm – untreated | | 6 months |
| ● Unruptured aneurysm treated by craniotomy | | 6 months |
| ● Subarachnoid haemorrhage due to AVM treated by surgery | | 12 months |
| *Cerebral infection* | | |
| ● Cerebral abscess treated by surgery (burr holes or craniotomy) | | 12 months |
| ● Acute encephalitis or meningitis (associated with seizures in acute phase) | | 6 months |
| ● Cerebral infarction, haemorrhage, and transient ischaemic attack | | |
| – single attack with satisfactory recovery | | 1 month |
| – recurrent attacks with satisfactory recovery | | 3 months |
| *Other conditions* | | |
| ● Serious head injury (operated acute intracerebral haematoma, or compound depressed fracture with > 24 h post traumatic amnesia, or dural tear | | 12 months |
| ● Intraventricular shunt (revision or insertion) | | 6 months |

*Notes*
If seizures have occurred in the above conditions, the epilepsy regulations must apply (an exception is for the occurrence of seizures during the acute phase of meningitis, encephalitis, stroke, head injury). In other conditions/treatments driving is not usually restricted (e.g. benign supratentorial cerebral tumour without surgical treatment, benign infratentorial tumour treated by surgery, chronic subdural haematoma, pituitary tumours treated by transphenoidal surgery, AVM treated by embolization, etc)

It must be stressed that there is a legal obligation in the UK for the person with epilepsy to inform the DVLA about the condition. This is the case regardless of clinical or domestic circumstances or extenuating factors. The obligation on the doctor is to inform the patient about the regulations and instruct the sufferer to inform the DVLA. This instruction should be recorded in the medical notes, to avoid claims of negligence.

### 7.2.2. Lifestyle restrictions and precautions

Doctors will be frequently asked about the suitability of certain leisure activities for people with epilepsy. There are, however, few findings from scientific studies that can act as a basis for decision making. It is difficult to provide clear-cut answers that are appropriate to every situation. Individual assessment of both the person concerned and the proposed activity is highly desirable but not always possible. Most sports that are undertaken competitively now have their own club medical advisors, who can be valuable sources of advice. The voluntary epilepsy associations can provide advice and guidance and the British Sports Association for the Disabled is another useful resource.

In a review of the effect of exercise on seizure frequency, there was no strong evidence to suggest physical exertion had an adverse effect on seizure frequency (Ellertson et al 1993). However, studies are few, particularly those which include adequate controls. In one recent study, the median number of seizures dropped during the exercise phase of a controlled trial. However, considerable individual variability was noted, with changes in seizures ranging from a decrease of 65% to an increase of 20%. The authors concluded,'physical training represented no danger and a number of positive effects in the group including a reduction in overall number of seizures. Physical training like the aerobic training programme presented can be recommended safely for people with epilepsy'.

One-off accidents can happen to anyone whether epilepsy is present or not. If a seizure occurs during an activity this does not mean something tragic will ensue and future participation must be barred. Nor should it be concluded that the activity precipitated the seizure. Anxiety on the part of family members and responsible professionals is entirely appropriate and understandable but it should not be allowed to lead to unreasonable restrictions and the psychological consequences these will produce. It is also quite reasonable to arrange a higher level of skilled supervision if a participant with epilepsy would be likely to sustain significant injury during an activity or where other participants could be in danger if a seizure occurred. For high-risk activities in which such supervision is not available, the freedom-from-seizure rule used to assess fitness to drive has been suggested as being applicable (Thompson & Oxley 1993).

The following guidelines for risk assessment have been adapted from Sonnen (1988). He recommends the following when advising parents and people with epilepsy.

- Point out the difference between safeguards appropriate to a short-term illness and those appropriate for a chronic condition such as epilepsy
- Assign each patient to a high- or low-risk group on the basis of the known factors about that patient

- Distinguish between restrictive measures, e.g. a ban on swimming, and non-restrictive measures, e.g. proper supervision during swimming
- Emphasize that leisure is as important an activity to the child's development as school work
- Avoid giving dogmatic 'yes' or 'no' answers to parents' enquiries, however much this is requested
- Outline the facts, those that exist, and the options which will allow patients to make their own judgements

*Participation in sports*

Boxing, wrestling and other contact sports where injury to the head is highly probable are not advisable for people with epilepsy. Exacerbation of a seizure disorder may occur should brain damage result from a blow to the head.

Team sports such as soccer, cricket, basketball and netball, which are undertaken in most schools, are generally appropriate for individuals with epilepsy. Recommendations regarding swimming should take into account the features of the person's epilepsy. When seizure control is good, the risks are reduced. Exploration of possible triggering factors such as cold water, stress and excitement need to be explored. In properly managed swimming pools there should be little extra risk for the person with epilepsy and minimal increase in the workload for swimming pool attendants. Every person with epilepsy should have the benefit of learning to swim. Swimming in the sea and rivers carries more hazard and should be avoided unless seizures are controlled.

There are no laws regarding cycling and epilepsy, but riders may be financially liable if they cause an accident and another person is injured. It has been suggested that a 2-month seizure-free period is a reasonable rule regarding going cycling (Thompson & Oxley 1993). Wearing a cycling helmet should be strongly advised for the person with epilepsy.

*Other social activities*

For a number of individuals, leisure involves the social milieu of the local cafe or bar. Medical opinion on drinking alcohol varies. Some physicians recommend total avoidance of alcohol and others suggest that it can be taken in moderation. If the person with epilepsy has good seizure control there is usually no contraindication to the moderate consumption of alcohol, up to 2 units per day. They need to be aware, however, that the acute effects of alcohol are potentiated by concomitant AEDs. In the end it comes down to the person with epilepsy weighing up the evidence, the risk of seizures, their confidence of keeping within the bounds of occasional drinking and their own experience. Some people with epilepsy choose not to drink alcohol at all and it is now increasingly socially acceptable to drink non-alcoholic or low-alcohol beverages. Alcohol-induced seizures usually occur in the withdrawal phase. Some patients experience marked exacerbation of seizures on alcohol withdrawal and these individuals should avoid the use of alcohol altogether (Mattson 1983). When drinking becomes excessive or occurs in binges, poor seizure control is more likely to arise. In part, this is because heavy drinking is often associated with late nights, missed meals and forgotten tablets.

Discotheques are a part of normal growing up and should not be needlessly avoided by the young person with epilepsy who seeks a full social life. Some people may find flashing, flickering lights unpleasant but generally it is only bright white strobe lights, operating at more than 10 flashes per second, that may, in some individuals with photosensitive epilepsy, induce seizures. It should be emphasized that the majority of those with epilepsy are not photosensitive. Many local authorities have rules governing the use of such lights, restricting the flash frequency to make the induction of seizures less likely. Should a person with epilepsy be exposed to such a light, however, turning away from the light source and covering one eye should be sufficient to prevent an attack. If a seizure should occur in a discotheque it may well be spontaneous or due to another cause.

A few people with epilepsy have seizures while watching television, but in view of the amount of time spent in this activity, this is likely to be by chance rather than a causal association. It is only individuals with photosensitive epilepsy who will have seizures provoked by television. In such patients, sitting 2–3 m away from the set, at a level with the screen and not below it, reduced screen contrast and brightness, and increased background illumination in the room reduce the risk of seizures. The susceptible person should also avoid approaching the set and use hand-held controls to make adjustments. Similarly, video games pose problems for only a minority of children (Fish et al 1994) (Ch. 4, 4.1.3).

*Holidays*

Having epilepsy should not be a reason for avoiding taking holidays. The type of the holiday and the activities involved must be considered on an individual basis. Most countries have no restrictions regarding entry of people with epilepsy. Restrictions regarding the carrying of antiepileptic drugs are variable and patients travelling abroad should take with them a written statement from their doctor that details the type and dosage of their treatment. It is advisable for the traveller with epilepsy to take sufficient medication with them for the entire vacation as replacements may be difficult to obtain and formulations may vary significantly. Patients should be warned that antimalarial prophylaxis may increase the risk of seizures in susceptible persons. The International Bureau for Epilepsy (IBE) has published a small book of guidelines for the traveller with epilepsy, which includes details of any restrictions imposed by 58 countries (International Bureau for Epilepsy 1989).

Most airlines do not have restrictions regarding persons with epilepsy. However, if seizures are likely to occur it is advisable to inform the airline in advance. Flying does not cause seizures but disrupted sleep and altered biological rhythms on long-distance flights may trigger seizures. A benzodiazepine, such as clobazam, may be usefully taken to cover a journey in these circumstances. Sleep deprivation should be minimized and individuals should try to compensate for any loss of sleep on arrival. Time changes due to long-distance travel may also effect taking medication. Changes necessitated by new time zones should be phased in gradually after arrival. The traveller with epilepsy abroad needs to know how and where to obtain medical help in the country they are visiting and in addition it may be useful to know how to get in touch with local epilepsy support organizations.

*Safety in the home*

Most accidents occur within the home and garden. Often they result from careless errors or oversight. Forethought and common sense will reduce the risk of injuries.

*Cooking*: There is a high risk of accidents in the kitchen. If seizures are frequent, the ideal solution to reduce the risk of burns when cooking is to use a microwave oven to prepare meals and hot drinks. Gas cookers have advantages and disadvantages. They can, for example, be easily turned off, but the naked flame can result in burns, particularly if contact is made with clothing during a seizure. Electric cookers avoid this problem but they do take longer to cool down when switched off and this too can result in burns. When cooking on a hob it is safer to use back burners with handles of saucepans pointing backwards, never sticking out where they may be knocked, causing spillage of food and accidents. When serving food it is safer to bring plates to the stove rather than bring a pan of hot food to the plate. The use of electric deep fat fryers for cooking chips and other such foods, electric toasters and coffee makers is also associated with less risk of burns than the use of kettles, open pans and saucepans.

*Bathing*: The possibility of a person with epilepsy having a seizure and drowning in a bath is a hazard that must be acknowledged. This risk may be avoided by the use of a shower or a shallow bath, with the taps turned off before getting into the tub. People with epilepsy should let somebody know when they are taking a bath. We would also recommend that, in order to improve access, people with uncontrolled seizures should not lock themselves into the bathroom or toilet but rather employ an engaged notice or use a lock that can be opened from the outside.

*Sleeping*: The risk of falling out of bed is probably not very great but it can be minimized by having low-level divans or mattresses on the floor. If individuals do not wish to adopt these options, they can reduce the risk of sustaining injury by having soft carpets or mats fitted around the bed. For individuals who have nocturnal seizures it may be sensible to invest in safety pillows. These reduce the risk of suffocation, but for the majority of people with epilepsy such precautions are unnecessary.

*Heating*: Central heating is probably one of the safest ways of heating houses if radiators are reasonably flush against the walls. In high-risk situations, low temperature radiators may be recommended. Fixed lighting is also sensible. Wall lights cannot be knocked over and also result in more space in the room. Trailing flexes should be avoided. If seizures are really poorly controlled, then windows and doors can be fitted with specially toughened glass.

*Outdoors*: Some safety precautions may be needed outside the home. If full seizure control has not been achieved, the wearing of a MedicAlert bracelet or necklace may be sensible. MedicAlert is a charitable organization which was founded almost 50 years ago. There is a once-in-a-lifetime membership fee. The cost covers a specially engraved bracelet or necklace which contains details of the person's medical problems and also a telephone number. People coming to the assistance of someone having a seizure outside their home are then in a position to phone the number and obtain more information.

For a minority of patients with frequent seizures in which sudden falls occur, protective headgear should be considered to reduce the risk of head injury. Understandably, patients often resent these helmets because of the visible label of epilepsy.

### 7.2.3. Schooling

This section is written with reference to the schooling system in the UK. The same general principles, however, are globally applicable. A substantial portion of a child's life is spent at school and, understandably, this environment will greatly influence the child's academic, emotional and social development. Sweeping statements about children with epilepsy are difficult to make. The majority of children with epilepsy now attend mainstream schools and the numbers so doing have increased substantially over the past two decades, particularly following the 1981 Education Act. This advocated that children, even with special needs, should be educated wherever possible in normal schools. Placing a child in a mainstream school, however, is no guarantee of educational success. There is evidence from a number of studies that a significant number of children with epilepsy do underachieve with respect to their overall ability.

Academic difficulties can arise for a number of reasons. Most research attention has focused on seizure-related factors, with poor educational prognosis associated with early age of onset and a long history of poorly controlled seizures (Seidenberg 1989). For children with complex partial seizures, the site of the epileptic discharge may influence the nature of the cognitive disturbance. Seizures arising from the left hemisphere, as this is for most people the primary language processing hemisphere, seem at greatest risk.

Other factors which should be considered as a possible cause of lack of achievement include the occurrence of nocturnal seizures, brief epileptic discharges which can result in transient cognitive impairment in the classroom and high levels of medication or polypharmacy (Ch. 9, 9.5). Psychosocial factors, however, are often the main culprits and, if recognized early, are easier to rectify. These include low expectations of both parents and teachers, frequent and prolonged absences from school, low self-esteem and anxiety of the child, possibly developing from bullying and teasing at school.

A minority of children with epilepsy may require some special educational input. This may range from a few classes within the ordinary school environment to a residential placement. The provision of specialized input will generally only be made after the child has been 'statemented'. This requires the educational authorities to conduct a multiprofessional assessment taking into account medical, educational, psychological and other factors, including the views of parents. If, following this assessment, the consensus is that the child has special educational needs, a written statement of such needs must be made and special education provision must be made to meet these needs. When placement in special schools is considered, this decision will often have been made because of the severity of an accompanying behavioural or learning problem and not on the basis of the epilepsy alone.

Inadequate communication can contribute to educational and social difficulties for the child with epilepsy. During the 1950s in the UK it was estimated that up to half of all children with epilepsy were unknown to the school authorities. It is to be hoped the situation has now improved; however, non-disclosure by parents definitely still occurs (Thompson 1987). If the school is unaware that a child has seizures, the impact of an attack during school hours is potentially devastating. Reports which have focused in part on the education of children with epilepsy have endorsed the need for openness and a full exchange of information between the primary health care service and school health services. When good communication channels exist they can exert a positive influence on treatment. Communication is of limited value and may even be counterproductive unless the exchange of information is accurate and the recipients have adequate knowledge to understand what is being said. The doctor must ensure that parents have an accurate and adequate understanding about epilepsy and must encourage them to pass this on to the school, as well as communicating directly with teachers. The DHSS Working Group (Department of Health and Social Security 1986) considered school nurses to have a pivotal role within the school health services, including 'allaying fears about epilepsy and promoting the ability of children with epilepsy'.

It is important that undue restrictions on sporting and other activities are not imposed as a result of faulty information. Such restrictions can have a negative impact on a child's self-image and their ability to relate to peers. For the child with epilepsy, minimizing time off school is important. Teachers with adequate knowledge will be able to ensure that a whole day's schooling is not lost because of a seizure occurring during the first lesson. Clinic appointments also can be scheduled to minimize time away from school. When hospitalization is required, the professionals involved should ensure that the period of in-patient treatment is limited and, if elective, is scheduled to occur during vacations. If a child is likely to miss several weeks from school, the possibility of providing education within the hospital setting should be explored. Careful, yet unobtrusive, observation and monitoring of educational progress and social development of the child with epilepsy is important. Unfortunately, problems are all too often perceived as an invariable consequence of the child having epilepsy. The earlier difficulties are observed, the sooner they can be addressed. Good communication from teacher to parents may result in a medical review, and possible medication changes and improvement in school performance may ensue. Similarly, the child's physician should regularly ask about how the child is progressing at school when medication reviews are taking place. If a child presents with poor academic progress, psychological or social difficulties, then a detailed psychological evaluation should be sought. It is possible that a child has cognitive deficits secondary to a specific cerebral dysfunction. These should be identified at an early an age as possible, so that appropriate remedial tuition may be commenced to mitigate their adverse effects and to capitalize on the child's strengths.

### 7.2.4. Employment

Dissatisfaction with employment represents one of the major concerns of people with epilepsy. It has been accepted that unemployment and underemployment are over-represented in people with epilepsy, as they are in other groups with disabilities. Difficulties with employment generally has financial repercussions but also can have a serious impact on the psychological and social adjustment of the individual.

Restrictions upon employment arise for a number of reasons. In the UK there are some legislative barriers. For instance, for certain occupations a history of epilepsy is sufficient to bar recruitment. This includes the armed services, diving, operational duties in the fire brigade, London regional transport and the merchant navy. For other occupations, a recent history may make some occupations untenable. This includes working in the prison service and the police force, traffic wardens and train drivers. For many professions, no specific legislation exists and each case will be considered individually. However, there may be difficulty in working as a teacher, a nurse, a doctor or a health visitor if seizures are not extremely well controlled.

In some cases, high levels of unemployment in epilepsy are attributable to prejudice and often ignorance on the part of the employer. Surveys of employers show that many hold a number of myths about people with epilepsy, for instance that people with epilepsy have high accident rates, place others in physical danger, have lower levels of performance, lower productivity rates, elevated absentee rates and require a considerably higher insurance premium (John & McLellan 1988). There is a lack of evidence to support these beliefs. The doctor may be in a position to support a person's application and dispel misconceptions which may exist, and thus assist the person gain employment. A number of voluntary organizations run workshops aimed at employers which focus on employment of people with epilepsy, the problems and misconceptions. The International Bureau for Epilepsy, which is the international body representing the voluntary agencies in various countries, has in an attempt to promote employment drawn up principles of good practice directed toward employers about employing people with epilepsy. This can be obtained from the voluntary epilepsy organizations (see Appendix).

In some instances, the reason for unemployment resides with the person themselves. Individuals may have unrealistic expectations, inadequate qualifications and others may harbour negative attitudes. There are a few studies which show that people with epilepsy expect a negative attitude from employers and therefore approach job application forms and interviews in an overtly hostile way. Some people with epilepsy may need to develop their job-seeking skills, e.g. the presentation of their epilepsy and when and how to disclose their seizures. Although superficially attractive, non-disclosure of active epilepsy is not to be recommended, as the occurrence of a seizure may be embarrassing or dangerous and can result in instant dismissal.

*Career advice*

Career advice needs to be geared to the strengths and weaknesses of each individual, with regard to their mental and physical attributes, and the local job opportunities. In the UK, for instance, large job centres have Disability Employment Advisors, who may provide practical advice. Aspirations need to be appropriate. If, for example, a patient has had epilepsy that has been difficult to control for many years and eventually achieves seizure control, it is sensible advice that they do not take a job for which a driving licence is crucial.

*Financial support*

Financial assistance from the State to support individuals out of work varies enormously between countries. In the UK, there may also exist considerable variation in entitlement to benefits. If people have had paid employment in the past and have accrued sufficient National Insurance they may be entitled to Invalidity Benefit. If they do not meet these requirements, then they may be eligible for Income Support. For all people under the age of 65 whose seizures result in difficulty in physically getting around and/or result in them needing personal care, application can be made for the Disability Living Allowance. Certification by a doctor must accompany such an application. For people with severe difficulties, most notably where epilepsy is combined with learning difficulties, there is also the Severe Disablement Allowance. When an individual is in receipt of Disability Living Allowance and the Severe Disablement Allowance, their 'carer' may be entitled to make a claim for Invalidity Care Allowance. For people in receipt of Income Support there are also other benefits, such as assistance with fares for visiting hospital for out-patient visits or in-patient admissions. For those on Income Support it is also possible they may get Housing Benefit to assist them in paying rent. For all low-income families in which the adult working income is low, there is the possibility of Family Credit.

Understanding Social Security benefits is by no means straightforward. It is often useful to have a Welfare Rights' Advisor, a social worker or some other person to assess an individual's circumstances and to offer assistance to complete the necessary paperwork.

## REFERENCES

Department of Health and Social Security 1986 Report of the working group on services for people with epilepsy: A report to the Department of Social Security, the Department of Education and Science and the Welsh Office. HMSO, London

Driving and Vehicle Licensing Agency 1994 At a glance guide to the current medical standards of fitness to drive. DVLA, Swansea

Ellertson B, Erikson HR, Mostofsky DI, Ursin H 1993 Exercise and epilepsy. In: Mostofsky DI, Loyning Y (eds) The neurobehavioural treatment of epilepsy. Lawrence Erlbaum, New Jersey, p 107–122

Espir M, Godwin-Austin RB 1985 In: Raffle A (ed) Medical aspects of fitness to drive. Medical Commission on Accident Prevention, London

Fish DR, Quirk JE, Smith SJM, Sander JWAS, Shorvon SD 1994 Videogames and epilepsy. Final Report. HMSO, London
Fisher RS, Parsonage M, Beaussart M et al 1994 Epilepsy and driving: an international perspective. Epilepsia 35: 675–684
Hansotia P, Broste SK 1991 The effect of epilepsy or diabetes mellitus on the risk of automobile accidents. N Engl J Med 324: 22–26
Hansotia P, Broste SK 1993 Epilepsy and traffic safety. Epilepsia 34: 852–858
International Bureau for Epilepsy 1989 A traveller's handbook for persons with epilepsy. IBE, The Hague
John C, McLellan L 1988 Employer's attitude to epilepsy. Br J Indust Med 45: 713–715
Mattson RA 1983 Seizures associated with alcohol use and alcohol withdrawal. In: Browne TR, Feldman RG (eds) Epilepsy, diagnosis and management. Little, Brown, Boston, MA, p 325–332
Parsonage M 1986 Fits and other causes of loss of consciousness while driving. Q J Med 58: 295–304
Seidenberg M 1989 Academic achievement and school performance in children with epilepsy. In: Hermann BP, Seidenberg M. (eds) Childhood epilepsies, neuropsychological, psychosocial and intervention aspects. John Wiley, Chichester, p 105–118
Shorvon SD 1994 Driving and epilepsy. A National Society for Epilepsy factsheet. National Society for Epilepsy, Chalfont St Peter
Sonnen AEH 1988 Practical guidelines for dealing with risk in patients with epilepsy. In: Canger R, Loeber JN, Castellano F (eds) Epilepsy and society: realities and prospects. Excerpta Medica (ICS 802), Amsterdam, p 165–168
Taylor JF 1983 Epilepsy and other causes of collapse at the wheel. In: Godwin-Austin RB, Espir ML (eds) Driving and epilepsy and other causes of impaired consciousness. Royal Society of Medicine, International Congress and Symposium Series 60. Royal Society of Medicine, London
Thompson PJ 1987 Educational attainment in children and young people with epilepsy. In: Oxley J, Stores G (eds) Epilepsy and education. Medical Tribune Group, London, p 15–24
Thompson PJ, Oxley JR 1993 Social aspects of epilepsy. In: Laidlaw J, Richens A, Chadwick D (eds) A textbook of epilepsy, 4th edn. Churchill Livingstone, Edinburgh, p 661–704
Van der Lugt PJM 1975 Traffic accidents caused by epilepsy. Epilepsia 16: 747–751

# 8 Prognosis, prevention, morbidity and mortality

## 8.1 THE PROGNOSIS OF EPILEPSY

The prognosis of epilepsy may be defined as the prospect of attaining terminal remission once an individual has established a pattern of recurrent epileptic seizures. 70–80% of people developing epilepsy will achieve this, while the remaining 20–30% will continue having seizures despite optimum drug treatment. Remission usually occurs within the first 5 years. Thus, for the majority of people, epilepsy is a short-lived condition (Sander 1993). Several aspects of prognosis deserve closer consideration. These include the risk of seizure recurrence after a first epileptic seizure, the natural history of the condition and the influence of aetiology and treatment on the long-term prognosis.

### 8.1.1 Recurrence after a single seizure

The traditional view that single seizures should not be equated with epilepsy originated from early studies which indicated that many patients with a single seizure had no further seizures. Hauser & Kurland (1975), however, found the incidence of epilepsy to be much greater than that of single seizures, suggesting that the great majority of patients with a single seizure will have a recurrence. Reported estimates of the risk of recurrence after a first seizure have varied from 27–81% (Hauser & Hesdorffer 1990, Hart et al 1990, Berg & Shinnar 1991, Sander 1993). The majority of hospital-based estimates have fallen in the lower end of the range while estimates from population-based studies and studies in which patients were enrolled within 24-h of a seizure lie at the top end. The reasons for this variation are likely to be methodological problems, particularly diagnostic accuracy, the interval to entry to the study, selection bias in the patient population chosen for a study and the method of analysis.

*Methodological problems*

*Diagnostic accuracy*: A primary issue in studies of the prognosis of epilepsy concerns the accuracy of diagnosis. Epilepsy remains a clinical diagnosis the reliability of which may vary depending on the observer. The diagnosis of epilepsy may be difficult in its early stages, particularly after a first seizure. In 21% of patients enrolled in a population-based study, the diagnosis was still unclear 6 months after entry (Sander et al 1990). In another study, the time from the first seizure to diagnosis exceeded 2 years in more than 30% of patients (Hauser & Kurland 1975).

In addition, it has been estimated that, in specialized clinics, as many as 10–20% of patients referred with seemingly intractable seizures do not have true epileptic attacks (Lesser 1985). Common sources of confusion are syncope or psychogenic attacks (Ch. 1). A further compounding factor is that some of these patients may also have epileptic seizures or have had epilepsy in the past.

*Time of entry into a study*: The risk of seizure recurrence is much higher in the first weeks or months after an initial seizure (Hauser & Hesdorffer 1990, Sander 1993). Consequently, if there is a long interval between the first seizure and registration into a recurrence study, a second seizure may have already occurred and the patient therefore will not be included; this will, inevitably, lead to an underestimation of the risk of recurrence. A large hospital-based study of the recurrence of single generalized tonic-clonic seizures clearly showed this: a recurrence rate of 15% was reported among patients registered after 8 weeks of their first seizure, compared with a recurrence rate of 50% in patients registered within the first 4 weeks (Hopkins et al 1988).

*Population bias*: In many recurrence studies patients have been recruited from EEG Department referrals and hospital clinic attenders. For instance, Saunders & Marshall (1975) and Camfield et al (1985) ascertained cases for their studies from patients attending for an EEG after a single seizure. Not everyone, however, is referred for an EEG after a first seizure. In one community-based British study, for instance, up to a third of patients developing seizures did not have an EEG in the first year after diagnosis (Duncan & Hart 1993). Similarly, patients recruited from hospital clinics (Cleland et al 1981, Hauser et al 1982, Hopkins et al 1988) form a selected sample. Elwes & Reynolds (1988) found that 32% of patients did not seek medical advice until after their second or subsequent seizures and would therefore not be considered for a study of seizure recurrence.

*Recurrence calculation methods*: The method of calculating recurrence rates may also be partly responsible for variations in reported findings. Two methods have been used: actuarial survival analysis and crude recurrence rates. Although some authors have suggested that actuarial analysis may produce an artificially high recurrence rate (van Donselaar & Geerts 1988), distortions are more likely to happen with the use of crude recurrence rates as they do not take into account incomplete follow-up.

*Recurrence rates*

In a prospective community-based study recurrence rates were determined by actuarial analysis for 564 unselected patients with non-febrile seizures (Hart et al 1990). Overall 67% of patients had a recurrence within 12 months of a first seizure and 78% had a recurrence within 36 months. Seizures associated with a neurological deficit, presumed present at birth, had a 100% rate of relapse within the first 12 months, whereas seizures associated with a central nervous system lesion acquired postnatally carried a risk of relapse of 75% by 12 months, and 85% by 36 months. Seizures occurring with an acute insult to the brain or in the context of an acute precipitant carried a risk of relapse of 40% by 12 months, and 46% by 36 months. The majority of recurrences occurred in the first 6 months and the risk decreased the longer a patient remains free from a further seizure.

*Risk factors*

It is likely, but not proven, that the aetiology of the seizure is an important determinant of the risk of recurrence. Patients with an abnormal neurological examination were more likely to have a recurrence after a first seizure than those with a normal examination (Camfield et al 1985). The presence of a family history has also been reported to increase the risk for seizure recurrence (Hauser et al 1982). Although the role of an abnormal EEG is controversial, a number of studies have suggested that it may be an important predictor of recurrence (Camfield et al 1985, Shinnar et al 1990, van Donselaar et al 1991).

*The impact of antiepileptic treatment*

The impact of AED treatment on the risk of recurrence has been assessed in only a few studies and only one of which involved randomization of patients. In the UK community study (Hart et al 1990), 86 patients were treated after a first seizure and their recurrence rate was 50% by 12 months and 57% by 36 months compared to 67% and 78% respectively for those untreated. Patients were not randomly assigned to treatment in this study and it is likely that treatment was started in patients in whom the risk of relapse was perceived to be high. In an Italian hospital-based study, 400 patients were randomized to treatment, or to no treatment after a first generalized tonic-clonic seizure (First Seizure Trial Group 1993). The treated group had a risk of recurrence at 24 months of 26%, compared to 51% for those who were untreated.

The reduction in the risk of recurrence by AEDs was similar in both studies. It is uncertain, however, whether early treatment has an impact on the long-term prognosis of epilepsy although preliminary findings from the Italian study suggest that it does not (Musicco et al 1994) (see below, 8.1.3).

In summary, the risk of a recurrence after a first seizure is greater than has been previously suggested; in about two out of three cases seizures will recur. This casts doubt on the value of distinguishing between single seizures and epilepsy. It may be that the distinction between single seizures and epilepsy is useful for acute symptomatic seizures, although even in this group a significant proportion of patients will have further seizures.

## 8.1.2 The natural history of treated epilepsy

*Newly diagnosed epilepsy*

Usually when a patient has had two or more unprovoked seizures a working diagnosis of epilepsy is made and AED treatment is started. There have been a number of hospital-based prospective interventional studies reporting the effect of treatment in newly diagnosed cases (Hauser & Hesdorffer 1990, Sander 1993). Outcome is usually discussed in terms of a seizure remission defined as 1, 2 or 5 years of freedom from seizures. Overall, the 1-year-remission rates reported in these studies have varied between 58% and 95%, with most studies reporting rates between 65% and 80%.

The prognosis for the control of partial seizures is less good than for generalized. In one large study, complex partial seizures were controlled in only 16–43% of patients, while in those with only secondarily generalized attacks control was achieved in 48–53% at 1 year (Mattson et al 1985). Most studies have reported outcome to be less favourable in patients with multiple seizure types, associated neurological deficit and behavioural or psychiatric disturbance. One study also associated a worse prognosis with a positive family history of epilepsy and a high frequency of tonic-clonic seizures before treatment (Elwes et al 1985).

Two retrospective population-based studies have been carried out looking into the remission of treated epilepsy. In Rochester, Minnesota, an analysis of the outcome of all patients with epilepsy registered by the Mayo Clinic record linkage system was performed (Annegers et al 1979). Remission was defined as a 5-year period without seizures. 12 months after diagnosis, 42% of patients entered a remission period, and by 10 years 65% were in remission. By 15 years after onset, 76% were in a 5-year remission. In a study of an unselected UK population, 73% of the patients were in remission, defined as 2 years seizure-free (Goodridge & Shorvon 1983). In both studies, most patients who entered remission did so in the first 2 years and, as time elapsed, the prospect of entering remission decreased. In the Rochester study, 42% of patients entered remission after the first year, a further 22% in the next 9 years and only a further 11% in the subsequent 10 years. In the UK study, the probability of a patient whose epilepsy was still active (defined as at least one seizure in the previous 2 years) at 5 years, being in a 2-year remission 5 years later was only 33%, and 38% 10 years later. In contrast, these percentages were 100% and 95% in patients who were seizure-free at 5 years.

There has been no report yet associating good outcome with any particular AED. Although there are individuals who do respond better to a particular agent, all first line drugs seem to be equally effective on a population basis.

*Chronic epilepsy*

In contrast to newly diagnosed patients, only 20% of chronic patients have periods of seizure freedom and even short-term remission is unlikely in the majority of these patients (Rodin 1968). The hope of patients with chronic epilepsy for full seizure control lies in novel AEDs or in surgical intervention. The latter approach is only possible in a small proportion of patients. Only a small percentage of people with chronic epilepsy have been rendered seizure-free by the addition of the recently developed AEDs and the likelihood is that some patients will be refractory to any medical treatment.

*Drug withdrawal and seizure relapse*

70–80% of newly diagnosed patients on AED treatment will eventually become seizure-free. To what extent this remission is due to drug therapy is often uncertain in any individual case. Nevertheless, because of the possible long-term adverse effects of AEDs, it is common clinical practice to consider drug withdrawal after a patient enters a substantial remission period (see also Ch. 4, 4.6). There are, however, risks of relapse in doing so. Several studies have addressed this issue (Aarts et al 1988, Callaghan et al 1988, Matricardi et al 1989, MRC Antiepileptic Drug Withdrawal Group 1991). The probability of relapse has varied between 11% and 41%. Most studies in children have reported rates at the lower end of this spectrum while studies in adults have given results at the upper end.

In the largest study, 1013 patients in long-term remission were randomized to either continuing treatment or the slow withdrawal of medication (MRC Antiepileptic Drug Withdrawal Group 1991). The risk of relapse was 41% within the first 2 years of withdrawing medication, whereas the probability of relapse in the group randomized to continuing treatment was 22% in the first 2 years after randomization. The differences between these two policies were maximal between 1 and 2 years and after this the risk of seizure relapse is actually greater in those continuing treatment. Some other factors (e.g. non-compliance, voluntary withdrawal of medication), however, may have played a role here and this should be interpreted with care.

A number of risk factors for seizure recurrence after discontinuation of treatment have been identified. These include a long history of seizures before remission started, the occurrence of more than one seizure type; the presence of a structural brain lesion, the presence of abnormal neurological signs or learning difficulties and a past history of remission and relapses. One study also identified juvenile myoclonic epilepsy as having a high risk of recurrence (MRC Antiepileptic Drug Withdrawal Group 1991). Whether an EEG is helpful in predicting recurrence remains controversial in adults. In children, however, the presence of slow background rhythms or frankly abnormal discharges in the record indicates an increased risk of recurrence (Ch. 4, 4.6.1).

### 8.1.3 The natural history of untreated epilepsy

The natural history of untreated epilepsy is largely unknown. Studies of the outcome of epilepsy in the developed world have almost invariably been of the treated condition since effective treatment became available in 1857, when bromide therapy was introduced. Consequently, two important questions remain unanswered: what is the possibility of spontaneous remission and what is the effect of early treatment on outcome? The answers to these questions are important in view of the suggestion that the failure to treat epilepsy in its early stages could lead to later intractability (Shorvon 1984, 1987, Reynolds 1987).

*The spontaneous remission rate in epilepsy*

Patients with epilepsy in developing countries may have had the condition, untreated, for long periods of time (Sander 1993). If these patients never remit, the prevalence rate for epilepsy in developing countries should be much higher than those usually found in the developed world (0.5–1%) and should approach the cumulative incidence rate (the difference being explained by differential death rates in the cases (Sander & Shorvon 1987)). In the developed world, the difference between the two rates is now largely attributed to drug-induced remission. Assuming that incidence rates for epilepsy are similar in both the developed and developing world (though there is some evidence that it is higher in the latter (Sander 1993)), and that failure to provide early treatment for epilepsy may facilitate the evolution of epilepsy into an intractable condition (Shorvon 1984, 1987, Reynolds 1987), one would expect higher prevalence rates in the developing world.

Some studies in developing countries have reported high prevalence rates for epilepsy. One problem with these, however, is that they were all small-scale studies of selected or isolated populations, which may have high rates of degenerative CNS disease, parasitic infestation or specific epileptic syndromes (Sander 1993). Generally, the prevalence rates reported in developing and developed countries do not differ widely. In a cross-sectional population-based study of 72 121 persons carried out in Ecuador the incidence of epilepsy was estimated to be 122/100 000/year and the lifetime prevalence rate to be 1.9%, but the prevalence rate for active epilepsy was only 0.67% (Placencia et al 1992). Only 15% of all cases identified were on treatment at the time of the survey and only 29% had ever received AED treatment. Regardless of this fact, 46% of the untreated cases were in long-term remission. Because of case ascertainment bias, patients in long-term remission are usually under-represented in this type of study and this should be seen as the minimum estimate of patients in remission in this community (Placencia et al 1994).

In a large population-study in Nigeria covering 18 954 people a similar prevalence rate (0.53%) for active epilepsy was found and only 4% of the prevalent cases were receiving treatment at the time of the survey (Osuntokun et al 1987). Similar data came from Ethiopia where, in a study of 60 820 people, a prevalence rate of 0.52% was established and only 1.6% of the 316 patients with active epilepsy identified had ever received AED treatment (Tekle-Haimanot et al 1990). Large scale population based studies in China (Li et al 1985) and in India (Bharucha et al 1988, Koul et al 1988) also found similar prevalence rates.

These rates in largely untreated populations are similar to the rates found in the developed countries. One explanation could be that epilepsy carries a higher mortality rate in the developing world, although it is very unlikely that this would account for the whole difference. Another explanation is that case ascertainment for active seizures was not optimal. It is common experience, however, that cases in remission rather than active cases are likely to be missed in such studies (Schoenberg 1983, Sander & Shorvon 1987, Sander 1993). A more plausible explanation would be that some patients enter spontaneous remission. Two small retrospective studies, one carried out in a hospital clinic in Finland (Keranen & Riekkinen 1993) and the other in a rural community in Southern India (Mani et al 1993), support this explanation: both reported a remission rate of 50% in untreated patients.

### *Effects of early AED treatment on prognosis*

Observations on the efficacy of treatment in 302 patients with chronic epilepsy who had not previously received AED treatment have come from a prospective study carried out in an area of rural Kenya (Feksi et al 1991). 249 patients completed the study, of whom 53% became seizure-free in the second 6 months of therapy when compared with the baseline pre-treatment 6-month period, and a further 26% of the patients had a substantial (50% or more) reduction in seizures. These findings were similar to those reported in newly diagnosed patients in the developed world. 202 (81%) of the patients completing the study were drug-naive, many were chronic cases (52% had had epilepsy for more than 5 years) and had frequent seizures (38% had had over 100 seizures). The outcome of treatment was found to be uniformly good in these cases and neither the duration of the condition nor number of seizures before treatment was a predictor of outcome.

Similar observations have also been made in Ecuador (Placencia et al 1993) and in Malawi (Watts 1992). These results offer some evidence against the view that, unless treatment is given early, chronic epilepsy will develop. The ideal method to test the hypothesis that AEDs influence the prognosis of epilepsy would be to randomly allocate patients developing cryptogenic epilepsy to two groups: early treatment (treatment after a first attack) and delayed treatment (withholding treatment as long as possible), and compare long-term prognosis. Preliminary results from an Italian study suggest that early treatment of epilepsy does not affect the long-term prognosis of the condition (Musicco et al 1994). A further multicentre study is in progress in the UK to address this issue (Chadwick D, personal communication).

### 8.1.4 Heterogeneity of epilepsy: prognosis of different epileptic syndromes

Many different conditions may result in recurrent epileptic seizures and 'epilepsy'. There have been few studies reporting outcome according to epileptic syndromes. Most studies of prognosis have reported results according to seizure type rather than syndromic classification.

In epilepsy the features that usually define a syndrome are the types of seizures that occur, the presence of characteristic structural lesions, the age at onset of the condition, the presence of a family history, the natural history and characteristic changes in the EEG. A classification scheme for epileptic syndromes and related disorders proposed by the International League against Epilepsy is presently used in most tertiary referral centres (Commission on Classification and Terminology of the International League Against Epilepsy 1989). This classifies epileptic syndromes in four groups: localization-related (partial or focal); generalized; undetermined; and special syndromes. Within these groups syndromes are further divided in three subgroups: idiopathic; secondary or symptomatic; and cryptogenic disorders. When epileptic seizures occur as the only symptom of an inherited or genetic disorder the syndrome is termed idiopathic; when they occur as symptoms of a condition associated with structural brain lesions the syndrome is termed secondary; when the aetiology of the condition is unknown the term cryptogenic is used (Ch. 2, 2.2).

Once the diagnosis of an epileptic seizure is firmly established, a syndromic diagnosis should always be attempted, although this may be difficult, particularly at the onset of the condition. Some of the epileptic syndromes are clear-cut. The majority, however, may have considerable overlap or may be based on a rather loose association of clinical features. There may be disagreement about the precise limits of a syndrome and there may be different aetiologies for the same syndrome. In addition, some syndromes may not yet have been defined: for example it is possible that there are patients with low concentrations of GABA in critical sites in the brain who may respond very well to vigabatrin and not to other AEDs.

*The prognosis of individual epileptic syndromes*

The following age-linked epileptic syndromes are well recognized and there is considerable knowledge about their natural history, although less is known about their aetiologies or physiopathology (Chs 2 and 4, 4.4).

*Neonatal convulsions*: Neonatal seizures are attacks occurring in the first 4 weeks of life and this syndrome is defined mainly by age of onset (Ch. 2, 2.6.1). Causes include infection, brain damage, metabolic and nutritional disturbances; in around a quarter of cases no aetiological factor is identified. About 0.5% of all infants have neonatal seizures and the overall prognosis is not good: 25% will die within their first year of life and half will either carry on having seizures into adult life or will have other impairments such as mental retardation or spasticity; only about one-quarter will make a full recovery.

Indicators of poorer prognosis include prematurity, early onset of seizures (i.e. first 2 days of life), focal cerebral lesion or malformation, intracranial bleeding and the presence of a very abnormal EEG. The prognosis is better in those infants in whom no aetiological factor is found. Two important subgroups can be identified, however: benign neonatal familial convulsions and the so-called 'fifth-day fits'. The former is transmitted as an autosomal dominant trait with variable expression; seizures usually start in the second day of life but stop spontaneously in the great majority of cases. In the latter, seizures usually start between the third and seventh day and have a benign course.

*Generalized (symptomatic or cryptogenic) epileptic syndromes*: These include West's syndrome (Ch. 2, 2.6.2) and the Lennox–Gastaut syndrome (Ch. 2, 2.6.8). In about half of cases development is normal until the seizures start, but then it becomes impaired. It is possible that a common physiopathological mechanism is responsible for both conditions; the differences in presentation being accounted by different stages of brain maturation. The onset of West's syndrome is usually around the age of 6 months (range: 3–9 months), and the child may have an identifiable aetiology (most commonly tuberous sclerosis, cortical dysplasias or anoxic–ischaemic insults), but in about one-third of cases no aetiology can be found. The outcome is bleak, with arrest of psychomotor development and the appearance of other seizure types in more than 90% of cases.

Lennox–Gastaut syndrome is characterized by multiple seizure types, including atonic seizures, complex absences, tonic-clonic and myoclonic seizures. It is a rare condition, accounting for perhaps 1% of all new cases of epilepsy, though it may account for as many as 10% of people with severe epilepsy. This syndrome is frequently associated with learning difficulties and neuropsychiatric disturbances. In about half the cases no aetiological factor can be identified. A past history of West's syndrome is the commonest identifiable factor. Other causes include perinatal CNS trauma, meningitis and encephalitis, tumour and severe head trauma.

The syndrome usually affects children between the ages of 1 and 8 years (typically between 3 and 5 years), but may start at later ages. Patients are at high risk of developing status epilepticus, both tonic-clonic and non-convulsive. It has a very poor prognosis with regard to seizure control and mental development.

*Severe myoclonic epilepsy in infancy*: This is a rare condition of the first year of life, with associated generalized tonic-clonic and myoclonic seizures (Ch. 2, 2.6.1). Antiepileptic drug treatment is not effective and the prognosis for seizure control, mental and motor development is gloomy.

*Idiopathic generalized epilepsies*: The syndromes in this group account for about one-third of all epilepsies in the younger age groups (Ch. 2, 2.7). Patients usually have a family history of generalized epilepsy; the onset of seizures in this group is usually between the ages of 5 and 15 years, affecting either sex, although sometimes they may start in the neonatal period. Benign neonatal familial convulsions, benign myoclonic epilepsy in infancy, childhood and juvenile absence epilepsy, juvenile myoclonic epilepsy and epilepsy with generalized tonic-clonic seizures on awakening are the commonest types. The prognosis for full seizure control and long-term remission in all these forms is usually very good, as treatment with specific AEDs is highly effective. Most patients may expect to come off AEDs successfully after a number of years in remission; the exception being juvenile myoclonic epilepsy which has a high relapse rate on the discontinuation of medication (Chs 2, 2.7 and 4, 4.6).

*Benign partial epilepsies*: The most common benign partial epilepsy of childhood is rolandic or centro-temporal epilepsy (Ch. 2, 2.6.5). Other types are benign occipital and benign frontal epilepsy. The onset of seizures is between the ages of 2 and 14 years, usually between 5 and 10 years. This syndrome accounts for about 10–15% of epilepsy in this age group. About 30% of children have a positive family history of epilepsy. There are no neurological or intellectual abnormalities associated with this condition and it has an excellent prognosis for complete seizure remission. Long term treatment is usually not required and sometimes there is no need for AED treatment.

*Epilepsia partialis continua*: This is a rare form of severe chronic epilepsy which starts in the first decade of life in more than half the patients. There are two different forms with regard to aetiology and clinical presentation. The first, which is the more prevalent of the two, is caused by a chronic unilateral encephalitis (Rasmussen's encephalitis) for which no infective agent has yet been positively identified, although a number of different viruses have been postulated. The second form, which may start at any age, is associated with static or progressive lesions such as dysplastic tissue, neoplasia or vascular malformations. The encephalitic form is progressive, with neurological deficits and mental impairment, while the focal form has a better prognosis. AED treatment is not very effective and surgical treatment should be considered (Ch. 5, 5.2.2).

*Acquired epileptic aphasia or Landau–Kleffner syndrome*: This is a rare epileptic syndrome in which persisting aphasia develops in association with seizures, usually between 4 and 7 years (Ch. 2, 2.6.7). The aetiology is unknown and the condition usually occurs in children with previously normal development. Prognosis for full seizure control is uncertain, although half of the cases seem to have a complete recovery; prognosis for the language disturbance is, however, guarded as up to 60% have persistent learning difficulty.

*Epilepsy with continuous spike-waves during slow wave sleep*: This is a rare form of childhood epilepsy which has as its hallmark almost continuous slow spike and wave discharges on the EEG during most of non-REM sleep (Ch. 2, 2.6.6). It usually starts during the first decade of life. The aetiology is unknown, although about 20–30% of cases are associated with identifiable brain pathology (e.g. previous meningitis, birth asphyxia, CMV infection). In most cases there is an arrest of mental development at the time of onset and severe behavioural disturbances may develop. The prognosis for full seizure control is good, although learning and behavioural disorders usually persist.

*Febrile convulsions*: Febrile seizures affect as many as 3% of children in the general population between the ages of 6 months and 6 years and there is often a family history of febrile convulsions or epilepsy (Ch. 2, 2.6.3). In the great majority of children presenting with febrile convulsions, even if recurrent, the overall prognosis is excellent, with no further seizures or other problems. In about 3%, non-febrile seizures may develop. Children who have prolonged convulsions (lasting more than 20–30 min), who previously had signs of neurological development delay or who present partial features in their seizures seem to be particularly at risk of developing temporal lobe epilepsy in later life, in association with hippocampal sclerosis.

*Prognostic groups according to background aetiology*

Epileptic syndromes may be classified in four prognostic groups (Sander 1993). Categorization into these broad groups is to a large extent permanent, and change from one group to another is unlikely unless new factors arise, e.g. exposure to a novel AED, surgical intervention or the progression of a cerebral lesion or damage.

1. *Excellent prognosis*: In this group syndromes and conditions are self-limiting and very benign. They may comprise about 20–30% of all people who develop epileptic seizures. Usually, only a few seizures occur. Patients commonly do not require AED treatment as spontaneous remission is the rule. Conditions include benign neonatal familial convulsions, fifth-day seizures, the benign partial epilepsies, benign myoclonic epilepsy of infancy and some of the epilepsies with precipitated seizures (acute symptomatic seizures, drug-induced and alcohol-withdrawal seizures, febrile convulsions).

2. *Good prognosis*: Epilepsies in this group are usually benign, are short-lived and may comprise about 30–40% of all people who develop epileptic attacks. Seizures are easily controlled with AEDs, although spontaneous remission in some cases can not be ruled out. Once remission is achieved this is permanent and AEDs can be successfully tapered. To

what extent AEDs act simply to suppress seizures in this group until the epileptic diathesis resolves spontaneously is uncertain. Conditions include childhood absence epilepsy, epilepsy with generalized tonic-clonic seizures on awakening, generalized tonic-clonic seizures in patients with no neurological signs and some of the localization-related epilepsies (both cryptogenic and symptomatic types).

3. *Uncertain prognosis*: In this group there is a long-term tendency to seizures. This comprises about 10–20% of people who develop epilepsy. AEDs in this group are suppressive of seizures rather than curative. Patients may achieve remission but have a tendency to relapse if AEDs are stopped. Conditions include juvenile myoclonic epilepsy, and the bulk of the localization-related epilepsies (both cryptogenic and symptomatic). Some patients in the latter group may, however, be amenable to surgical intervention, with a subsequent improvement in prognostic group.

4. *Bad prognosis*: This group comprises up to 20% of all people who develop epilepsy. AEDs in this group are palliative and there is a continuous tendency for seizures despite intensive treatment with all AEDs, although occasional patients may respond to a novel AED. Some patients in this group may also be amenable to surgical intervention with subsequent improvement in prognostic group. Conditions include seizures associated with a neurological deficit present from birth (tuberous sclerosis, Sturge–Weber syndrome, malformations, cerebral palsy, etc), epilepsia partialis continua, progressive myoclonic epilepsies and other progressive neurological diseases, West's syndrome, Lennox–Gastaut syndrome, localization-related seizures associated with gross structural lesions and some of the localization-related cryptogenic epilepsies.

The concept that aetiology is the main determinant of the prognosis is not universally accepted and it has been suggested that epilepsy itself is a progressive biological process (Elwes et al 1988). While this is possibly the case in some individuals the evidence for it as a general phenomenon is not persuasive.

In conclusion, the outcome of epilepsy is determined to a large extent by its aetiology. Studies reporting outcome should classify cases according to epileptic syndromes rather than seizure type. Not all epileptic syndromes are clearly delineated yet, however, and efforts are needed to improve this situation.

## 8.2 PREVENTION OF EPILEPSY

In a significant number of cases of epilepsy no cause can be found; in such cases prevention is obviously not possible. Furthermore, in the majority of symptomatic cases, the identified aetiology is also currently unpreventable. This includes cases with epilepsy due to cerebral tumour, cerebral dysgenesis or malformations, most epilepsies with a genetic basis and most epilepsies associated with mental retardation. In a proportion of cases, however, a potentially preventable cause exists, e.g. those due to poor perinatal care, cerebral infection, neonatal or early childhood infectious diseases, infantile dehydration, uncontrolled febrile seizures and head trauma.

### 8.2.1 Head injury and neurosurgery

Head trauma is an important cause of neurological morbidity and of symptomatic partial seizures; post-traumatic epilepsy accounts for up to 10% of all cases of chronic epilepsy. The likelihood of developing epilepsy following a head injury depends on the severity of the trauma and the presence of complicating factors, including prolonged loss of consciousness, post-traumatic amnesia, intracranial bleeding, dural tear or skull fracture (Annegers et al 1980) (Ch. 2, 2.5.1, 2.5.2).

Mild head injury (amnesia or loss of consciousness for less than 30 min and no cranial fracture), which accounts for the great majority of episodes of head trauma, carries a very slight risk (< 2%). A head injury with a non-depressed skull fracture or which results in loss of consciousness or amnesia from 30 min–24 h leads to a risk of 2–5%. Severe head injury (intracranial bleed, brain contusions, dural tear, unconsciousness, or amnesia for more than 24 h) increases the risk to 12–15%, while survivors of penetrating or missile head injuries have a risk as high as 50% of developing epilepsy (Salazar et al 1985). The incidence is higher in the first year but will still be slightly increased for the next 9 years after the injury, particularly those caused by severe head trauma or by missiles (Annegers et al 1980). Early seizures occurring immediately after the injury or within the first week do not usually presage the development of chronic epilepsy.

It has been common policy in many neurosurgical centres to use prophylactic AED treatment after head trauma in an attempt to prevent the development of late epilepsy. This practice, however, is not supported by controlled studies and indeed these have suggested that there is no difference in the incidence of post-traumatic epilepsy between people treated with AEDs or with placebo (Temkin et al 1990, Young et al 1983) (Chs 2, 2.5.1 and 4, 4.1.1).

Supratentorial neurosurgical procedures are associated with the development of epileptic seizures in about 10% of cases. The incidence, however, varies according to the location and the condition for which the craniotomy was performed. In patients with uncomplicated aneurysm surgery it may be as low as 5%, while it can be as high as 90% following surgery for cerebral abscess. The seizures are usually partial, and occur within the first year in the majority of cases. Prophylactic AED treatment after craniotomy has been advocated although there is little evidence that it reduces the risk of developing epilepsy (Foy et al 1992) (Chs 2, 2.5.2 and 4, 4.1.1).

### 8.2.2 Preventive measures

The following actions might be effective in reducing the incidence of epilepsy (although some of these propositions have not yet been formally tested in practice) (Ch. 2, 2.5):

*Trauma*

The incidence of head trauma is potentially reducable through improved safety at work, firearm control and safer driving, including the use of seat belts, and helmets for cyclists. For instance, in Italy in the year following the application of a law which required all motorcyclists to wear crash helmets the incidence of severe head injury decreased by more than a third (Nurchi et al 1987).

*Neonatal*

Adverse perinatal events occurring during labour may cause symptomatic epilepsy, either as a result of direct trauma or because of anoxia. The outcome is variable and to a large extent dependent on the severity of the injury. Birth injury and hypoxia was a common cause of epilepsy in the past, but this has improved with improvements in antenatal and obstetric care. Further falls in the incidence of fetal hypoxia, perinatal haemorrhage, eclampsia and toxaemia may subsequently reduce the incidence of secondary epilepsy.

*Infection*

Intracranial infection can cause persistent seizures. For instance, postnatal meningitis, brain abscess and encephalitis increase the risk of epilepsy 3–10-fold, depending on the severity, the extent of the damage and the age at infection (Annegers et al 1988) (Ch. 2, 2.5.6). Early diagnosis and aggressive treatment of infections may reduce the risk of cerebral damage and consequent epilepsy.

*Parasitic diseases*

Cysticercosis, malaria, schistosomiasis and hydatid disease are important causes of epilepsy in the developing world. For instance, in one hospital series in Ecuador, over 50% of all patients with epilepsy had the condition as a result of neurocysticercosis (Del Bruto et al 1992). Most of these parasitic diseases are preventable through improved sanitation and hygiene. Efforts directed towards their prevention would decrease the incidence of epilepsy in the endemic areas.

*Vaccines*

An allergic reaction to vaccine components very occasionally leads to an acute encephalopathy, which may result in chronic epilepsy. Such a reaction has been reported following vaccination against rabies, smallpox and whooping-cough (pertussis). It is, however, extremely rare, and is becoming even more uncommon as more purified and less antigenic vaccines are used. It is likely that children are presently more at risk of developing epilepsy as result of infectious diseases themselves than from the vaccines used to prevent them. Immunization should, therefore, be encouraged.

*Febrile convulsions*

Temporal lobe epilepsy with hippocampal sclerosis is strongly associated with a history of prolonged febrile convulsions in childhood. The prompt treatment of high fevers with measures to lower body temperature may prevent the occurrence of febrile convulsions. Additionally, the rapid and appropriate treatment of febrile convulsions lasting more than 10 min may prevent the late development of temporal lobe epilepsy.

*Cerebrovascular disease*

Thromboembolic events and cerebral haemorrhage are important causes of symptomatic epilepsy starting in later life and are responsible for as many as 50% of cases in this age-group (Sander et al 1990) (Ch. 2, 2.5.3).

Seizures are almost always partial, and usually start within a year of the cerebrovascular event, although sometimes they may precede the stroke, suggesting previous silent ischaemic episodes. Seizures occurring during or immediately after a stroke are not predictive of the late development of epilepsy. It has been estimated that 5–15% of people with a stroke will eventually develop epileptic seizures. The risk of stroke can be reduced by controlling hypertension, avoiding smoking and attention to diet.

*Neuronal migration defects*

Abnormalities of neuronal migration during embryogenesis may result in cerebral malformations and cortical dysplasias, which are being recognized with increasing frequency with high resolution MRI. Underlying causes can include a genetic predisposition, intrauterine infection, maternal illness or exposure to toxins and drugs, but in many cases no cause is identified. It is presently uncertain whether it will be possible to reduce the incidence of cortical dysplasia.

In the last two decades there has been a decrease in the incidence of epilepsy among young children in developed countries (Sander et al 1993, Hauser et al 1993). The explanation of this decrease is not certain. It could be related to an improvement in prenatal care and the adoption of healthier life style by expectant mothers, leading to a decrease in neuronal migration defects, and to a reduction in the incidence of birth hypoxia.

## 8.3 MORBIDITY OF EPILEPSY

Epilepsy carries both social and medical morbidity. The majority of patients diagnosed as having epilepsy have only a few seizures, each usually lasting only minutes, yet the consequences of the diagnosis are enduring, particularly in the areas of employment and education (Ch. 7, 7.2).

The medical morbidity associated with epilepsy may be caused by the underlying aetiological process, or the treatment, or it may occur as a direct result of the epileptic seizures. Seizures may cause head injury, cervical trauma, limb fractures, burns, scalds or drowning. Status epilepticus causes considerable neurological morbidity if not promptly treated (Ch. 5, 5.3.3).

### 8.3.1 The prevention of secondary morbidity

Complete seizure control reduces the number of accidents and head injuries in people with epilepsy, thus reducing secondary morbidity. Patients with continuing seizures should be encouraged to avoid dangerous situations. For instance, by using a microwave oven for cooking or boiling water rather than a conventional cooker or kettle will reduce the risk of scalding should a seizure occur.

The frequency and sequelae of head injury due to seizures have been estimated in a study from a residential centre for epilepsy. Out of a total of 27 934 consecutive recorded seizures, there were 12 626 falls and 766 significant head injuries. 341 head injuries required suturing. There was one confirmed skull fracture, one extradural haemorrhage and one subdural haematoma. Thus, minor injury is relatively common, but serious injury is rare (Russell-Jones & Shorvon 1989). In the rare cases of uncontrollable seizures that involve falls to the ground with head injury, protective measures such as the use of helmets to cushion the head on impact should be encouraged (Ch. 7, 7.2.2). It is also important that the acute and chronic side effects of AEDs should be recognized and minimized (Ch. 4, 4.5).

### 8.3.2 Secondary cerebral damage

A small minority of patients with uncontrolled seizures experience a progressive decline of their cognitive functions, which may also sometimes be accompanied by physical impairment such as cerebellar ataxia. The aetiology of this deterioration is usually uncertain and it is likely that multiple factors may be operating: prolonged exposure to AEDs sometimes at toxic levels, frequent seizures, subclinical seizure activity, head injuries and the underlying aetiology may all be relevant. It is difficult to judge if this deterioration is preventable, but attempts should be made to control seizures with the minimum effective doses of AEDs, avoiding chronic toxicity (Ch. 9, 9.5).

Suggestions that the chronic use of some AEDs, particularly phenytoin, may cause cerebellar dysfunction still need clarification. Another controversial area relates to the extent to which seizure activity itself causes progressive neuronal damage. It has been suggested that chronic epileptic discharges can lead to secondary epileptogenesis (kindling). Evidence for this in some experimental models of partial seizures is convincing but similar evidence is lacking in humans, in whom the hypothesis is difficult to test. It is generally true, though, that short, uncomplicated seizures cause no permanent or progressive neurological dysfunction in humans. In contrast, prolonged generalized tonic-clonic status epilepticus is associated with a high incidence of neurological morbidity and may result in permanent brain damage (Ch. 5, 5.3.3).

### 8.3.3 Social consequences

Many people with epilepsy, particularly if seizures are continuing, may face problems within society and may encounter negative attitudes in many areas, including family, schooling, adult society and employment. The intensity of these problems is partly determined by the severity of the condition and the level of disability associated with or secondary to the epilepsy. There is often lack of information and understanding about epilepsy in the community at large and this may often result in prejudice or even hostility. These issues are considered in more detail in Chapter 7 (7.2).

## 8.4 THE MORTALITY OF EPILEPSY

Epilepsy is often assumed to be a benign condition with a low mortality. There is, however, increased mortality in patients with epilepsy, which is relatively high among younger patients and those with severe epilepsy (Hauser et al 1980, Hauser & Hersdorffer 1990, Nashef et al 1995a).

Age, sex, race, socioeconomic status, interval from diagnosis, seizure frequency and seizure type are also variables that affect mortality rates.

Estimates of this mortality have varied from study to study. Case ascertainment, selection bias and diagnosis pose a number of methodological difficulties. Two methods are used to compare death rates in patients and control populations.

*Proportional mortality ratio (PMR)*: This ratio gives the proportion of death due to a specific cause among a study population and compares it to a control group. It is not a direct measure of the death rate.

*Standardized mortality ratio (SMR)*: This is the ratio of deaths observed in a group to the numbers of deaths that would be expected to have occurred during a follow-up period if the group in question had experienced the same age- and sex-specific death rates as the control population.

### 8.4.1 Mortality rates and variables affecting excess mortality

In a retrospective community study overall SMRs were two to three times higher than those of the general population and this increased risk seems also to be largely limited to the first 10 years after diagnosis (Hauser et al 1980). In this study the SMR was 3.8 in the first year after diagnosis, falling to 1.4 20 years after the diagnosis. However, cryptogenic generalized convulsions also carried a higher mortality ratio (SMR of 2.4 overall but 3.5 in the first year after diagnosis).

In a prospective population-based study of 564 newly diagnosed patients with epilepsy, followed for between 6 and 9 years, there were 114 deaths compared to an expected number of 37 (Cockerell et al 1994). The overall SMR was 2.5, and it was 7.6 in those aged under 50 years at diagnosis. The death rate was highest in the first year (SMR 6.6), falling to 2.3 by the third year and 1.7 in the fifth year. The basis of this pattern is that death soon after the diagnosis of epilepsy is usually due to the underlying aetiology (e.g. tumour, stroke) and not to the epilepsy itself. Even in idiopathic epilepsy, however, the SMR was elevated at 1.6, and it was 2.9 in acute symptomatic epilepsy and 4.3 in remote symptomatic epilepsy.

Mortality rates are often higher in patients with chronic severe epilepsy, being an SMR of 5.1 among attendees at a specialist epilepsy clinic (Nashef et al 1995a,b). The majority (75%) of deaths were epilepsy-related, in marked contrast to the situation in newly diagnosed epilepsy. The highest epilepsy-related mortality rates were found in patients with frequent seizures, in those with generalized tonic-clonic seizures, young age, mental retardation and a long duration of epilepsy.

A higher SMR for males than females has consistently been reported but to date no convincing explanation has been advanced for this. The highest reported SMRs are in the under 40 years age-group, a group which has the smallest mortality in the general population.

Seizure type is also relevant. In a retrospective community study, the SMR of patients with absence seizures only was no different from the general population while myoclonic seizures carried a SMR of 4.1 (Hauser et al 1980). Complex partial seizures, with or without secondary generalization, were not associated with a significantly elevated SMR. Other studies have also shown increased mortality in patients with idiopathic epilepsy (Hauser & Hersdorffer 1990, Cockerell et al 1994, Nashef et al 1995a).

In one study an SMR of 3.8 was reported in patients with severe epilepsy. This was significantly higher than the SMR of 1.8 for those who were seizure-free, which was in itself an excess mortality (Henriksen et al 1970). Another study also reported an excess mortality in patients with well controlled or in long-term remission (Hauser et al 1980). Higher mortality rates for non-whites of either sex, both for deaths due to and related to epilepsy, have been reported in the USA (Chandra et al 1984). This might, however, be due to socioeconomic factors.

### 8.4.2 Causes of death

The commonest causes of death in people with epilepsy include: chest infections, cancers, accidents, suicide and epilepsy-related death.

*Chest infections*

Reported SMRs for bronchopneumonia have varied between 1.7 and 7.9. Bronchopneumonia is an important cause of death of patients with epilepsy, especially, but not only, in the elderly age-group (Hauser et al 1980, Zielinski 1974, Klenerman et al 1993). A predisposing factor might be pneumonias secondary to aspiration during seizures although this hypothesis has not yet been formally tested.

*Cancers*

The SMRs and PMRs for cancer have been uniformly elevated, whether or not primary brain tumours were included, in all studies and it is likely that death due to cancer is more frequent in patients with epilepsy than in the general population (Hauser et al 1980, Klenerman et al 1993, White et al 1979). Some studies have, however, reported that this excessive number of deaths appears to be related to a diagnosis of a neoplasm prior to the diagnosis of epilepsy rather than the other way around (Hauser et al 1980, Zielinski 1974, Chandra et al 1984).

*Accidents*

Traumatic death rates are uniformly elevated, which strongly suggests that accidents and trauma are a more frequent cause of death in patients with epilepsy than in the general population (Henriksen et al 1970, Zielinski 1974, Iivanainen & Lehtinen 1979, White et al 1979, Hauser et al 1980, Chandra et al 1984, Hashimoto et al 1989). Patients with epilepsy may die as result of drowning more often than the general population (Iivanainen & Lehtinen 1979, Hashimoto et al 1989). In countries where bathing is favoured over showering there might be a higher death rate of drowning, although this has never been properly investigated.

*Suicide*

Patients with epilepsy are at a higher risk of committing suicide than the general population (Henriksen et al 1970, Zielinski 1974, White et al 1979, Hauser et al 1980, Hashimoto et al 1989). Patients with temporal lobe epilepsy and severe epilepsy, or epilepsy with a handicap, have a much greater risk of suicide: 25 times greater in the cases of temporal lobe epilepsy and five times greater for severe epilepsy (Hawton et al 1980, Barraclough 1987). There is some evidence that risk declines with duration of the condition (Barraclough 1987).

### 8.4.3 Epilepsy-related death

Epilepsy as a cause of death is usually subdivided into different categories: status epilepticus, seizure-related and sudden unexpected death.

*Status epilepticus*

Status epilepticus is more common in children than in adults but mortality is higher in adults. Death is usually due to the underlying disease, with only a small percentage of cases directly attributable to status, and this appears to have declined more recently. In a recent study of institutionalized patients, fewer than 1% of deaths were due to status, compared to 11% in the same setting 20 years earlier (Klenerman et al 1993). Prompt and better treatment of serial seizures and early status stage may be responsible for this important decrease, although more accurate certification may also have contributed (Ch. 5).

*Seizure-related and sudden unexpected deaths in epilepsy (SUDEP)*

Seizure-related deaths and SUDEP are common in people with chronic epilepsy but are generally under-recognized.

The term 'death due to a seizure' or 'seizure-related death' is used when the patient dies during or shortly after a seizure, when there is no evidence for status epilepticus and when after autopsy no other explanation is found. SUDEP is defined as a non-traumatic unwitnessed death occurring in a patient with epilepsy who had been previously relatively healthy and for whom no cause is found even after a thorough post-mortem examination (Neuspiel & Kuller 1985, Leestma et al 1989, Lathers & Schraeder 1990). A common scenario is that of a patient found dead in or off the bed; evidence for an associated seizure is found in half of the cases.

Most SUDEP cases are likely to be seizure-related. Pulmonary oedema, well documented in seizures, with or without congestion of other organs, is a frequent finding in cases of SUDEP (Leestma et al 1989). Marked autonomic changes occur during seizures and recent studies of ictal recordings show a high frequency of central apnoea during complex partial and generalized tonic-clonic seizures. The central apnoea preceded cardiac rhythm changes in most cases, and in others was complicated by an obstructive component (Nashef et al 1995a,c). The hypothesis that SUDEP is due to central apnoea, possibly consequent on endogenous opioid release, is a plausible explanation. Other possibilities include suffocation during a seizure, a deleterious action of AEDs, non-compliance with AED treatment and autonomic seizures leading to cardiac arrythmias.

A high rate of SUDEP in young people with severe epilepsy, with an SMR of 15.9, was recently found in a study from a residential school (Nashef et al 1995d). Procedures at this school ensured that patients were attended to immediately should a seizure occur, during both wakefulness and sleep, and all deaths occurred when the children were away from the school. This investigation suggests that immediate attention after a seizure may prevent SUDEP (Nashef et al 1995d).

PMRs of 7.5–17% in patients with epilepsy have been ascribed to seizure-related death and to SUDEP (Lathers & Schraeder 1990). The rates are highest in cohorts with more severe epilepsy and a history of generalized tonic-clonic seizures (either primary or secondarily generalized) (Nashef et al 1995a). It has been suggested on the basis of low post-mortem AED plasma levels that the abrupt cessation of or non-compliance with AED treatment could be a precipitating factor in SUDEP (Lund & Gormsen 1985). Post-mortem determination of AED levels is, however, of questionable reliability and, furthermore, SUDEP was recorded well before the introduction of the modern AEDs (Nashef et al 1995a).

An annual mortality rate of one SUDEP in every 370–1100 people with epilepsy in the community has been suggested in one American study (Leestma et al 1989) and one in 740–1800 in a Canadian survey (Tennis et al 1995). In a sample of adults with severe epilepsy in residential care at the Chalfont Centre, the rate was one death in every 260 persons per year (Klenerman et al 1993), while the rate in a cohort of attenders at the epilepsy clinic at Queen Square was 1/200/year (Nashef et al 1995b). This is even higher in the 20–40-year age group, and still higher if only patients with uncontrolled seizures are selected.

SUDEP also occurs in children and in one study it was responsible for 10% of total deaths among children with epilepsy aged 2–20 years (Keeling & Knowles 1989). In another study, 12% of 93 deaths among young children with epilepsy were sudden and unexpected (Harvey et al 1993).

### 8.4.4 The role of antiepileptic drugs

Idiosyncratic side-effects of AEDs have been sometimes associated with the death of patients. Fatal hepatic failure has been documented with phenytoin, phenobarbitone, sodium valproate and lamotrigine. Other examples include blood dyscrasias with carbamazepine and felbamate, sinus arrest with carbamazepine and disseminated intravascular coagulation following treatment with lamotrigine. Comparative estimates of the rates of the occurrence of such deaths per treatment year are not available, and it is difficult to estimate the exact magnitude of the risk. These seem, however, to be very rare events and usually happen in the early stages of treatment rather than in the long term.

It has been suggested that long-term use of barbiturates and phenytoin could have oncogenic potential (Clemmensen 1974). This, however, needs clarification and further long-term studies are necessary.

### 8.4.5 The mortality of epilepsy: key points for clinical practice

Epilepsy carries an increased risk of death that is not always recognized. This excess mortality is mainly due to the underlying disease, accidents or suicide, or is directly attributable to epilepsy, although deaths due to AED therapy may also occasionally occur. Accidental death and suicide are potentially preventable and attempts should be made to minimize possible risks.

Although much remains to be learnt about seizure-related death and about SUDEP, current knowledge can be summarized as follows: patients with epilepsy, particularly young adults, are at risk of SUDEP at a rate of one per 200–1000/year. Young patients and those with frequent seizures, generalized seizures and mental retardation have a higher risk, although deaths can occur in patients with relatively well controlled seizures. The relatively high incidence in selected groups needs to be taken into consideration in clinical management. Physicians need to acknowledge this entity and ensure that bereaved relatives are given adequate support (Nashef et al 1995a). At present it is unknown to what extent and how these cases may be preventable.

## REFERENCES


Aarts WFM, Visser LH, Loonen MC et al 1988 Follow-up of 146 children with epilepsy after withdrawal of antiepileptic therapy. Epilepsia 29: 244–250

Annegers JF, Hauser WA, Elveback LR 1979 Remission of seizures and relapse in patients with epilepsy. Epilepsy 20: 729–737

Annegers JF, Grabow JD, Groover RV 1980 Seizures after head trauma: a population study. Neurology 30: 683–639

Annegers JF, Hauser WA, Beghi E et al 1988 The risk of unprovoked seizures after encephalitis and meningitis. Neurology 38: 1407–1410

Barraclough BM 1987 The suicide rate of epilepsy. Acta Psychiat Scand 76: 339–345

Berg AT, Shinnar S 1991 The risk of recurrence following a first unprovoked seizure: a quantitative review. Neurology 41: 965–972

Bharucha NE, Bharucha EP, Bharucha AE, Bhishe AV, Schoenberg BS 1988 Prevalence of epilepsy in the Parsi community of Bombay. Epilepsia 29: 111–115

Callaghan N, Ganett A, Goggin T 1988 Withdrawal of anticonvulsant drugs in patients free of seizures for two years. N Engl J Med 318: 942–946

Camfield PR, Camfield CS, Dooley JM 1985 Epilepsy after a first unprovoked seizure in childhood. Neurology 35: 1657–1660

Chandra V, Bharucha N, Schoenberg B, Feskanich D 1984 National mortality data for death due to, and all death related to, epilepsy in the United States. In: Porter R et al (eds) Advances in epileptology. XVth Epilepsy International Symposium. Raven Press, New York, p 531–534

Cleland PG, Mosquera I, Steward WP, Foster JB 1981 Prognosis of isolated seizures in adult life. Br Med J 283: 1364

Clemmensen J 1974 Are anticonvulsants oncogenic? Lancet 1: 705–707

Cockerell OC, Johnson AL, Sander JWAS, Hart YM, Goodridge DMG, Shorvon SD 1994 Mortality from epilepsy: results from a prospective population-based study. Lancet 334: 918–921

Commission on Classification and Terminology of the International League Against Epilepsy 1989 Proposal for revised international classification of epilepsies, epileptic syndromes and related seizure disorders. Epilepsia 30: 389–399

Del Bruto OH, Santibanez R, Noboa CA, et al 1992 Epilepsy due to neurocysticercosis: analysis of 203 patients. Neurology 42: 389–392

Duncan JS, Hart YM 1993 The Services for people with epilepsy. In: Richens A, Chadwick D, Laidlaw J (eds) A textbook of epilepsy, 4th edn. Churchill Livingstone, Edinburgh, p 705–722

Elwes RDC, Reynolds EH 1988 First seizure in adult life. Lancet 2: 36

Elwes RDC, Chesterman P, Reynolds EH 1985 Prognosis after a first untreated tonic-clonic seizure. Lancet 2: 752–753

Elwes RDC, Johnson AL, Reynolds EH 1988 The course of untreated epilepsy. Br Med J 297: 948–950

Feksi AT, Kaamugisha J, Sander JWAS, Gatiti S, Shorvon SD 1991 Comprehensive primary health care antiepileptic drug treatment programme in rural and semi-rural Kenya. Lancet 337: 406–409

First Seizure Trial Group 1993 Randomized clinical trial on the efficacy of antiepileptic drugs in reducing the risk of relapse after a first unprovoked tonic-clonic seizure. Neurology 43: 478–483

Foy PM, Chadwick DW, Rajgopalan N, Johnson AL, Shaw MDM 1992 Do prophylactic anticonvulsant drugs alter the pattern of seizures after craniotomy. J Neurol Neurosurg Psychiat 55: 753–757

Goodridge DMG, Shorvon SD 1983 Epilepsy in a population of 6000. Br Med J 287: 641–647

Hart YM, Sander JWAS, Johnson AJ, Shorvon SD 1990 National General Practice Study of epilepsy: recurrence after a first seizure. Lancet 336: 1271–1274

Harvey AS, Nolan T, Carlin JB 1993 Community-based study of the mortality in children with epilepsy. Epilepsia 34: 597–603

Hashimoto K, Fukushima Y, Saito F, Wada K 1989 Rehabilitation and Sociology. Jpn J Psychiat Neurol 43: 546–547

Hauser WA, Hesdorffer DC 1990 Epilepsy: frequency, causes and consequences. Demos Publications, Maryland

Hauser WA, Kurland LT 1975 The epidemiology of epilepsy in Rochester, Minnesota 1935 through 1967. Epilepsia 16: 1–66

Hauser WA, Annegers JF, Elveback LR 1980 Mortality in patients with epilepsy. Epilepsia 21: 339–412

Hauser WA, Anderson VE, Loewenson RB, McRoberts S 1982 Seizure recurrence after a first unprovoked seizure. N Eng J Med 307: 522–528

Hauser AW, Annegers JF, Kurland LT 1993 Incidence of epilepsy and unprovoked seizures in Rochester, Minnesota 1935–1984. Epilepsia 34: 453–468

Hawton K, Fagg J, Marsack P 1980 Association between epilepsy and attempted suicide. J Neurol Neurosurg Psychiat 43: 168–170

Henriksen B, Juul-Jensen P, Lund M 1970 The mortality of epileptics. In: Brackenridge RD (ed) Proceedings of the 10th International Congress of Life Assurance Medicine. Pilomen, London, p 81–86

Hopkins A, Garman A, Clarke C 1988 The first seizure in adult life: value of clinical features, electroencephalography, and computerised tomographic scanning in prediction of seizure recurrence. Lancet 1: 721–726

Iivanainen M, Lehtinen J 1979 Causes of death in institutionalised epileptics. Epilepsia 20: 485–492

Keeling JW, Knowles SA 1989 Sudden death in childhood and adolescence. J Pathol 159: 221–224

Keranen T, Riekkinen PJ 1993 Remission of seizures in untreated epilepsy. Br Med J 307: 483

Klenerman P, Sander JWAS, Shorvon SD 1993 Mortality in patients with epilepsy: a study of patients in long term residential care. J Neurol Neurosurg Psychiat 56: 149–152

Koul R, Razdan S, Motta A 1988 Prevalence and pattern of epilepsy (Lath/Mirgi/Laran) in Rural Kashmir, India. Epilepsia 29: 116–122

Lathers CM, Schraeder PL 1990 Epilepsy and sudden death. Dekker, New York

Leestma JE, Walczak T, Hughes JR, Kalelkar MB, Teas SS 1989 A prospective study of sudden death in epilepsy. Ann Neurol 26: 195–203

Lesser RP 1985 Psychogenic seizures. In: Pedley T, Meldrum BS (eds) Recent advances in epilepsy 2. Churchill Livingstone, Edinburgh, p 273–296

Li SC, Schoenberg BS, Bolis CL, et al 1985 Epidemiology of epilepsy in urban regions of the People's Republic of China. Epilepsia 26: 391–394

Lund A, Gormsen H 1985 The role of antiepileptic drugs in sudden death in epilepsy. Acta Neurol Scand 72: 444–446

Mani KS, Rangan G, Srinivas HV, Narendran S 1993 Natural history of untreated epilepsy: a community based study in Rural South India. Epilepsia 34(suppl 2): 166

Matricardi M, Brinciotti M, Benedetti P 1989 Outcome after discontinuation of antiepileptic drug therapy in children. Epilepsia 30: 582–589

Mattson RH, Cramer JA, Collins JF et al 1985 Comparison of carbamazepine, phenobarbital, phenytoin and primidone in partial and secondarily generalized tonic-clonic seizures. N Engl J Med 313: 145–151

MRC Antiepileptic Drug Withdrawal Group 1991 Randomised study of antiepileptic drug withdrawal in patients in remission. Lancet 337: 1175–80

Musicco M, Beghi E, Solari A et al 1994 Effects of antiepileptic treatment initiated after the first unprovoked seizure in the long term prognosis of epilepsy. Neurology 44(S2): A337–338

Nashef L, Sander JWAS, Shorvon SD 1995a Mortality in epilepsy. In: Pedley TA, Meldrum BS (eds) Recent advances in epilepsy 6. Churchill Livingstone, Edinburgh (in press)

Nashef L, Sander JWAS, Fish DR, Shorvon SD 1995b Incidence of sudden unexpected death in an outpatient cohort with epilepsy at a tertiary referral centre. J Neurol Neurosurg Psychiat 58: 462-464

Nashef L, Walker F, Sander JWAS, Fish DR, Shorvon SD 1995c Apaoea and bradycardia during epileptic seizures: relation to sudden death in epilepsy. Neurology 45 suppl 4: A424

Nashef L, Fish DR, Garner S, Sander JWAS, Shorvon SD 1995d Sudden death in epilepsy: a study of incidence in a young cohort with epilepsy and learning difficulty. Epilepsia: in press

Neuspiel DR, Kuller LH 1985 Sudden and unexpected natural death in childhood and adolescence. JAMA 254: 1321–1325

Nurchi GC G, Golino P, Flaris F et al 1987 Effect of the law on compulsory helmets in the incidence of head injuries among motorcyclists. J Neurosurg Sci 31: 141–143
Osuntokun BO, Adeuja AO, Nottidge AJ et al 1987 Prevalence of the epilepsies in Nigerian Africans. Epilepsia 28: 272–279
Placencia M, Shorvon SD, Paredes V, Sander JWAS et al 1992 Epileptic seizures in an Andean region of Ecuador: incidence and prevalence and regional variation. Brain 115: 771–782
Placencia M, Sander JWAS, Shorvon SD et al 1993 Antiepileptic drug treatment in a community health care setting in Northern Ecuador: a prospective 12 month assessment. Epilepsy Res 14: 237–244
Placencia M, Sander JWAS, Roman M et al 1994 The characteristics of epilepsy in a largely untreated population in Rural Ecuador. J Neurol Neurosurg Psychiat 57: 320–325
Reynolds EH 1987 Early treatment and prognosis of epilepsy. Epilepsia 28: 97–106
Rodin EA 1968 The prognosis of patients with epilepsy. Charles C Thomas, Springfield, IL
Russell-Jones D, Shorvon SD 1989 The frequency and sequelae of head injury in epilepsy. J Neurol Neurosurg Psychiat 52: 659–662
Salazar AN, Jabbari B, Vance SC et al 1985 Epilepsy after penetrating head injury. Clinical correlates: a report of the Vietnam Head Injury Study. Neurology 35: 1406–1415
Sander JWAS 1993 Some aspects of prognosis in the epilepsies: a review. Epilepsia 34: 1007–1016
Sander JWAS, Shorvon SD 1987 Incidence and prevalence studies in epilepsy and their methodological problems: a review. J Neurol Neurosurg Psychiat 50: 829–839
Sander JWAS, Hart YM, Johnson AJ, Shorvon SD 1990 National General Practice Study of epilepsy: newly diagnosed seizures in a general population. Lancet 336: 1267–1271
Sander JWAS, Cockerell OC, Hart YM, Shorvon SD 1993 Is the incidence of epilepsy falling in the UK? Lancet 342: 874
Saunders M, Marshall C 1975 Isolated seizures: an EEG and clinical assessment. Epilepsia 16: 731–733
Schoenberg BS 1983 Epidemiological aspects of epilepsy. In: Nistaco G, Di Perre R, Meinardi H (eds) Epilepsy: an update on research and therapy. Alan R Liss, New York, p 331–343
Shinnar S, Berg AT, Moshe SL et al 1990 Risk of seizure recurrence following a first unprovoked seizure in childhood: a prospective study. Pediatrics 85: 1076–1085
Shorvon SD 1984 The temporal aspects of prognosis in epilepsy. J Neurol Neurosurg Psychiat 47: 1157–1165
Shorvon SD 1987 Do anticonvulsants influence the natural history of epilepsy? In: Warlow C, Garfield J (eds) More dilemmas in the management of the neurological patient. Churchill Livingstone, Edinburgh, p 8–13
Tekle-Haimanot R, Forsgren L, Abebe M et al 1990 Clinical and electroencephalographic characteristics of epilepsy in rural Ethiopia: a community-based study. Epilepsy Res 7: 230–239
Temkin NR, Dikmen S, Wilensky AJ et al 1990 A randomized, double-blind study of phenytoin for the preventation of post-traumatic seizures. N Engl J Med 323: 497–502
Tennis P, Cole TB, Annegers JF, Leestma JE, McNutt M, Rajput A 1995 Cohort study of incidence of sudden unexplained death in persons with seizure disorder treated with antiepileptic drugs in Saskatchewan, Canada. Epilepsia 36: 29–36
van Donselaar CA, Geerts AT 1988 First seizure in adult life. Lancet 2: 36
van Donselaar CA, Geerts AT, Schimsheimer R 1991 Idiopathic first seizure in adult life: who should be treated? Br Med J 302: 620–623
Watts AE 1992 The natural history of untreated epilepsy in a rural community in Africa. Epilepsia 33: 464–468
White S, McLean A, Howland C 1979 Anticonvulsant drugs and cancer. A cohort study in patients with severe epilepsy. Lancet 2: 458–461
Young B, Rapp R, Norton JA et al 1983 Failure of prophylactically administered phenytoin to prevent late posttraumatic seizures. J Neurosurg 58: 236–241
Zielinski JJ 1974 Epilepsy and mortality rate and causes of death. Epilepsia 15: 191–201

# 9 Psychological and psychiatric aspects of epilepsy

Before consideration of the psychiatric consequences of epilepsy, it is necessary to examine some of the conditions that simulate epilepsy and are a diagnostic trap for the unwary (Ch. 1). Many of these attacks may be confused with epilepsy and may uncritically be diagnosed as the latter, leading to confusion and inappropriate treatment.

## 9.1 NON-EPILEPTIC ATTACKS

### 9.1.1 Definition and frequency

The term pseudoseizure has enjoyed popularity but is not a good term; synonyms have included pseudoepileptic seizures, non-epileptic attack disorder and non-epileptic seizures. The seizures in these patients are very real, both to patients, third-party observers and physicians. Indeed, so real are they that it is estimated that some 20% of patients attending chronic epilepsy clinics do not have epilepsy, but have some form of non-epileptic disorder (Jeavons 1977). Alternative terms, including hysterical seizures and psychogenic seizures, are also inadequate, the former being pejorative, the latter defining a form of reflex seizure induced by mental activity (Fenwick 1981).

Conversion symptoms are common in medical practice, and seizures, as a conversion symptom, occur in approximately 10–40% of patients. In the stable form of hysteria, Briquet's hysteria (see below), it is estimated that non-epileptic seizures occur in 12% of patients.

It is important to note that, although patients with established epilepsy may also have non-epileptic attacks, the latter frequently occur in the absence of epilepsy. Definite epilepsy was noted in 12% and possible epilepsy in 24% of over 300 reported cases of non-epileptic attacks (Lesser 1985).

### 9.1.2 Differential diagnosis and aetiology of non-epileptic attacks

The principal medical, and psychiatric conditions to be considered are shown in Tables 9.1 and 9.2 (see also Ch. 1). Obvious cardiovascular causes, e.g. vasovagal attacks, frequently present in adolescence and often lead to the development of non-epileptic attacks. It is important that they are not retrospectively thought to be epileptic seizures. Metabolic conditions, e.g. hypoglycaemia, should always be included in the differential diagnosis.

Sleep disorders are a common area of misdiagnosis (Ch 1, 1.10). Both REM and non-REM disorders can be misdiagnosed as epilepsy, as can

**Table 9.1** Medical differential diagnosis of seizures

*Neurological*

- Epilepsy
- Migraine
- Movement disorders: dystonia, tic, myoclonus
- Vestibular disorders
- Hyperekplexia
- Transient ischaemic attack
- Tonic spasms of multiple sclerosis
- Sleep disorders
  - Parasomnias
  - Hypersomnias: narcolepsy, cataplexy

*Metabolic*

- Hypoglycaemia
- Hypocalcaemia
- Drug use and abuse
- Acute encephalopathy

*Cardiological/pulmonary*

- Vasovagal, syncope
- Arrhythmia
- Outflow obstruction, pulmonary hypertension

**Table 9.2** Psychiatric differential diagnosis of seizures

- Anxiety
  - Generalized anxiety disorder
  - Panic disorder (hyperventilation, depersonalization)
- Depression (fugues)
- Schizophrenia
- Conversion disorder
- Somatization disorder
- Episodic dyscontrol
- Malingering

some of the hypersomnolent conditions. Night terrors arise out of stage 4 sleep, as opposed to the nightmares of REM sleep. They are associated with the sudden onset of restless motor activity, sometimes with a vocalization of fear.

REM behaviour disorder, which occurs in patients who have subtle brainstem damage and no longer have the characteristic REM muscle paralysis, can present with kicking around, self-injury and aggression. Cataplexy, if the other elements of the narcolepsy–cataplexy syndrome (narcolepsy, sleep paralysis and either hypnagogic or hypnopompic hallucinations) are absent, can look deceptively like an epileptic drop attack, and the crucial history of the precipitation by emotional events should be asked for.

Of the psychiatric conditions, anxiety-related disorders are the most commonly misdiagnosed as epilepsy. In particular, panic attacks, especially if associated with episodes of déjà vu, depersonalization or autoscopy, are deceptive. The onset of the panic may be sudden, not obviously triggered by environmental events, and it may last a relatively short time. Some patients have all of the autonomic elements of a panic attack, without the subjective sense of fear.

Clues in the history include past episodes of an anxiety-related condition, the environmental triggers, associated agoraphobia and the classical features of the panic attack, which rarely occurs as an epileptic seizure. Panic involves palpitations, sweating, rising apprehension and fear and difficulty in breathing. Many patients reach a point at which they black out, and have an amnesia for the episode.

Less severe anxiety disorder can also present with paroxysmal episodes of sensory or motor change, which to the unwary may be mistaken for epilepsy.

A depressive illness often underlies a diagnosis of non-epileptic attacks. Clues in the history include a past history of depression, recent significant life events, e.g. a bereavement, which might have precipitated a depressive illness, and the central features of depression, which, unless they are asked for, may not be volunteered by a patient. The latter include appetite and sleep changes, anhedonia, suicidal thoughts and social withdrawal.

The importance of recognizing a depressive illness is obvious, since it is a readily treatable cause of non-epileptic attacks.

Schizophrenia rarely presents with non-epileptic attacks: occasional patients with catatonic outbursts of motor activity, which are misinterpreted as paroxysmal epileptic events, are encountered. These episodes were well described in the older textbooks but are seen less frequently these days. Clinical observation of such attacks will reveal their nature, but on occasions video-EEG telemetry is required.

Conversion disorder, presenting either as dissociative symptoms or as conversion hysteria, is still seen quite frequently in specialist practice and must always be considered. Secondary gain may be readily discerned but is an unreliable clinical feature. A past history of conversion phenomena and associated clinical findings such as hemianaesthetic areas and visual field defects with corkscrew patterns should be noted.

Conversion involves the mechanism of dissociation, which implies that patients will be amnesic for their attack. However, patients who seem to know absolutely nothing about their seizures, especially after a history of several years of frequent episodes, rarely have epilepsy. Sexual abuse is often found in the background history and has important treatment implications.

Briquet's hysteria, or somatization disorder, is another condition in which non-epileptic attacks occur. Patients are typically female and polysymptomatic. They characteristically have a history of an excessive number of surgical operations and hospitalizations, and present with numerous somatic complaints. There may be sociopathic personality traits and alcoholism in the family history.

The condition typically starts in early childhood, and by definition is chronic. It is estimated that some 1–2% of consecutive female patients attending hospital for investigations, and up to 10% of psychiatric in-patients, have Briquet's hysteria. The diagnosis can be made by careful history taking and noting the abnormal illness behaviour in the patient's background.

In the differential diagnosis of non-epileptic attacks, it is essential to take an adequate history, taking note of both psychiatric and neurological background features. In addition, information regarding such obvious factors as seizure-precipitating events should be sought, paying particular attention to the setting and timing of the very first attack. Seizures occurring many times a day in the presence of a normal interictal EEG are likely to be non-epileptic, as are seizures with talking, screaming and displays of emotional behaviour immediately after the attack.

The presence of paroxysmal abnormalities on the EEG does not necessarily confirm a diagnosis of epilepsy, and there are several patterns of EEG abnormality seen in psychiatric patients that may be misreported as epileptiform (Ch. 3, 3.2), which can be very misleading. These include the small sharp spikes, which may be temporal in distribution, seen with affective disorder, and rhythmic mid-temporal discharges, which arise in drowsiness and may be mistaken for bitemporal theta. Further, theta waves, sometimes paroxysmal, and even sharp waves, are often seen in patients with extreme anxiety disorders and schizophrenia. The diagnosis of epilepsy should never be based on a reporting of such 'epileptiform features' on an electroencephalogram.

Self-injury is not unusual in non-epileptic attacks. The siting of the self-injury is often different from that in epilepsy; in particular, carpet burns, caused by rubbing the skin on the floor, may commonly be seen on the elbows or face. Patients with non-epileptic attacks sometimes even break bones.

Pseudostatus epilepticus is quite common. If patients present in apparent status and have a normal EEG, the diagnosis is unlikely to be epilepsy (Ch. 3, 3.2.7). Patients with pseudostatus are at particular risk for further morbidity, including respiratory depression from excessive amounts of sedative medication, which in some cases leads to artificial ventilation (Ch. 5, 5.5).

Measurement of prolactin can be helpful in the differential diagnosis of seizures. Significant elevations of this neurohormone occur for up to 20 mins, after a generalized convulsion. The test is less reliable in patients with complex partial seizures and not reliable in patients with simple partial seizures or in patients who have status epilepticus. The prolactin elevation needs to be a significant one (probably over 1000 IU/l to be sure of an epileptic seizure) in the setting of a normal baseline (Trimble 1978). Although other neurohormones are also altered by seizures, including arginine vasopressin, LH and FSH, prolactin is the most reliable diagnostic test in this setting.

### 9.1.3 Management and prognosis of non-epileptic attacks

The diagnosis of non-epileptic seizures carries with it certain responsibilities. First, many patients are unhappy about it. They have been told, often by several specialists, in the past that they have epilepsy. Further, they have usually taken antiepileptic drugs (AEDs) for many years and suffered side-effects, including sedation. They will have stopped driving and will probably have been barred from vocational and occupational development.

One response, quite naturally, is disbelief. This is often combined with anger, and the latter may be related to an acute deterioration of the clinical state and an exacerbation of the frequency of seizures.

As a general principle, confrontation is not a good approach. The possibility that epilepsy may not be the cause of a patient's seizures should be tactfully brought up at an early stage and psychiatric evaluation should be seen as part of a routine set of clinical investigations, like the EEG, that the patient may require.

The next stage in management depends on the results of investigations. If the patient has both epileptic and non-epileptic seizures, then AEDs will need to be continued. It is important to teach the patient to distinguish between the different seizure types, and emphasize how they each may require different modes of treatment. It is often the non-epileptic attacks that are causing the most distress and disruption.

If there is underlying psychopathology, then this needs investigation and treatment in its own right. Depression, panic attacks, generalized anxiety disorder and psychoses will need, in varying proportions and combinations, psychotropic drugs, psychotherapy and behaviour therapy. The latter is often aimed at anxiety management. Panic attacks, with or without accompanying agoraphobia, usually respond well. It is sometimes necessary to combine this intervention with anxiolytics such as a benzodiazepine or a tricyclic drug. Antidepressants should be tailored to the patient's needs and prescribed in therapeutic doses. Often, patients are given these drugs in doses that are too low to be effective and are given compounds such as sedative tricyclics with unpleasant side-effects that put them off further courses.

Psychotherapy should be available to all those patients in whom it is deemed necessary. It is of especial value in those patients who have been traumatized or abused, and in this setting requires therapists accustomed to handling such patients. They can be very difficult and demanding on therapists' time, especially if the patient has an underlying personality disorder.

In these circumstances, AEDs should be slowly withdrawn. This process alone often improves patients' wellbeing. The practice of keeping patients on small doses 'just in case' is to be deprecated. A different, but common, situation is that of patients who have both epileptic seizures and non-epileptic attacks. These individuals need a combination of AEDs and psychological treatment. Management is difficult and the relative proportion of different types of seizure needs to be kept under review.

The prognosis of non-epileptic attacks depends on the underlying mechanisms. However, as with epilepsy, there is a hard core of patients who fail to respond to any therapeutic intervention. Occasionally this is financially motivated, and may amount to malingering. Much more often it is related to an underlying personality disorder. Briquet's hysteria has a poor prognosis. The longer the time of the misdiagnosis the worse the outcome, which is more positive for adolescents than for adults but is also dependent upon whether or not the patient has been offered treatment and how appropriate that has been. A diagnosis of non-epileptic seizures needs to be the beginning of appropriate therapy and not the end of medical attention.

## 9.2 PERSONALITY AND BEHAVIOUR DISORDER IN EPILEPSY

The relationship between epilepsy and personality disturbances has been controversial, although reference to behaviour problems in patients with epilepsy stems back to the early history of the subject. The first systematic observations and investigations of this disorder were made in the 19th century. Falret (1824–1902) recognized both peri-ictal disorders and interictal problems, defining patients who entered a prolonged abnormal mental state,'folie épileptique', in which slight epileptic paroxysms could be unrecognized or were substituted for by the abnormal mental state (Trimble & Schmitz 1992)

Morel (1809–1879) developed the concept of the epileptic character. He noted,'Il est dans la nature des maladies nerveuses d'imprimer à l'idiosyncrasie physique et morale des malades un chachet tout à fait particulier' (Reynolds 1861). From these ideas grew the concept of larval or masked epilepsy, and it was only a short step to suggesting the existence of epilepsy without seizures, identified by behavioural features only. This legacy still influences clinical practice, with concepts such as episodic dyscontrol.

Many studies have attempted to assess whether patients with epilepsy, when rated on personality rating scales, show different profiles to patients without epilepsy. By and large the results support the hypothesis that patients with epilepsy have abnormal personalities. However, this finding may be attributed to many factors. These include biological variables, for example, head injury following recurrent seizures, or the prescription of long-term AEDs, which may lead to behavioural change. It may also relate to psychosocial variables such as stigmatization, and a low expectancy of achievement by the family or by teachers.

Psychiatric disturbances in epilepsy are often linked to abnormalities of the temporal lobe. This link was postulated at a time when the biological basis of behaviour was being explored through the understanding of the limbic system. Behavioural problems such as the Kluver–Bucy syndrome, produced by bilateral extirpation of the amygdala, were described and the recognition of an integrated neuronal circuit which helped modulate emotions was recognized. Gibbs and Stamps (1953) stated: 'The patient's emotional reactions to his seizures, his family and his social situation are less important determinants of psychiatric disorder than the site and type of the epileptic discharge'. These views were based on observations that anterior temporal foci were common in patients with epilepsy who had associated psychiatric disorder, the latter including not only psychosis but also personality change.

The rating scale most commonly used for scientific investigations has been the Minnesota Multiphasic Personality Inventory (MMPI). The subscale scores that are most commonly abnormal are depression, paranoia, schizophrenia and psychaesthenia. Hermann et al (1980) noted an association between adolescent age of onset of seizures and a high frequency of reporting on these psychotic subscales and, in a separate study, noted that patients with an aura of ictal fear scored more highly on the MMPI profiles of paranoia, psychaesthenia, schizophrenia and psychopathic deviation (Hermann et al 1991). The link of abnormal profiles to an aura of fear is of interest as the latter suggests a seizure focus in the region of the amygdala.

The controversial Bear–Fedio scale was developed by bringing together characteristics described in prior clinical reports of personality in epilepsy. In the original paper, patients with unilateral temporal lobe epilepsy were compared to normal subjects and a group with neuromuscular disorders (Bear & Fedio 1977). Patients with epilepsy had abnormal profiles, particularly in regard to such features as humourlessness, dependence, circumstantiality and increased sense of personal destiny. Further, some laterality differences were noted; patients with left temporal lobe epilepsy described more anger, paranoia and dependence, while those with right temporal foci reported more elation. The Bear–Fedio Inventory does not suggest that all patients with temporal lobe epilepsy suffer from a distinctive personality profile and several authors have contended that the scale does no more than assess non-specific psychopathology.

The view that there is indeed an interictal behaviour syndrome of epilepsy, associated largely with temporal lobe epilepsy, was strongly supported by Gastaut et al (1953) and Geschwind (Waxman & Geschwind 1975). These reports highlighted changes in sexual behaviour, hypergraphia (a tendency to compulsive and extensive writing) and religiosity. They also highlighted stickiness or viscosity, patients showing a striking preoccupation with detail and concerns over moral or ethical issues. Estimates of the frequency with which such a profile occurs, from cluster analysis studies using MMPI and other clinical variables, vary from 7% (Rodin et al 1984) to 21% (Mungas 1992).

Although the controversy over the association between epilepsy and personality disorder continues, those dealing with patients with chronic epilepsy are quite familiar with these personality clusters, which sometimes dominate the clinical picture. In other cases, the features are used creatively, (an artistic example may be Van Gogh, literary examples may be Flaubert or Dostoievski). In other patients the tone of the personality is suggestive and the features are more apparent at times of seizures and seizure clusters. Although the evidence supporting the view that these abnormalities are commoner in patients with temporal lobe epilepsy is far from conclusive, the number of positive studies far outweighs the negative ones.

## 9.3 DEPRESSION

Depression is a clinically important concomitant of epilepsy. A link between the two states was described by Hippocrates: 'Melancholics ordinarily become epileptics, and epileptics melancholics: of these two states what determines the preference is the direction the malady takes; if it bears upon the body, epilepsy, if upon the intelligence, melancholy' (Lewis 1934). This association has continued to intrigue observers through the ages (Temkin 1971). In his textbook on epilepsy written in 1861, at the beginning of the scientific approach to the treatment of epilepsy, Reynolds (1861) discussed the interactions between mental state and seizures. More recently a number of reviews have documented the nature of the association between depression and epilepsy (Barraclough 1981, Dodrill & Batzel 1986, Robertson 1988, 1989, Blumer 1991, Devinsky & Bear 1991).

### 9.3.1 Prevalence

Although most authors accept that depression is more often seen in epilepsy than in the population at large, the significance of the association depends on the population studied. There have been very few studies investigating the absolute prevalence of psychiatric morbidity in epilepsy in the community. Two studies in England have assessed all the patients with epilepsy registered with a number of primary health care family doctors. In a sample of 218 patients, psychological difficulties were recorded in 29% (Pond et al 1960). In half of these the difficulties were 'neurotic' in nature. In a similar community-based survey of 88 patients, neurotic depression was noted in 22% (Edeh & Toone 1985). Hence, psychiatric disturbances are often seen in epilepsy but in the absence of a similarly assessed community control population the significance of this frequency is difficult to interpret.

In a study of patients with temporal lobe epilepsy, 19% were found to have clinically apparent anxiety while 11% were depressed (Currie et al 1971).

The importance of understanding depression in epilepsy is highlighted when the frequency of suicide and parasuicide in this population is considered. In a series of 11 studies there was a suicide rate five times of that in the general population (Barraclough 1981). In a further eight studies a suicide rate in epilepsy of 5% in patients with epilepsy compared to 1.4% in control populations was noted (Mathews & Barabas 1981). In patients with temporal lobe epilepsy the relative risk is even greater, as is the risk of parasuicide, particularly of overdoses.

Mania is rare in association with epilepsy. Williams (1956) described elation in just 3 of 2000 patients. The few cases reported in the literature are in the form of anecdotal accounts of individual cases (Hurwitz et al 1985, Barczak et al 1988).

### 9.3.2 Aetiology of depression in epilepsy

There are no clearly established mechanisms by which epilepsy may bring about clinical depression. Just as depression is a heterogenous condition, so it is likely that various factors combine in different ways in different patients with epilepsy to generate particular forms of associated depressive illness. It is possible, however, to explore possible aetiological elements common across patients.

Unfortunately, although a number of studies have examined depression in epilepsy, the data from these investigations are not strictly

**Table 9.3** The associations of depression in epilepsy (studies providing data: Williams 1956, Reynolds et al 1966, Currie et al 1971, Shorvon & Reynolds 1979, Trimble et al 1980, Kogeorgos et al 1982, Thompson & Trimble 1982, Perini & Mendius 1984, Edeh & Toone 1985, Mendez et al 1986, Brent et al 1987, Kramer et al 1987, Robertson et al 1987, Hermann & Wyler 1989, Mendez et al 1989, Altshuler et al 1990, Moller & Froscher 1990, Hermann et al 1991, Naugle et al 1991)

| Association | Number of studies finding association | No association |
|---|---|---|
| *Seizure characteristics* | | |
| Seizure type | 1 | 4 |
| Temporal focus | 3 | 1 |
| Left focus | 3 | 7 |
| Seizure frequency | 1 | 4 |
| Seizure duration | 1 | 4 |
| *Treatment-related* | | |
| Polypharmacy | 3 | 3 |
| Phenobarbitone | 3 | |
| Low serum folate | 3 | |
| *Personal factors* | | |
| Male preponderance | 2 | 3 |
| Loss of control | 1 | 1 |
| Family history of depression | 1 | 1 |

comparable. Patients were recruited from various sources, ranging from the community to specialist neuropsychiatric clinics. Some were well controlled on antiepileptic medication while others were being considered for surgical treatment following a long period of inadequate response to AEDs. In addition, numerous assessment techniques were utilized, including clinical examination, structured interviews and self-completed questionnaires, and the information obtained was interpreted using different diagnostic criteria and groupings. However, an overview of a large number of studies permits some tentative conclusions to be drawn (Table 9.3).

*Psychological factors*

The social sequelae of having epilepsy were relevant more than 2000 years ago when Hippocrates referred to the condition as 'the sacred disease'. Since that time much has been written on the social stigmatization of those with epilepsy. Even now, there is evidence that stigmatization persists (Betts 1993). The most powerful means of reducing this prejudice is education of the patients, their families and the public about epilepsy.

The adverse effects of stigma, discrimination, vocational difficulties and attendant strains of often unpredictable losses of consciousness have been evaluated using the psychological construct of locus of control (Hermann & Wyler 1989). In a population of patients awaiting temporal lobe surgery for epilepsy it was concluded that there was a significant association between an external locus of control, indicating a feeling of loss of personal control over life, and depression.

In addition, for many patients there will be more general social difficulties associated with problems of living with a chronic and, at times, disabling illness. Turner and Beiser (1990) interviewed more than 700 people chronically disabled by various conditions, most frequently heart disease or arthritis. They found that the disabled group suffered several disadvantages, regardless of their precise diagnosis. They were more likely to have a lower income and to be depressed. The increased depression was felt to be a reaction to chronic stress associated with the difficulties of chronic illness. It is likely that these non-specific factors also operate for those with epilepsy, even though these patients generally have fewer physical difficulties.

The contribution of psychosocial factors may be the critical factor that determines those with a particular biological state who will go on to develop depression.

*Seizure-related factors*

Several studies (Table 9.3) suggest that neither seizure type (complex partial with or without secondary generalization or primary generalized seizures) nor frequency, nor duration of epilepsy influence the occurrence of depression. Many studies, however, report an association between interictal depression and temporal lobe epilepsy. The situation regarding the laterality of the epileptic focus is more equivocal. Several studies have shown that major depression is more often associated with left, as opposed to right hemisphere lesions, for example after a stroke. Post-stroke mania is strongly associated with a right hemisphere lesion in a limbic-connected area (Starkstein & Robinson 1989). In epilepsy there is a link to the left hemisphere with depression (Robertson 1988) and hypomania has been related to seizures arising from the right temporal lobe (Barczack et al 1988, Byrne 1988).

A study by Hermann et al (1991) suggests a possible complex association between temporal lobe epilepsy and the presence of depression. These authors observed that in their patients with left (but not right) temporal lobe epilepsy there was a significant correlation between the degree of frontal lobe dysfunction, measured using a frontal lobe cognitive task, the Wisconsin Card Sorting Test, and the presence of a self-reported dysphoric mood state. Although acknowledging the limited value of self-reported ratings of mental states and the relatively mild nature of the mood disturbance, the authors concluded that the presence of concomitant frontal lobe dysfunction was important in the aetiology of affective disturbance associated with temporal lobe epilepsy. Such a suggestion is compatible with observations from imaging studies of depression and with the literature on post-stroke depression.

The role of the temporal lobes in the generation of affective states may also be investigated by considering the effects of temporal lobe surgery performed for the control of epilepsy.

In a minority of patients with chronic epilepsy, depression has worsened or developed de novo after temporal lobectomy, often acutely (Devinsky & Bear 1991). Of 72 patients followed postsurgically for 1–2 years, six made suicide attempts and in every case this was in the first month after the operation (Jensen & Larsen 1979). An increase in depression following anterior temporal lobectomy was also described by Bruton (1988) in an analysis of the series of patients from the Maudsley Hospital. In this group of 249 patients only one was considered depressed at the time of surgery, but during postsurgical follow-up the incidence of depression rose to 10% and six patients committed suicide. The mechanism of this effect is unknown although the postsurgical increase in depression may in part be a statistical artefact of comparing rates at a single point in time with those obtained over a prolonged follow-up period. It may also be a reflection of 'forced normalization' in some cases.

*Biochemical factors*

Biochemical links between epilepsy and depression remain to be established. Animal studies have suggested that limbic seizures may alter the functioning of cerebral corticotrophin releasing hormone (CRH) pathways. It has been suggested that these changes can increase vulnerability to stress-precipitated psychopathology (Adamec 1991). However, there is currently no evidence that this occurs in humans and as yet there are no treatment implications.

Another potential biochemical mechanism is folate depletion. The latter has been observed in patients on polytherapy (Reynolds 1991) and a relationship between mental illness and folate deficiency has been reported (Carney 1967). Phenytoin and barbiturates can both lead to falls in folate concentration in serum, red blood cells and cerebrospinal fluid. In epilepsy a link between low folate and depression has been noticed in several patient groups (Trimble et al 1980, Robertson et al 1987). Serum and red blood cell folate levels in a community sample of patients with epilepsy were significantly lower in those on polytherapy and in those achieving psychiatric 'caseness' using the Clinical Interview Schedule (Edeh & Toone 1985). This was true for the depressive neurosis subgroup but not the anxiety subgroup. The association, however, does not imply causality and the links between folate deficiency and mood change are not clear. In addition, therapeutic trials of folate have not been effective in treating depression, although early studies of methyl donors such s-adenosyl methionine are more promising.

## 9.3.3 Diagnosis of depression in epilepsy

The association between epilepsy and affective disturbance differs in the prodromal, peri-ictal and interictal periods.

*Prodromal phenomena*

In a prospective study, 27 patients with epilepsy self-rated their moods using personal feelings scales and recorded life events on a daily basis for at least 56 days (Blanchet & Frommer 1986). During this time, 13 patients had at least one seizure. In these patients the mean ratings of mood on eight of the 10 scales showed a decline on the day(s) preceding the seizure and an increase after the seizure. In four patients the mean Depression Scale rating on the day preceding the seizure was significantly lower than the mean rating on normal days.

There are several possible explanations for the association between lowered mood ratings and the subsequent occurrence of seizures. Lower mood may be a symptom of the prodromal phase of seizure activity, initiated by the same biological processes that bring about the seizure. Alternatively, it may be that the mood change itself precipitates a seizure. The question remains without a definitive answer since in this study the relationship of life events and mood to seizures appeared to be independent.

*Peri-ictal phenomena*

The aura is the earliest stage of subjective awareness of seizure activity. Many different sensations have been recorded (Lennox & Cobb 1933). Of 215 auras of various complexities and types in 88 patients with temporal lobe epilepsy there were 24 experiences of 'epigastric fear'; there were no reports of any other affective states (Taylor & Lochery 1987).

Williams (1956) investigated emotional phenomena in 2000 patients with epilepsy and found that 100 of them reported an emotion as part of the 'epileptic experience'. The most commonly reported emotion was fear, occurring in 61% of the 100 patients with emotional phenomena. On some occasions this fear was severe, with psychic and somatic features. In contrast to this, depression was reported less often, in just 21 cases (i.e. in 1% of the whole group). However, Williams observed that when depression did occur it tended to last for longer than other peri-ictal phenomena, persisting for up to several days after the ictus. This is akin to naturally occurring depression, which also tends to be self-sustaining.

Although of short duration, postictal depression may be severe and at times include suicidal ideation. Case descriptions give a clear impression that the depressive phase is more than purely an emotional reaction to the advent of a seizure, suggesting instead a biological link with the seizure process (Blumer 1992).

Thus peri-ictal depression, though it does occur, is not common but is characterized by a greater persistence than other postictal emotional phenomena. It is interesting to note that depressive auras appear to be rare.

*Interictal phenomena*

Several recent studies have investigated the phenomenology of interictal depression. Mendez et al (1986) compared 20 depressed epileptic in-patients to 20 non-epileptic depressed subjects. Both groups met DSM-III criteria for major depression. All the patients had features of endogenous depression, anergia, anhedonia, appetite and sleep disturbance, but the major distinguishing characteristics of the depressed patients with epilepsy with respect to the non-epileptic group were a chronic dysthymic background, a relative lack of neurotic traits such as somatization or self-pity and a history of periods of agitated peri-ictal psychotic behaviour.

The depressive phenomenology of a larger group of epileptic patients meeting research diagnostic criteria for major depressive disorder was described by Robertson et al (1987). These authors assessed 66 patients using clinical examination and a number of standardized rating scales. In this study patients obtained very high state and trait anxiety scores. The authors suggested that the high level of state anxiety may have been due to the depression, since it decreased significantly during a 6-week double-blind placebo-controlled trial of an antidepressant (Robertson & Trimble 1985).

## 9.3.4 Management of depression in epilepsy

Multiple factors may contribute to the development of depression in epilepsy and any treatment approach should address all these areas. In the first instance a clinical assessment of the severity of depression should be made, since there is an increased risk of suicide. Subsequent actions will be determined by the result of this assessment. Epilepsy, AED and psychosocial variables should all be examined.

*Seizures*

Seizure control should be optimized. A recent increase in seizure frequency or the development of secondarily generalized seizures in a patient with partial epilepsy may be associated with the development of depression by virtue of the increased disruption to the daily life of the patient. Conversely, depression may lead to increased seizures as a result of sleep deprivation or failure of compliance.

*Antiepileptic drugs*

Polytherapy is often associated with depression. Improvements in psychological test performances and a reduction in depression scores on the Middlesex Hospital Questionnaire were observed following a reduction in the number of different AEDs prescribed (Thompson & Trimble 1982).

The use of phenobarbitone is linked to the development of depression in adults (Robertson et al 1987), and in children (Brent et al 1987). A much higher prevalence of major depressive disorder (40% versus 4%) and suicidal ideation (47% versus 4%) was noted in children treated with phenobarbitone compared with carbamazepine, especially in those who had a family history of depression. Phenobarbitone enhances GABA-mediated postsynaptic inhibition as part of its antiepileptic activity both experimentally and in patients (Engel 1989). Vigabatrin results in elevated brain GABA concentrations and increased stimulation of GABA receptors. A minority of patients prescribed vigabatrin have become depressed in association with this treatment (Ring & Reynolds 1991) (Ch 4, 4.5.15).

Carbamazepine, which is structurally related to the tricyclic antidepressants, may be antidepressant (Dalby 1975, Thompson & Trimble 1982). Carbamazepine has also been demonstrated to be antidepressant in non-epileptic depressed patients and has a role as a prophylactic agent in the control of manic-depressive illness (Post et al 1986).

Thus, when treating depression, consideration should be given to reducing polytherapy and, if patients are receiving phenobarbitone or vigabatrin, withdrawing these and introducing carbamazepine.

*Specific antidepressant treatments*

Depression in patients with epilepsy can be successfully treated with antidepressants (Robertson & Trimble 1985, Blumer 1991). It is important to bear in mind the possibility of drug interactions between antidepressants and AEDs (Richens et al 1983). Fluoxetine, a selective serotonin-uptake-inhibiting antidepressant, results, in animal studies, in an increase in antiepileptic potency, producing a dose-related increase in the antiepileptic activity of phenytoin and carbamazepine against experimental seizures (Leander 1992).

All antidepressants, however, may lower the seizure threshold, although the risk is least with monoamine uptake inhibitors (Robertson 1988). Although seizures have often been reported in depressed patients taking therapeutic doses of tricyclic antidepressants, a causal relationship is difficult to establish (Edwards 1985). A prospective study of the incidence of antidepressant-induced seizures found that seizures requiring treatment with an AED occurred in less than 1 case in 1000 (Jick et al 1983). These observations were made in patients without epilepsy and the implications for those who have the condition are not clear. While Edwards (1985) suggested that a family history of epilepsy was relevant, Blumer (1991) concluded that a lowering of the seizure threshold with modest doses of a tricyclic antidepressant was rarely of clinical significance. In general, caution is advised in giving tricyclic agents to patients with epilepsy. Of the antidepressants, tricyclics, particularly clomipramine, the tetracyclic maprotiline, mianserin and buproprion (in higher doses) seem more likely to provoke seizures than some of the new selective 5-HT uptake inhibitors (e.g. fluvoxamine, paroxetine and fluoxetine); however, seizures have been described with all of these compounds. Lithium also has a pro-convulsant potential. Nevertheless, many patients with epilepsy and depression benefit from antidepressant medication and provided the small risk of exacerbating seizures is acknowledged there is no general contraindication to their usage.

Although there is limited experience of the use of electroconvulsive therapy in epilepsy, Betts (1981) reports that it causes no problems and points out that in severe drug-resistant depression, with the attendant risk of suicide, it may be life-saving.

In view of the interplay of psychosocial and biological factors in the genesis of depression, several authors have pointed out the importance of including appropriate psychotherapy within the overall management plan (Robertson 1988, Devinsky & Bear 1991).

## 9.4 PSYCHOSES OF EPILEPSY

### 9.4.1 Postictal psychosis

There are few who doubt that psychotic states can be associated with epilepsy. Most neurologists are familiar with the acute ictal and postictal psychosis that occurs in patients, either during complex partial seizure status, or more commonly following a cluster of seizures. In these settings the psychosis is dominated by confusion, associated with hallucinations and delusions. The mental state fluctuates over the course of time, and the psychosis is usually cleared within an hour or two. In many cases it is much more short-lived. However, there are patients who enter prolonged phases of psychosis, with signs of disorientation and confusion, following clusters of seizures.

The frequency of postictal psychoses is unknown, but is almost certainly less than it used to be before the era of effective antiepileptic therapy. Its high prevalence in the 19th century is one explanation of the frequent reporting of severe disturbances of the mental state in patients with chronic intractable seizures.

*Phenomenology*

Postictal psychoses present with confusion, automatisms, wandering and inappropriate behaviour. In a series of 52 cases, the patients were older than cases 'without clouded states', and hallucinations, mainly auditory, were reported in 36%, with delusions (mainly persecutory) in a quarter. The abnormal mental state developed within 24 hours of the seizure in 17 of 23 cases, but in four it was 1–2 days later, and in two it was 2–7 days. In 14 of 21 cases, two or more seizures heralded the disorder (Levin 1952).

Logsdail and Toone (1988) have provided a more detailed phenomenological account of the postictal psychosis, which they defined as follows.

- An episode of confusion or psychosis manifested immediately upon a seizure, or emerged within a week of the return of apparently normal mental function
- A minimum duration of 24 h, and a maximum of 3 months
- A mental state characterized by one of the following:
  1. clouding of consciousness, disorientation or delirium
  2. delusions, hallucinations in clear consciousness
  3. a mixture of 1 and 2
- No evidence of the following extraneous factors which might have contributed to the abnormal mental state:
  1. antiepileptic drug toxicity
  2. a previous history of interictal psychosis
  3. EEG evidence of non-convulsive status
  4. recent history of head injury, or alcohol or drug intoxication

Five of their patients had one psychotic episode, six had two to four and three had several recurrences. Three patients had idiopathic generalized epilepsy but the rest had complex partial seizures with intermittent secondary generalization. In 86% of cases there was a clear history of an increase in generalized seizure frequency prior to the onset of the psychosis, usually in a cluster. In 78% there was an obvious lucid interval, lasting from 1–6 days, in which the mental state was normal after recovery from the seizures, prior to the sudden onset of the psychosis.

The psychosis itself has pleomorphic phenomenology, some patients displaying obvious confusion. 50% had paranoid delusions, while auditory and visual hallucinations were both common. These authors commented on the relative frequency of affective change, observations supported by the reporting of five cases of hypomania following temporal lobe seizures (Barczak et al 1988, Byrne 1988). In two, religiosity was a prominent part of the mental state. Interestingly, all were male, had had a flurry of seizures and had a right-sided focus.

### 9.4.2 Interictal psychosis

In some patients it may be difficult to distinguish a postictal from an interictal state. In clinical practice, the psychoses that emerge postictally sometimes continue for several weeks, and it would be appropriate to then refer to them as interictal. Some patients initially have recurring bouts of postictal psychoses that then gradually become fixed. Occasionally, following clusters of seizures, patients will develop a postictal psychosis that fails to resolve.

*Epidemiology*

There are no reliable epidemiological surveys giving the prevalence of these psychoses. Gudmundsson (1966) personally examined adult epileptic patients in a comprehensive study in Iceland, and in this sample 7.1% were psychotic. In a recent epidemiological survey of general practice patients, four patients (4.5%) were identified who were currently psychotic (Edeh & Toone 1987).

Several authors have suggested that patients with temporal lobe epilepsy are more likely than those with other focal epilepsies or generalized epilepsies to present with severe psychopathology. In a meta-analysis of MMPI studies a total of 809 patients with epilepsy from 10 studies were compared with over 1000 patients from 15 other studies who had non-neurological illness (Whitman et al 1984). In addition there were 870 subjects with neurological, non-epileptic conditions. Patients with epilepsy manifested more severe psychopathology than both the neurological or the illness control groups.

*Relationship with temporal lobe epilepsy*

In a review of the world literature (Trimble 1991) the incidence of psychosis in temporal lobe epilepsy was 17%, and 2% in other focal epilepsies. When patients with psychosis and epilepsy were classified according to the type of seizure disorder, 217 (76%) of 287 patients had a temporal lobe disturbance.

The studies that failed to note an increase in psychosis with a temporal lobe focus derived largely from one group (Small et al 1966, Small & Small 1967; Stevens 1966). However, in some of these studies nearly two-thirds of the patients having psychotic episodes had a diagnosis of 'psychomotor temporal epilepsy' (Stevens 1966).

One of the more convincing links between psychosis and temporal lobe epilepsy emerged from a long-term follow-up study of 100 children with temporal lobe epilepsy, of whom nine developed a schizophrenia-like illness. Several additional patients had psychotic symptoms (Ounsted & Lindsay 1981).

As noted above, an aura of ictal fear is associated with more abnormal profiles on the MMPI, including the psychotic subscales, and similar findings were replicated by Devinsky et al (1991). Stark-Adamec et al (1985) have shown a link between psychiatric disturbance in epilepsy and limbic auras, and other studies using EEG localization (Nielsen & Kristensen 1981), or neuro-hormone profiles (Dana-Haeri & Trimble 1984) suggest that there is a subgroup of patients with medial temporal or limbic seizures who are the most susceptible to developing a psychosis. This is consistent with the known anatomical associations of the limbic system to behavioural changes.

*Phenomenology*

Phenomenologically interictal psychoses are similar to, but differ in part from the classical psychiatric syndromes. Slater and Beard (1963) collected 69 cases and noted three major groups: chronic psychoses with recurrent confusional episodes, chronic paranoid states and hebephrenic states. The onset was usually insidious, with the gradual appearance of delusions, especially in the chronic paranoid subgroup. In 17, the chronic psychoses appeared as a sequel to a series of epileptic confusional episodes, and in a further 20, short-lived psychotic episodes lasting from 11–38 days occurred immediately before the onset of the more chronic disorders. Delusions were present in all but two of the patients, and in many these were religious or mystical. Passivity feelings were prominent, and many attributed significant feelings and special significance to commonplace events. A number of patients claimed special powers, for example of healing. Hallucinations, visual and auditory, were present in many patients, the latter often being persecutory voices, but classical first-rank Schneiderian hallucinations were also frequent (Table 9.4). Thought disorder was shown by half of the patients, but in addition there were thought-blocking, neologisms and evidence of disturbed syntax. The point was made that motor disturbances were rare and that affective symptoms were prominent.

**Table 9.4** The first-rank symptoms of Schneider

- The hearing of one's thoughts spoken aloud in one's head
- The hearing of voices commenting on what one is doing at the time
- Voices arguing in the third person
- Experiences of bodily influence
- Thought withdrawal and other forms of thought interference
- Thought diffusion
- Delusion perception*
- Everything in the spheres of feeling, drive and volition which the patient experiences as forced on him or influenced by others

*An abnormal significance attached to a real perception without any cause that is understandable in rational or emotional terms

The psychosis associated with temporal lobe epilepsy more often presents with typical first-rank symptoms of Schneider and with less evidence of personality deterioration and negative symptoms than do psychoses associated with other forms of epilepsy, for example generalized epilepsies. The latter tend to be more associated with evidence of organic brain syndromes and intellectual handicap. Classical manic depressive pictures are rare, and depressive psychoses often present as a paranoid state.

*Risk factors*

Many patients develop psychosis in their late teens or early 20s, several years after the onset of complex partial seizures (Table 9.5). This has led some to suggest that a biological mechanism exists similar to kindling, leading to the development of a psychotic illness. Studies with MRI do not reveal any underlying structural changes that distinguish psychotic from non-psychotic epileptic patients (Conlon et al 1990). However, studies with positron emission tomography (Gallhofer et al 1985) have shown widespread changes of function, not only in patients with epilepsy but also in patients with epileptic psychosis, that involve areas of the brain removed from the temporal lobe focus, in particular other limbic areas, the basal ganglia and the frontal cortex.

**Table 9.5** Risk factors associated with psychosis of epilepsy

- *Age of onset:* Early adolescence
- *Interval – onset of seizures to onset of psychosis:* is approx. 14 years
- *Sex:* Bias to females
- *Seizure type:* Complex partial – automatisms
- *Seizure frequency:* Diminished, especially temporal lobe
- *Seizure focus:* Temporal, especially left-sided
- *Neurological findings:* Sinistrality
- *Pathology:* Gangliogliomas, hamartomas
- *EEG:* Mediobasal temporal lobe focus

Complex partial seizures are the most frequent seizure type associated with psychoses. Some patients appear to manifest less frequent seizures for the duration of any psychotic episode. This is related to the phenomenon of forced normalization (see below).

Flor-Henry (1969) was the first to discuss the issue of laterality in relationship to the psychoses of epilepsy. In many patients being evaluated for epilepsy surgery, he noted that if patients had temporal lobe epilepsy and were psychotic, those with a right-sided focus tended to be manic depressive while those with schizophrenia-like psychoses tended to have a left-sided focus.

Several other groups have looked at this relationship, and of a total of 341 patients from 14 studies it was shown that, where a left- or right-sided focus could be discerned, in 65% it was left-sided (Trimble 1991). Trimble and Perez (1982) noted a more exclusive association between nuclear schizophrenia, presenting with first-rank symptoms of Schneider, and left hemisphere lesions. The association of manic depressive illness with right-sided lesions has failed to receive further confirmation, although a link between affective disturbance and the right temporal lobe has been noted above in the literature on the ictal psychoses. An increased incidence of sinistrality in patients with epilepsy and psychosis has been noted, possibly implying abnormal organization of cerebral function (Taylor 1975).

In summary, the interictal psychoses of epilepsy take forms similar to but not identical with classical psychiatric syndromes and are seen more frequently in association with temporal lobe epilepsy than with seizures arising from other sites. They are thought to be related to the gradual development of functional change within the brain. Their prevalence is such that they form an important part of practice for those dealing with patients with chronic epilepsy, and their treatment becomes an integral part of that practice.

### 9.4.3 Forced normalization

Earlier this century it was suggested that there existed an antagonism between epilepsy and psychosis. In the 1950s Landolt (1953, 1958) published a series of papers on patients who had epilepsy who became psychotic when their seizures were under control, and proposed the concept of forced normalization: 'Forced normalization is the phenomenon characterized by the fact that, with the recurrence of psychotic states, the EEG becomes more normal, or entirely normal as compared with previous and subsequent EEG findings.'

Forced normalization is thus essentially an EEG phenomenon. The clinical counterpart of patients becoming psychotic when their seizures are controlled, and their psychosis resolving with return of seizures, is referred to as alternative psychoses (Tellenbach 1965).

These phenomena have now been well documented clinically, and further observations have been made. First, the EEG does not need to become 'normal', but the interictal disturbances decrease and in some cases disappear.

Second, the clinical presentation need not necessarily be a psychosis. In childhood, or in the mentally handicapped, aggression and agitation are common. Other manifestations include non-epileptic seizures or other conversion symptoms, depression, mania and anxiety states.

Third, the psychotic episodes may last days or weeks and can be terminated by a seizure, with the return of EEG abnormalities.

Fourth, although originally associated with partial epilepsies, with the introduction of the succinimide drugs Landolt also noted an association with generalized epilepsy. Certainly, forced normalization may be provoked by the administration of AEDs, and has been reported with barbiturates, benzodiazepines, ethosuximide and vigabatrin.

The literature on antagonism between epilepsy and psychosis has been held to be incompatible with the suggestion that there is an increased association between epilepsy and psychosis. This issue has been resolved by more careful understanding of the original literature, in that there may be an antagonism of symptoms, namely between seizures and the symptoms of psychosis such as hallucinations and delusions (Wolf & Trimble 1985).

Forced normalization is less common than suggested by Landolt, however, but to ignore the fact that some patients manifest these problems can lead to the continuation of severe behaviour disturbances, with all of the social disruption that then emerges and with failure to treat the epilepsy appropriately.

### 9.4.4 Psychosis following surgery

Ever since its introduction, the possibility that temporal lobe surgery itself may be associated with the development of psychiatric disturbance, in particular psychosis, has been discussed. Some of the best evidence comes from the Maudsley series (Taylor 1975, Bruton 1988). Most centres have stopped operating on floridly psychotic patients, based on the observation that psychoses generally do not improve with the operation. The extent of the problem, however, is unclear as few centres regularly include a psychiatric evaluation as part of their preoperative assessment or postoperative follow-up. Assessment of psychosocial adjustment is rarely performed, in contrast to the often scrupulous recording of neuropsychological deficits.

The Maudsley series shows that some patients develop new psychosis postoperatively, and there is an increased reporting of depression. Suicide was reported in 2.4% of the sample, but accounted for 22% of the post-operative deaths.

Bruton has suggested that the development of postoperative psychoses may be commoner with certain pathologies (gangliogliomas), and patients with right-sided temporal lobectomies may be more prone to these psychiatric disturbances (Mace & Trimble 1991). In some cases, the sudden relief of seizures that occurs following surgery may suggest a mechanism similar to forced normalization, although no persistent clear relationship emerges between the success of the operation and the development of psychotic postoperative states.

In the series from the National Hospitals, analysis of 50 patients assessed psychiatrically preoperatively and then followed for at least 3 months postoperatively revealed that 16% developed depression requiring psychiatric intervention. One patient became psychotic. With potential suicide rates up to 5%, these data emphasize the need for continuing psychiatric observations in patients who have received temporal lobectomy. There is some evidence that a transient affective or psychotic disorder is most likely to develop in the first year after surgery and that the long-term psychiatric outcome is good.

## 9.4.5 Treatment of psychosis

The management of psychosis in patients with epilepsy is generally similar to that in patients without epilepsy. Patients with interictal and postictal psychoses may need treatment with neuroleptic medications, although these can lower the seizure threshold. Of the neuroleptics, phenothiazines are more likely to provoke seizures than the butyrophones, and of the available drugs, pimozide is perhaps the least likely to precipitate seizures. Patients most likely to have their seizure control disturbed are those with overt cerebral damage and patients given large initial doses or sudden changes of dose. Lithium also has a pro-convulsant potential.

Ictal psychoses occasionally need neuroleptic drugs, although they usually settle rapidly. It is important to prevent patients from damaging themselves or causing harm to others, and regular haloperidol or pimozide may control behaviour satisfactorily. The interictal paranoid or schizophrenia-like states need to be evaluated in terms of their relationship to seizure frequency. Thus, in patients who stop having seizures in association with the onset of psychosis, a neuroleptic that decreases the seizure threshold is reasonable, for example chlorpromazine.

Where patients with epilepsy have no alteration of the seizure frequency, or the psychosis is occurring in the setting of increased seizure frequency, a neuroleptic that is less likely to precipitate seizures, such as haloperidol, sulpiride or pimozide, is logical.

Patients receiving AEDs that increase hepatic metabolism will have lower serum levels of neuroleptics, and may therefore require higher doses than patients not on these medications to achieve a similar clinical effect. Occasionally the prescription of an antidepressant or a neuroleptic may lead to increases in serum AED concentrations. Although the addition of carbamazepine or sodium valproate to the regimen of psychotic patients does not influence the psychosis it is important in patients who have epilepsy and behaviour disturbances to attempt to use drugs that may have beneficial psychotropic effects, and to avoid barbiturates and, if possible, polytherapy.

As with all psychiatric problems, psychopharmacological management alone is not sufficient. Although the role of psychotherapy in the management of psychotic conditions has not been proved to be of any substantial value, it is important to acknowledge that epileptic patients with psychosis bear the burden of epilepsy in addition to their psychosis. Patients with intermittent psychotic states are often perplexed and embarrassed about what has happened to them while psychotic, and fear further continuing bouts, with a descent into insanity. Patients with continuous psychosis require the skills of paramedical intervention, and the full resources of community care may be needed to help rehabilitation and to assist their families in coping with their difficulties. In many patients with chronic psychoses of epilepsy, the preservation of affect and lack of personality disintegration over years sustains them well in their communities and may enable them to live with their families and to marry. Maintaining these patients and bringing support to them is important, keeping them in the community and preventing their recurrent admission into hospital. Further, a good family environment with adequate medical facilities and follow-up care enhances compliance and minimizes the problems associated with non-compliance.

## 9.5 IMPAIRMENT OF COGNITION AND MEMORY

### 9.5.1 Cognitive function

Impairment of cognitive abilities and a decline of intellectual function have been recognized as a complication of epilepsy since the mid 19th century. In recent years the factors underlying neuropsychological deficits and the types of psychological deficit associated with varying seizure types have been further clarified.

Several investigators have noted that patients with symptomatic epilepsy are more likely to have impaired intellect than those with epilepsy of no known cause (Bourgeois et al 1983). Pre-existing brain damage, however, does not completely explain the neuropsychological deficit and other epilepsy-related factors contribute to cognitive change in addition to underlying structural lesions (Klove & Matthews 1966).

An early age of onset of epilepsy has a poorer prognosis with regard to intellectual abilities. Patients with generalized seizures tend to show more deficits of attention and concentration compared to patients with focal seizures. Patients who have seizures arising from the temporal lobes are most likely to have memory impairments. Patients with typical absences show impaired cognitive function for the duration of the bursts of spike wave discharges, and generally have minimal interictal impairments. If absences are frequent, however, impairment of performance in the classroom setting may lead to educational underachievement. Binnie (1986) and his colleagues have pointed out that subclinical focal discharges may also have clinical significance, noting transient, usually subtle, cognitive impairment (TCI) on selective tasks at times of focal EEG discharges.

Seidenberg et al (1981) compared, longitudinally, a group of patients whose seizure frequency decreased during a test–retest interval on psychological tests with another group in which it remained unchanged or was increased. Those with a decreasing seizure frequency showed improvements in intellectual quotients. Dodrill (1986) examined the effect of estimated lifetime seizures on psychological tasks and noted that a lifelong history of more than 100 individual convulsions was associated with decreased functioning in a variety of areas.

In some patients a significant decline akin to a dementia occurs (Ch 3, 3.7.2–4). Retrospective studies (Trimble & Corbett 1980, Trimble 1989) have suggested that generalized tonic-clonic seizures with recurrent head injury, and the prescription of certain AEDs, notably phenytoin and primidone, are associated with cognitive decline.

The role of phenytoin in the causation of an encephalopathy has been discussed for some time (Rosen 1966). This picture affects only a minority of patients and a link with metabolic disturbances, e.g. folate deficiency, has been suggested. Patients with mental handicap, severe intractable epilepsy and recurrent head injuries are most susceptible to this encephalopathy, which may be partially reversed by discontinuing phenytoin and reducing polytherapy.

*Effects of antiepileptic drugs on cognitive function*

The effects of AEDs on cognitive function have been an area of intense investigation in recent years. Extensive reviews are available (Trimble & Thompson 1986), and only a brief summary is given here. In patients on polytherapy, reduction of AED intake improves cognitive function over a wide range of cognitive abilities (Thompson & Trimble 1982).

There has been a debate as to whether or not there are significant differences between individual AEDs. Generally, data favour the newer agents, carbamazepine, sodium valproate, vigabatrin and lamotrigine, and emphasize more cognitive impairments in association with phenytoin and phenobarbitone treatment (Thompson et al 1981, Thompson & Trimble 1982, Smith 1991). A controversy that has recently emerged is whether the cognitive impairments associated with AEDs are a reflection of purely motor impairments, rather than of some effect on higher cognitive function (Dodrill & Temkin 1989, Dodrill & Troupin 1991). Data bearing on this issue support the view that most AEDs may bring about some motor slowing, which is reflected in cognitive tasks. However, differences can be discerned, particularly between carbamazepine and phenytoin, in terms of higher cognitive tasks, with carbamazepine being associated with less impairment (Duncan et al 1990).

Several new AEDs have recently been introduced to clinical practice, but information on their cognitive effects is rather limited. Vigabatrin appears to have no significant influence on cognitive abilities (Mumford et al 1990, McGuire et al 1992, Gillham et al 1993), or a slowing of motor function and slight impairment of visual memory (Grunewald et al 1994). Further work with this and other new AEDs, such as lamotrigine and gabapentin, in the area of cognitive function is needed.

### 9.5.2 Memory

Patients with epilepsy frequently complain of memory difficulties. In some cases this is secondary to problems of concentration and attention, and may therefore not be a memory defect per se. For other patients, particularly in those with temporal lobe abnormalities, memory may be selectively affected. Most of the work in this area has been undertaken on patients undergoing temporal lobectomy, in whom careful testing of memory function prior to surgery is mandatory, and deficits may occur following removal of the offending temporal lobe.

Memory function is usually improved by improving control of seizures. The role of AEDs in exacerbating memory problems has yet to be clearly defined since the impairments associated with the drugs tend to reflect more on concentration, attention and psychomotor abilities than on memory function per se. Recent studies have suggested that the poor memory of patients with temporal lobe epilepsy does not correlate with seizure frequency. Seizures may have an acute effect on memory but this is usually transient and does not affect prospective memory (Bergin 1994). In large measure, the memory loss associated with epilepsy seems to be more related to the underlying pathology than to the seizures themselves.

## 9.6 OPTIMIZATION OF PSYCHOSOCIAL POTENTIAL

### 9.6.1 Measurement of psychosocial effects of epilepsy

Studies of quality of life (QOL) have come to prominence in recent years, although definition is problematic. However, in recognition of the fact that epilepsy is more than just seizures, and that the optimization of psychosocial potential requires attention to the many aspects of a patient's life that go towards making their own internal concept of their wellbeing, QOL has become an important management goal.

The World Heath Organization (1980) proposed three levels at which disease can impact upon an individual: impairment, disability and handicap. Impairment relates to abnormalities of body structure and organ systems, and disability is seen as the impact of the illness on a person's functional abilities and activity levels. Handicap most closely relates to quality of life, defining disadvantage due to disease or treatment which an individual experiences in relation to their peers and others in society.

Studies of QOL applied to epilepsy address physical, cognitive, affective, social and economic aspirations of patients. The word 'aspiration' is used here to emphasize an important conceptual aspect of QOL research. Thus, future expectations are a major component of perceived quality of life, actual abilities being less important than a discrepancy between the patient's position as they are now and their expected situation.

The diagnosis of epilepsy brings with it many psychosocial problems, including stigmatization, social isolation, psychological problems and education and employment difficulties (Thompson & Oxley 1988). Societal attitudes play a major role in determining QOL of patients with epilepsy, and discrimination and non-acceptance of patients are all too common. There are obvious ways that patients' psychosocial potential can be optimized. This begins at diagnosis, allowing patients fully to explore the concept of epilepsy and discuss their fears and myths about the condition.

From a medical point of view, it is important to provide constant contact with known individuals, who will look after them throughout their career of being a patient with epilepsy and also offer non-medical help and intervention (see below).

Measurement of QOL, and scientific study of improvements of QOL with various treatments (for example monotherapy versus polytherapy, or surgery, or even the introduction of new drugs) is in its infancy. There is a lack of appropriate measures for patients with epilepsy, existing QOL scales being developed for people with other specific physical illnesses, such as cancer. Several different approaches, including questionnaires (Trimble & Dodson 1994, Vickrey et al 1992) and repertory grid techniques are now being used. Using such techniques it is apparent that, while seizures are of central importance to some patients in determining QOL, this is not so for all. Cognitive and emotional factors rate highly, as do social isolation and lack of friendships. These data highlight the need for a broader management of epilepsy, recognizing that the condition involves more than having seizures. Such studies serve to emphasize one of the goals of increasing the awareness of all who look after epilepsy to the importance of psychosocial variables in patient management. In addition, such evaluations are necessary to determine the benefits of attempts at psychosocial rehabilitation.

### 9.6.2 Psychosocial rehabilitation

The goals of management in epilepsy go far beyond suppression of seizures, especially in those unfortunate patients who do not respond to medication. Often patients have difficulty coming to terms with the diagnosis, even after many years of attacks. Individual counselling by those experienced in epilepsy management is then required. Similar support should be available, through specialist clinics, for patients at any stage of their management in whom the condition has presented seemingly insurmountable problems. In some cases, more formal psychotherapy should be offered. Equivalent facilities are sometimes required for carers, and there is a continuing need to educate the general public about epilepsy.

Other personnel that are required as part of a team approach to management of a broad spectrum of patients are social workers, occupational therapists, psychologists and those with employment rehabilitation skills. Help offered includes assessment of patients' potential for daily independent living skills, education and occupations. Some severely disabled patients require day-centre placement, or even more prolonged care at one of the special residential centres for epilepsy.

A good example where such extended management teams are useful, but rarely applied, is following temporal lobectomy. It is no doubt a positive endeavour to relieve a patient of seizures, but this is the initiation of a new lifestyle for that person. They may have lost many years of ordinary social and vocational life, and are suddenly expected, now seizure-free, to live a 'normal' life. They require habilitation, as opposed to rehabilitation, a process of socialization that includes learning to live *without* seizures. Relatives and carers also need to be informed of the problems that may arise postoperatively, and how to help the patient cope. These patients need to have careful postoperative planning of their goals and expectations, and follow-up at regular intervals to update and reconcile their achievements. Initially, at least, this needs to be a structured process, with realistic aims being established and a timetable for progress being set.

## REFERENCES


Adamec RE 1991 Corticotrophin releasing factor – a peptide link between stress and psychopathology associated with epilepsy ? J Psychopharmacol 5: 96–104

Altshuler LL, Devinsky O, Post RM, Theodore W 1990 Depression, anxiety, and temporal lobe epilepsy: Laterality of focus and symptoms. Arch Neurol 47: 284–288

Barczak P, Edmunds E, Betts T 1988 Hypomania following complex partial seizures; A report of three cases. Br J Psychiat 152: 137–139

Barraclough B 1981 Suicide and epilepsy. In: Reynolds EH, Trimble MR (eds) Epilepsy and psychiatry. Churchill Livingstone, Edinburgh, p 72–76

Bear DM, Fedio P 1977 Quantitative analysis of interictal behaviour in temporal lobe epilepsy. Arch Neurol 34: 454–467

Bergin PS 1994 Memory and epilepsy. University of Otago, Dunedin, MD thesis

Betts T A 1981 Depression, anxiety and epilepsy. In: Reynolds E H, Trimble M R (eds) Epilepsy and psychiatry. Churchill Livingstone, Edinburgh, p 60–71

Betts T A 1993 Neuropsychiatry. In: Laidlaw J, Richens A, Chadwick DW (eds) A textbook of epilepsy, 4th edn. Churchill Livingstone, Edinburgh, p 397–458

Binnie CD 1986 Monitoring seizures. In: Trimble MR, Reynolds EH (eds) What is epilepsy? Churchill Livingstone, Edinburgh, p 82–7

Blanchet P, Frommer GP 1986 Mood change preceding epileptic seizures. J Nerv Ment Dis 174: 471–476

Blumer D 1991 Epilepsy and disorders of mood. In: Smith D, Treiman D, Trimble M (eds) Neurobehavioral problems in epilepsy. Advances in neurology 55. Raven Press, New York, p 185–195

Blumer D 1992 Postictal depression: Significance for the treatment of the neurobehavioral disorder of epilepsy. J Epilepsy 5: 214–219

Bourgeois BFD, Prensky AL, Palkes HS, Talent BK, Busch SG 1983 Intelligence in epilepsy: a prospective study in children. Ann Neurol 14: 438–444

Brent DA, Crumrine PK, Varma RR, Allan M, Allman C 1987 Phenobarbital treatment and major depressive disorder in children with epilepsy. Pediatrics 80: 909–917

Bruton CJ 1988 The neuropathology of temporal lobe epilepsy. Maudsley Monographs. Oxford University Press, Oxford

Byrne A 1988 Hypomania following increased epileptic activity. Br J Psychiat 153: 573–574

Carney M W P 1967 Serum folate values in 423 psychiatric patients. Br Med J 4: 512–516

Conlon P, Trimble MR, Rogers D 1990 A study of epileptic psychosis using MRI. Br J Psychiat 156: 231–235

Currie S, Heathfield KWG, Henson R A, Scott DF 1971 Clinical course and prognosis of temporal lobe epilepsy: A survey of 666 patients. Brain 94: 173–190

Dalby MA 1975 Behavioural effects of carbamazepine. In: Penry JK, Daly DD (eds) Complex partial seizures and their treatment. Raven Press, New York, p 331–344

Dana-Haeri J, Trimble MR 1984 Prolactin and gonadotrophin changes following partial seizures in epileptic patients with and without psychopathology. Biol Psychiat 19: 329–336

Devinsky O, Bear DM 1991 Varieties of depression in epilepsy. Neuropsychiat Neuropsychol Behav Neurol 4: 49–61

Devinsky O, Cox C, Witt E 1991 Ictal fear in temporal lobe epilepsy: association with interictal behaviour changes. J Epilepsy 4: 236–238

Dodrill C 1986 Correlates of generalised tonic-clonic seizures with intellectual, neuropsychological, emotional and social function in patients with epilepsy. Epilepsia 27: 191–197

Dodrill CB, Batzel LW 1986 Interictal behavioural features of patients with epilepsy. Epilepsia 27(suppl 2), S64–S76

Dodrill CB, Temkin NR 1989 Motor speed is a contaminating factor in evaluating the 'cognitive' effects of phenytoin. Epilepsia 30: 453–457

Dodrill CB, Troupin AS 1991 Neuropsychological effects of carbamazepine and phenytoin: a reanalysis. Neurology 41: 141–143

Duncan JS, Shorvon SD, Trimble MR 1990 Effects of removal of phenytoin, carbamazepine and valproate on cognitive function. Epilepsia 31: 584–591
Edeh J, Toone BK 1985 Antiepileptic therapy, folate deficiency, and psychiatric morbidity: A general practice survey. Epilepsia 26: 434–440
Edeh J, Toone BK 1987 Relationship between interictal psychopathology and the type of epilepsy. Br J Psychiat 151: 95–101
Edwards JG 1985 Antidepressants and seizures: Epidemiological and clinical aspects. In: Trimble MR (ed) The psychopharmacology of epilepsy. John Wiley, Chichester, p 119–139
Engel J JR 1989 Seizures and Epilepsy. FA Davis, Philadelphia, PA
Fenwick P 1981 Precipitation and inhibition of seizures. In: Reynolds EH, Trimble MR (eds) Epilepsy and psychiatry. Churchill Livingstone, Edinburgh, p 306–321
Flor-Henry P 1969 Psychosis and temporal lobe epilepsy: a controlled investigation. Epilepsia 10: 363–395
Gallhofer B, Trimble MR, Frackowiak R, Gibbs J, Jones T 1985 A study of cerebral blood flow and metabolism in epileptic psychosis using PET and oxygen-15. J Neurol Neurosurg Psychiat 48: 201–206
Gastaut H, Roger J, Lefevre N 1953 Différenciation psychologique des épileptiques en function des formes électrocliniques de leur maladie. Rev Psychol 3: 237–249
Gibbs FA, Stamps FW 1953 Epilepsy handbook. Charles C Thomas, Springfield, IL
Gillham RA, Blacklaw J, McKee PJW, Brodie MJ 1993 Effect of vigabatrin on sedation and cognitive function in patients with refractory epilepsy. J Neurol Neurosurg Psychiat 56: 1271–1275
Grunewald RA, Thompson PJ, Corcoran RS, Corden Z, Jackson GD, Duncan JS 1994 Effects of vigabatrin on partial seizures and cognitive function. J Neurol Neurosurg Psychiat 57: 1057–1063
Gudmundsson G 1966 Epilepsy in Iceland. Acta Neurol Scand (suppl 25)
Hermann BP, Wyler AR 1989 Depression, locus of control, and the effects of epilepsy surgery. Epilepsia 30: 332–338
Hermann BP, Schwartz MS, Karnes WE, Valda TP 1980 Psychopathology in epilepsy: relationship of seizure type and age of onset. Epilepsia 21: 15–23
Hermann BP, Seidenberg M, Haltiner A, Wyler AR 1991 Mood state in unilateral temporal lobe epilepsy. Biol Psychiat 30: 1205–1218
Hurwitz TA, Wada JA, Kosaka BD, Strauss EH 1985 Cerebral organization of affect suggested by temporal lobe seizures. Neurology 35: 1335–1337
Jeavons PM 1977 Choice of drug therapy in epilepsy. Practitioner 219: 541–546
Jensen I, Larsen JK 1979 Mental aspects of temporal lobe epilepsy: Follow-up of 74 patients after resection of a temporal lobe. J Neurol Neurosurg Psychiat 42: 256–265
Jick H, Dinan BJ, Hunter JR et al 1983 Tricyclic antidepressants and convulsions. J Clin Psychopharmacol 3: 182–185
Klove H, Matthews CG 1966 Psychometric and adaptive abilities in epilepsy with different aetiology. Epilepsia 7: 330–338
Kogeorgos J, Fonagy P, Scott DF 1982 Psychiatric symptom patterns of chronic epileptics attending a neurological clinic: A controlled investigation. Br J Psychiat 140: 236–243
Kramer LD, Fralin C, Berman NG, Locke GE 1987 Relationship of seizure frequency and interictal depression. Epilepsia 28: 629
Landolt H 1953 Some clinical EEG correlations in epileptic psychoses (twilight states). EEG and Clin Neurophysiol 5: 121
Landolt H 1958 Serial EEG investigations during psychotic episodes in epileptic patients and during schizophrenic attacks. In: AM Lorentz De Haas (ed) Lectures on epilepsy. Elsevier, Amsterdam, p 91–133
Leander JD 1992 Fluoxetine, a selective serotonin-uptake inhibitor, enhances the anticonvulsant effects of phenytoin, carbamazepine and ameltolide (LY201116) Epilepsia 33: 573–576
Lennox WG, Cobb S 1933 Epilepsy. XIII. Aura in epilepsy: a statistical review of 1359 cases. Arch Neurol Psychiat 30: 374–387
Lesser RP 1985 Psychogenic seizures. In: Pedley T, Meldrum BS (eds) Recent advances in epilepsy 2. Churchill Livingstone, Edinburgh, p 273–296
Levin S 1952 Epileptic clouded states. J Nerv Ment Dis 116: 215–225
Lewis AJ 1934 Melancholia: a historical review. J Ment Sci 80: 1–42
Logsdail SJ, Toone BK 1988 Post-ictal psychoses. Br J Psychiat 152: 246–252
Mace C, Trimble MR 1991 Psychosis following temporal lobe surgery: a report of six cases. J Neurology, Neurosurgery and Psychiatry 54: 639–644
McGuire A, Duncan JS, Trimble MR 1992 Effects of vigabatrin on cognitive function and mood when used as add-on therapy in patients with intractable epilepsy. Epilepsia 33: 128–134

Mathews WS, Barabas G 1981 Suicide and epilepsy: A review of the literature. Psychosomatics 22: 515–524

Mendez MF, Cummings JL, Benson F 1986 Depression in epilepsy: significance and phenomenology. Arch Neurology 43: 766–770

Mendez MF, Lanska DJ, Manon-Espaillat R, Burnstine TH 1989 Causative factors for suicide attempts by overdose in epileptics. Arch Neurol 46: 1065–1068

Moller AA, Froscher W 1990 Depressive disorder of the epilepsy patient – symptoms and factors of influence. Schweiz Arch Neurol Psychiatr 141: 139–148

Mumford JP, Beaumont D, Gisselbrecht D 1990 Cognitive function, mood and behaviour in vigabatrin treated patients. Acta Neurol Scand 82(suppl 133): 15

Mungas DM 1992 Behavioural syndromes in epilepsy: A multivariate, empirical approach. In: Bennett TL (ed) The neuropsychology of epilepsy. Plenum Press, New York, p 139–180

Naugle RI, Rodgers DA, Stagno SJ, Lalli J 1991 Unilateral temporal lobe epilepsy: An examination of psychopathology and psychosocial behavior. J Epilepsy 4: 157–164

Nielsen H, Kristensen O 1981 Personality correlates of sphenoidal EEG foci in temporal lobe epilepsy. Acta Neurol Scand 64: 289–300

Ounsted C, Lindsay J 1981 The long term outcome of temporal lobe epilepsy in childhood. In: Reynolds EH, Trimble MR (eds) Epilepsy and psychiatry. Churchill Livingstone, Edinburgh, p 185–215

Perini G, Mendius R 1984 Depression and anxiety in complex partial seizures. J Nerv Ment Dis 172: 287–290

Pond D, Bidwell B, Stein L 1960 A survey of 14 general practices. Part 1: medical and demographic data. Psychiat Neurol Neurochirurg 63: 217–236

Post RM, Uhde TW, Roy-Byrne PP, Joffe RT 1986 Antidepressant effects of carbamazepine. Am J Psychiat 143: 29–34

Reynolds JR 1861 Epilepsy: Its symptoms, treatment and relation to other chronic convulsive diseases. John Churchill, London

Reynolds EH 1991 Interictal psychiatric disorders. Neurochemical aspects. In: Smith D, Treiman D, Trimble M (eds) Neurobehavioral problems in epilepsy. Advances in neurology 55. Raven Press, New York, p 47–58

Reynolds EH, Chanarin I, Milner G, Mathews DM 1966 Anticonvulsant therapy, folic acid and vitamin $B_{12}$ metabolism and mental symptoms. Epilepsia 7: 261–270

Richens A, Nawishy S, Trimble M 1983 Antidepressant drugs, convulsions and epilepsy. Br J Clin Pharmacol 15: 295–298

Ring HA, Reynolds EH 1991 Vigabatrin. In: Pedley T & Meldrum BS (eds) Recent advances in epilepsy 5. Churchill Livingstone, Edinburgh, p 177–195

Robertson MM 1988 Depression in patients with epilepsy reconsidered. In: Pedley TA, Meldrum BS (eds) Recent advances in epilepsy 4. Churchill Livingstone, Edinburgh, p 205–240

Robertson MM 1989 The organic contribution to depressive illness in patients with epilepsy. J Epilepsy 2: 189–230

Robertson MM, Trimble MR 1985 The treatment of depression in patients with epilepsy. a double-blind trial. J Affect Disord 9: 127–136

Robertson MM, Trimble MR, Townsend HRA 1987 Phenomenology of depression in epilepsy. Epilepsia 28: 364–372

Rodin E, Schmaltz S, Twitty G 1984 What does the Bear–Fedio Inventory measure? In: Porter RJ, Mattson RH, Ward AA Jr, Dam M (eds) The XVth Epilepsy International Symposium. Raven Press, New York, p 551–555

Rosen JA 1966 Dilantin dementia. Trans Am Neurol Assoc 93: 273

Seidenberg M, O'Leary DS, Berent S, Boll T 1981 Changes in seizure frequency and test re-test scores on the WAIS. Epilepsia 22: 75–83

Shorvon SD, Reynolds EH 1979 Reduction in polypharmacy for epilepsy. Br Med J 2: 1023–1025

Slater E, Beard AW 1963 The schizophrenia-like psychoses of epilepsy: V. Discussion and conclusions. Br J Psychiat 109: 143–150

Small JG, Small IF 1967 A controlled study of mental disorders associated with epilepsy. Rec Adv Biol Psychiat 9: 171–181

Small JG, Small IF, Hayden MP 1966 Further psychiatric investigations of patients with temporal and non-temporal lobe epilepsy. Am J Psychiat 123: 303–310

Smith DB 1991 Cognitive Effects of Antiepileptic Drugs. In: Smith D, Treiman D, Trimble M (eds) Neurobehavioral problems in epilepsy. Advances in neurology 55. Raven Press, New York, p 197–224

Stark-Adamec C, Adamec RE, Graham JM, Hicks RC, Bruun-Meyer S E 1985 Complexities in the complex partial seizures personality controversy. Psych J Univ Ottawa 10: 231–236

Starkstein SE, Robinson RG 1989 Affective disorders and cerebral vascular disease. Br J Psychiat 154: 170–182

Stevens J R 1966 Psychiatric implications of psychomotor epilepsy. Arch Gen Psychiat 14: 461–471

Taylor DC 1975 Factors influencing the occurrence of schizophrenia-like psychosis in patients with temporal lobe epilepsy. Psychol Med 5: 249–254

Taylor DC, Lochery M 1987 Temporal lobe epilepsy: origin and significance of simple and complex auras. J Neurol Neurosurg Psychiat 50: 673–681

Tellenbach H. 1965 Epilepsie als Anfallsleiden und als Psychose. Nervenarzt 36: 190–202

Temkin O 1971 The falling sickness. Johns Hopkins Press, Baltimore, MD

Thompson PJ, Oxley J 1988 Socio-economic accompaniments of severe epilepsy. Epilepsia 29 (suppl S9): S18

Thompson PJ, Trimble MR 1982 Anticonvulsant drugs and cognitive functions. Epilepsia 23: 531–544

Thompson PJ, Huppert F, Trimble MR 1981 Phenytoin and cognitive functions; effects on normal volunteers and implications for epilepsy. Br J Clin Psychol 20: 151–62

Trimble MR 1978 Prolactin in epilepsy and hysteria. Br Med J 2: 1682

Trimble MR 1989 Cognitive hazards of seizure disorders. In: Trimble M R (ed) Chronic epilepsy: its prognosis and management. John Wiley, Chichester, p 103–111

Trimble MR 1991 The psychoses of epilepsy. Raven Press, New York

Trimble MR, Corbett JA 1980 Behavioural and cognitive disturbances in epileptic children. Irish Med J 73(suppl): 21–28

Trimble MR, Dodson WE 1994 Epilepsy and quality of life. Raven Press, New York

Trimble MR, Perez MM 1982 The phenomenology of the chronic psychoses of epilepsy. In: Koella WP, Trimble MR (eds) Temporal lobe epilepsy, mania and schizophrenia and the limbic system. S Karger, Basel, p 98–105

Trimble MR, Schmitz B 1992 Epileptic equivalents in psychiatry: Some 19th century views. Acta Neurol Scand(suppl): 122–126

Trimble MR, Thompson PJ. 1986 Neuropsychological aspects of epilepsy. In: Grant I, Adams KM (eds) Neuropsychological assessment of neuropsychiatric disorders. Oxford University Press, Oxford, p 321–46

Trimble MR, Corbett JA, Donaldson D 1980 Folic acid and mental symptoms in children with epilepsy. J Neurol Neurosurg Psychiat 43: 1030–1034

Turner RJ, Beiser M 1990 Major depression and depressive symptomatology among the physically disabled. J Nerv Ment Dis 178: 343–350

Vickrey BG, Hays RD, Graber J, Rausch R, Engel J, Brook RH 1992 A health-related quality of life instrument for patients evaluated for epilepsy surgery. Med Care 30: 299–319

Waxman SG, Geschwind N 1975 The interictal behaviour syndromes of temporal lobe epilepsy. Arch Gen Psychiat 32: 1580–1586

Whitman S, Hermann BP, Gordon A 1984 Psychopathology in epilepsy: how great the risk. Biol Psychiat 19: 213–236

Williams D 1956 The structure of emotions reflected in epileptic experiences. Brain 79: 29–67

Wolf P, Trimble MR 1985 Biological antagonism and epileptic psychosis. Br J Psychiat 146: 272–276

World Heath Organization 1980 International classification of impairments, disabilities and handicaps. World Heath Organization, Geneva

# 10 Epilepsy surgery

## 10.1 INTRODUCTION

### 10.1.1 History

The first epilepsy surgery of the modern era was performed in the 1880s by Victor Horsley at the hospital which is now called the National Hospital for Neurology and Neurosurgery, Queen Square, London. In the pioneering years of Victor Horsley and his successors, localization was mainly dependent on the focal ictal motor phenomena and/or the presence of a fixed neurological deficit. Consequently, many of the early patients had neocortical abnormalities, for instance in the region of the primary motor cortex.

The second era of epilepsy surgery commenced in the 1930s, largely with the work of Penfield at the Montreal Neurological Institute. From the late 1930s onwards the introduction of EEG offered a new method of localization. Recording techniques evolved in complexity and sophistication over the years. The introduction of video-EEG telemetry permitted the simultaneous recording of both the clinical behaviour and EEG changes and became of paramount importance from the late 1970s.

In the 1990s a new era of epilepsy surgery was ushered in, with the development of MRI (Ch. 3, 3.3, 3.4). The advent of high-resolution MRI, providing sufficient resolution to detect the underlying pathological changes responsible for most seizure disorders, has completely changed the nature of epilepsy surgery evaluation (see below).

### 10.1.2 The extent of the need for epilepsy surgery

In line with the expansion of investigative techniques there has been a considerable increase in the proportion of patients for whom surgery is a realistic option: 5–10% of patients with chronic medically refractory epilepsy may be potential surgical candidates. Realization that the prognosis of such a chronically disabling condition can be radically improved by surgical intervention has led to a marked increase of this form of treatment in Europe, North America and other developed countries.

Although there has been an expansion of epilepsy surgery in recent years, there is still an unmet need. In the UK, for example with a population of 56 million there is an estimated backlog of 10 000 cases and an annual *recurring* need for 600–2000 cases. A consultant neurologist in the UK has an average referral population of 300 000 and so would expect to have in that population 50 patients who were candidates for surgical treatment and an annual recurring need for 3–12 cases. A neurologist in the USA or some western European countries, with an average referral population of 30 000, may expect to have five potentially suitable patients, and a further patient becoming suitable every year.

### 10.1.3 Types of epilepsy surgery

Surgical approaches for the treatment of epilepsy can be divided into three broad strategies:

- Focal resections
- Lobar and multilobar resections
- Functional procedures to interrupt pathways of seizure spread

The overwhelming majority of cases, more than 90%, of epilepsy surgery involve localized resections. Currently, 70% of operations are directed towards the temporal lobe, while 23% are extratemporal cortical resections and lesionectomies. Hemispherectomies comprise approximately 3% and corpus callosal section and multiple subpial transection make up 4% of procedures.

## 10.2 PRESURGICAL EVALUATION

The aims of presurgical evaluation are:

1. To establish that the patient has medically intractable epilepsy, and would have an improved quality of life if the seizures were stopped or alleviated
2. To define the nature of the underlying pathology of the seizure disorder and the extent of the epileptogenic zone
3. To determine the likelihood of the patient becoming seizure-free or deriving significant benefit from surgery
4. To determine the risks to the patient of epilepsy surgery in terms of neurological, psychological, psychiatric or social effects

### 10.2.1 In which patients should surgery be considered?

Surgical treatment should be considered in all patients with partial seizures that have continued despite medical therapy with AEDs that do not cause significant adverse effects (Table 10.1). This includes simple, partial and secondarily generalized seizures. In judging intractability it is important to take into account the nature and severity of the seizure disorder. Patients who come to epilepsy surgery have usually been having repeated seizures over a period of at least 3–5 years, with a minimum of one to two complex partial seizures per month, or less frequent but more severe secondary generalized seizures. Patients with only simple partial seizures or whose life is relatively unimpaired by their attacks are unlikely to be suitable candidates for surgery, given the risk: benefit ratio, unless these seizures are very distressing for the patient or very frequent. There is no doubt, however, that as investigatory and surgical techniques have become more sophisticated and confident, the threshold for undertaking presurgical evaluation has come down.

A stereotyped onset of seizures is a favourable feature, regardless of the degree of secondary spread, although the occurrence of frequent

**Table 10. 1** Patients in whom to consider epilepsy surgery

- Partial seizures: simple and/or complex and/or secondary generalized
- Stereotyped onset
- Not having non-epileptic seizures
- No contraindication to neurosurgery
- Active epilepsy for > 2–3 years despite intensive medical treatment; trials of carbamazepine, phenytoin, valproate, vigabatrin to maximum tolerated doses
- Failure of adequate seizure control taking AEDs that do not cause side-effects
- Rule of thumb: at least two complex partial seizures per month
- Patient acceptance of best risk/benefit ratio
- Bitemporal EEG changes not a contraindication

secondarily generalized seizures is an adverse prognostic factor. Conversely if a patient has a variety of different modes of onset of seizures, more than one seizure focus may be implied and the prospects for a good result from surgery are reduced.

The continuing occurrence of non-epileptic attacks (Ch. 9, 9.1) is generally a contraindication to surgical treatment for concomitant epileptic seizures as, in this setting, the non-epileptic attacks may worsen dramatically after the removal of the epilepsy. This is a difficult area, however, and surgery could be entertained in a patient with a past history of non-epileptic attacks in whom the episodes had resolved following psychological therapy.

Patients need to be able to withstand prolonged anaesthesia and neurosurgery. There is no absolute age criterion, but in general surgery for epilepsy would not be common in patients aged over 40 years, as the gain in quality of life after this age is generally low.

It is important that patients understand from the outset that presurgical evaluation is demanding, time-consuming and arduous and may result in a decision not to operate. Further it must be made clear to them and their relatives that, even if all the clinical and investigatory data are optimal, there cannot be more than a 70–80% chance of being rendered completely seizure-free, and a minimum risk of significant postoperative neurological deficit of 1% and that these odds can only be made less attractive when the results of the presurgical evaluation are known.

In addition to explaining the risks of epilepsy surgery to the individual patient and their family it is important also to consider the risks of not operating. Chronic medically intractable epilepsy carries a poor prognosis with a mortality rate of approximately 1/200/year as a direct consequence of the seizures (Ch. 8, 8.4), in addition to the mortality that may relate to the underlying structural pathology, and the neurological and social morbidity of refractory epilepsy (Chs 7, 7.2 and 8, 8.3).

Adequate therapeutic trials of each of the major antiepileptic drugs (AEDs) should normally have been undertaken sequentially using monotherapy and at least one trial of combined drug therapy. However, there are an ever-increasing number of available AEDs. It may not be necessary for a patient to have taken all of the newer agents before they are deemed to be medically intractable. There is a law of diminishing returns such that when numerous drugs have been tried alone and in combination it becomes increasingly unlikely that an additional agent will cause a cessation of seizures, particularly if the epilepsy is due to an underlying structural abnormality. Furthermore, it must be recognized that drugs are not without their own hazards, especially if idiosyncratic reactions are severe. In patients who may be considered for epilepsy surgery it is important to evaluate the impact of each new agent reasonably quickly (over a period of a few months), because of the hazards posed by the seizure disorder itself.

If surgical intervention is likely to be appropriate there are cogent reasons for considering this option at the earliest reasonable opportunity in order to reduce:

- The impact of the seizure disorder on education and social development
- The risks of secondary injury or death from the seizures
- The possibility of secondary epileptogenesis (either through kindling or cerebral injuries)
- The possibility of progressive cognitive decline secondary to ictal activity, cerebral injury and chronic drug intake

Some patients who are candidates for surgical treatment may have their seizures partially controlled by AEDs, but at the cost of adverse effects of the medication. For these patients, surgery may be appropriate in order to reduce or eliminate their drug load.

With the greatly enhanced ability to demonstrate the underlying pathological substrate by MRI, the nature of the lesion itself influences the decision to operate, irrespective of intractability or otherwise of the seizures to AEDs. For example, the finding of a glioma or a vascular abnormality may increase the argument for surgical intervention. In addition consideration might also be given to early epilepsy surgery in patients with very severe life-threatening seizures in whom there is a particular risk of sudden death or injury in a seizure, or in female patients on polytherapy who are considering having a family.

The presence of a chronic psychosis is usually considered to be a contraindication to surgery, although well defined episodes of postictal psychosis are not. Other psychiatric disorders may be exacerbated by neurosurgery and operations should not be carried out on patients who are unlikely to benefit from them for reasons of their personality. Patients with an IQ less than 70 are often considered unsuitable for temporal lobe surgery, largely because the low IQ may reflect more widespread cerebral disturbance. This is not an invariable rule, however, and many patients with low IQs have a good result from epilepsy surgery.

If surgery is shown to be feasible in childhood or adolescence, a strong case can be made for operating at this stage in order to allow development into adult life to be unaffected by the epilepsy (Fish et al 1993). In some cases, such as the infant with frequent seizures and a structural abnormality shown with neuroimaging, radical surgery such as hemispherectomy is appropriate early on in the course of the epilepsy (see below, 10.3.5).

## 10.2.2 The nature of the epileptogenic zone

The epileptogenic zone is a hypothetical construct that is a useful descriptive term when evaluating patients for epilepsy surgery (Engel 1993) (Fig. 10.1). This zone is regarded as the area of brain that is responsible for generating the seizures, the removal of which is associated with cessation of attacks, and can be broken down into three components:

- The pathological lesion responsible for the seizure disorder
- The anatomical distribution of various electroclinical features (interictal spiking, seizure onset and those areas which become active in order to generate the typical ictal semiology)
- The area of functional deficit defined by psychometry or functional imaging associated with a seizure disorder (Fig. 10.1)

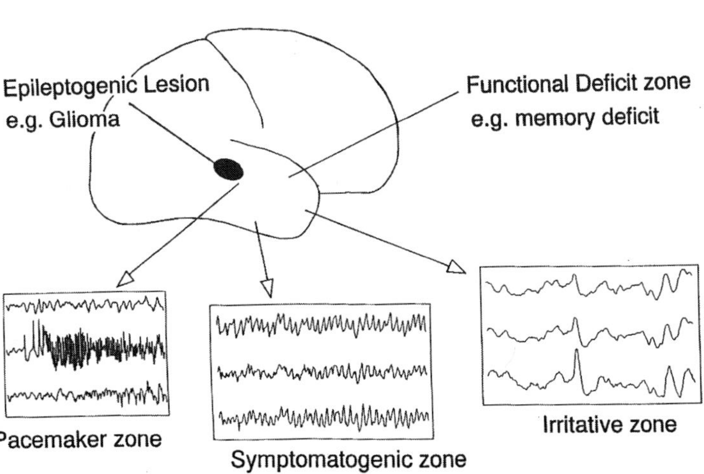


**Fig. 10.1** The key modalities of information that may be important in defining the epileptogenic zone

Of these components the nature of the pathological substrate and the extent of its removal are the key prognostic factors. It remains uncertain to what degree the other regions need to be excised in order to optimize outcome. A strategy that is not yet fully evaluated is to perform minimal resections of the pathological substrate ('lesionectomy'), accepting that, if this proves inadequate to control the seizures, a more extensive functional procedure can be performed as a second procedure.

## 10.2.3 Presurgical investigation strategy

Complementary data is acquired from many different sources when assessing whether a patient is suitable for surgical treatment and the optimal approach (Table 10.2). The principal components are in the fields

**Table 10. 2** Components of presurgical evaluation

- Looking for convergence of data, implying one epileptogenic and dysfunctional area, and rest of brain intact
- Discordant data, multifocal abnormalities, give less good prognosis

*Clinical*

- History of early childhood seizures, epilepsy, current seizure pattern, emotional state, social support
- Neurological and physical examination

*EEG*

- Interictal (awake and asleep) epileptiform activity, background rhythm
- Ictal onset

*Imaging*

- Structural neuroimaging
  High-resolution MRI: quantitative hippocampal volumes and T2 relaxation times, reformatting of cortex, 3D reconstruction
  Non-standard sequences
- Functional imaging
  FDG-PET, SPECT, if structural imaging unclear

*Neuropsychology*

- Focal deficits, especially language, verbal and non-verbal memory

*Neuropsychiatry*

- Personality, depression, psychosis, social support

of clinical history, neurological and general physical examination, EEG, imaging, neuropsychology and psychiatry. The general principle is to try to establish whether these different modalities provide data that is concordant and indicates that a single area of brain is the source of the epilepsy, that its removal would not impair the patient and that the rest of the patient's brain is normal. The finding of discordant data or widespread pathology or dysfunction reduces the chance of a good result from surgery.

It is important that presurgical evaluation is carried out in a programmed way, so that data acquisition and analysis is complete and efficient. Different units have evolved different strategies according to local needs; the National Hospital approach is summarized in Table 10.3.

*Neurology*

It is a fundamental requirement to establish both the history of the seizure disorder and any potential aetiological factors. Aetiologies which are likely to cause diffuse cerebral injury (e.g. blunt trauma, encephalitis) are usually associated with a less favourable surgical outcome. It is of crucial importance to verify that the clinical nature of the seizure disorder is compatible with the site of the underlying structural lesion in order to avoid the pitfall of operating on a coincidental or secondary lesion.

*Non-invasive EEG*

At the present time this evaluation includes prolonged interictal EEG recordings, and video-EEG telemetry on the vast majority of presurgical candidates, in order to document their habitual seizure symptomatology. It is likely in the future, however, that guidelines will evolve that allow

**Table 10. 3** National Hospital approach to presurgical evaluation

*1. Out-patient neurological assessment*
- Clinical review, discussion of investigations, risks and benefits, emotional state, social support
- MRI, neuropsychology, EEG

*2. Initial admission*
- 5 days video-EEG telemetry, neuropsychology, psychiatry
- Review of results, organize further tests (e.g. further MRI, FDG PET) if needed

*3. Carotid amytal (30% of TLE cases)*
- 2-day admission
- Lateralization of language and basic memory
- Review of all data

*4. Depth EEG (5–10% of patients)*
- 2-week admission

*5. Surgery*
- 7-day admission

certain groups, such as those patients with a concordant structural abnormality shown on MRI, clinical semiology and interictal EEG, to proceed to epilepsy surgery without the requirement to record seizures on telemetry. It is likely that the relative importance of EEG will depend upon the nature of the MRI findings (Fish & Spencer 1995) (Fig. 10.2).

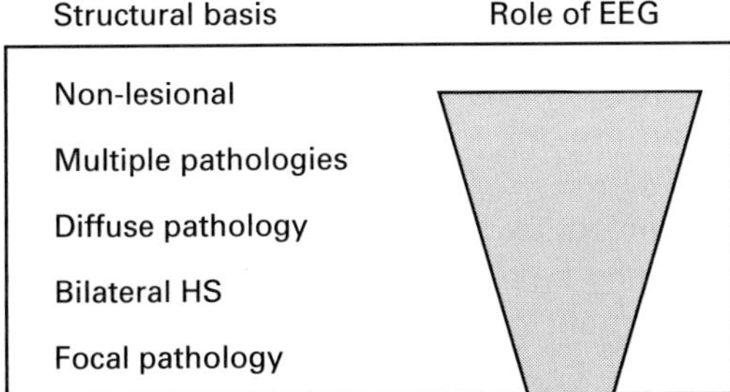


**Fig. 10.2** The role of EEG in relation to the neuro-imaging findings in presurgical evaluation

Many patients being considered for surgical treatment have seizures occurring less than once a week when they are taking AEDs. Video-EEG is a very expensive and labour-intensive investigation, and patients often find being recorded for 24 h per day for more than a week disturbing. For these reasons it is common practice to reduce the AEDs when a recording session starts, to hasten the occurrence of seizures. It is generally regarded that it is ideal to record three or more seizures. On average 5 days of video-telemetry is required to record three seizures when patients are undergoing presurgical evaluation (Todorov et al 1994).

The rate of drug reduction in these circumstances is controversial.

There is a risk of causing a flurry of seizures that may be harmful for the patient, and of precipitating seizures that are not of the patient's habitual type and onset. In our practice AEDs, with the exception of phenobarbitone or primidone, are halved on the first day of the recording and halved again on the second day, and then maybe withdrawn if no seizures have occurred. If three partial seizures or one secondarily generalized seizure occur, the tapered drug is reinstated, with a loading dose and a benzodiazepine, if necessary.

*Neuroimaging*

Structural neuroimaging with MRI is fundamental to presurgical evaluation, to identify an abnormality that is likely to be giving rise to the seizures, to predict its pathological nature and to determine if the rest of the brain is normal (Ch 3, 3.3). If there is a good clinical indication of an underlying focal pathology, it is appropriate to pursue MRI with imaging of the highest quality, post-acquisition processing of the data and the use of non-standard sequences. The place of functional imaging with PET and SPECT (Ch 3, 3.4) has to be re-evaluated in the light of advances in MRI. At present, functional imaging has an important role if structural imaging with MRI is unremarkable, and acts as a guide to further investigation.

*Neuropsychology*

Neuropsychometric tests are routinely performed on patients undergoing an evaluation for epilepsy surgery, in order to document that the area of functional deficit is broadly compatible with the underlying structural pathology. In addition, psychometric testing is important to verify the likely neuropsychological consequences of surgery. In particular, if there is evidence of bilateral memory impairment then this may not only be a poor prognostic factor from the point of view of seizure control but also raises the possibility of a serious memory impairment following temporal lobe surgery (Ch 3, 3.5.5).

Sodium amytal tests are indicated if it is necessary to determine the side of cerebral dominance (e.g. for operations being performed in the left inferior frontal gyrus or posteriorly in the left temporal lobe). In addition, they may be necessary in patients with evidence of bilateral memory impairment in order to confirm that the remaining hippocampus and temporal lobe are able to sustain adequate memory (Ch 3, 3.5.5).

*Neuropsychiatry*

A detailed neuropsychiatric assessment is essential, and most appropriate at an early stage of the presurgical evaluation. The patient's mood and mental state, expectations and fears and support need to be evaluated. The patient and their family also need to be counselled about the possible psychological and psychiatric sequelae of surgery so that any post-operative problems are identified early on and managed appropriately. However, the psychiatric features which are predictive of a good or bad outcome are not yet fully understood.

*Intracranial EEG*

In some centres a heavy reliance has been placed on intracranial EEG recordings to determine the site of seizure onset, particularly prior to the advent of current MRI techniques. In our practice, intracranial EEG recordings are carried out in less than 10% of operated cases.

Whilst such recordings allow information to be obtained from otherwise functionally inaccessible cortex, depth electrodes can only obtain EEG data from small areas of brain. This limitation is often forgotten, but is crucial. In consequence, electrode placements need to be carefully planned and invasive studies should only be used to test specific hypotheses, such as:

1. In patients with temporal lobe epilepsy and evidence of bilateral hippocampal sclerosis on MRI, are seizures arising from the left or the right hippocampus?
2. Patients in whom imaging shows dual pathology and the scalp EEG is indeterminate
3. Patients with relatively large neocortical lesions adjacent to or involving eloquent cortex in whom a partial resection of the lesion with sparing of functionally crucial cortex is planned
4. Patients with discordance of other structural and functional data

In view of the morbidity of intracranial EEG recordings it would generally be our policy to perform a sodium amytal test beforehand in patients who may require a temporal lobe resection, to determine language dominance and whether the implicated temporal lobe would be able to sustain adequate memory.

If non-invasive studies do not localize an extratemporal focus accurately, it may be necessary to carry out invasive recordings using subdural strips or grids of electrodes that are placed subdurally, over the surface of the brain, and/or implantation of intracerebral electrodes. While subdural strips and grids can cover a larger area than depth electrodes, the recordings obtained may not allow such precise localization. The implantation of subdural grids also allows stimulation of the cortical surface, facilitating preoperative functional mapping of the cortex, but involves a craniotomy and carries significant risks of morbidity, principally in the form of intracranial infection and damage to the cortex.

Intracerebral electrodes with multiple contacts only sample from a very limited (< 1 cm) core of brain tissue (Figs 10.3, 10.4). The risk of the procedure increases with the number of electrodes inserted and may be several per cent for complex implantations with many electrodes. Morbidity arises mainly from haemorrhage or infection. In consequence, there is no place for insertion of multiple electrodes without there being any prior idea about the most likely sites of seizure onset. Electrode placement is usually performed stereotactically. A combination of depth electrodes and subdural strip electrodes may be used, to combine recording from the surface cortex and also from inaccessible areas such as the medial temporal lobes.

As the main risk of intracranial EEG recordings comes from the insertion, intracranial recordings should be continued until a satisfactory number of habitual seizures have been recorded. During this time the patient is carefully monitored for developing complications, particularly an intracranial infection.

Foramen ovale electrodes have had proponents (Wieser et al 1985) as a means of recording from the medial temporal lobe to determine whether

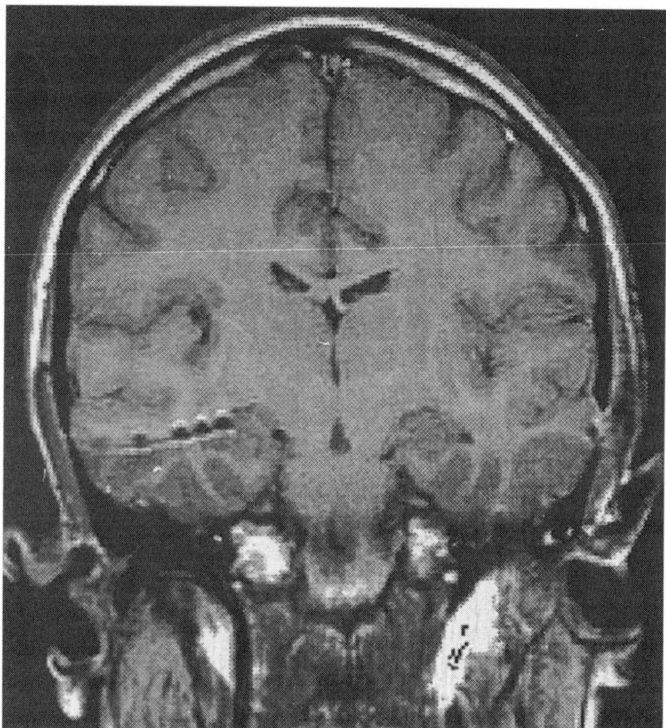

**Fig. 10.3** Coronal MRI scan showing multicontact intracerebral EEG electrode in right temporal lobe and anterior hippocampus

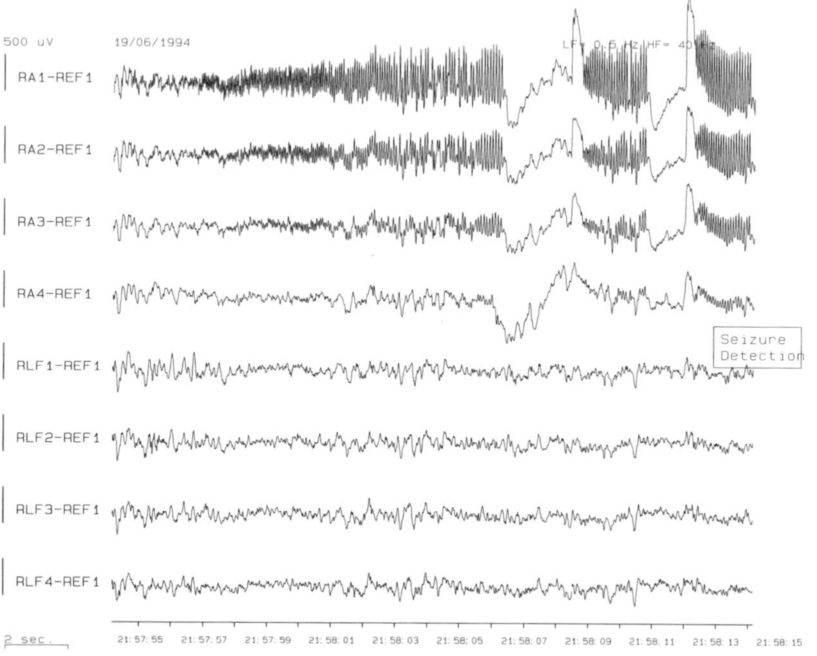


**Fig. 10.4** Intracerebral EEG recording showing onset of ictal activity (rhythmic fast) in the right medial temporal contacts (RA1, RA2, RA3) in a patient in whom the question had been: right medial temporal or right frontal onset of seizures?

temporal lobe seizures are commencing on the left or the right side, but they cannot distinguish temporal from extratemporal onset with certainty. This investigation was developed in the era prior to adequate MRI detection of hippocampal sclerosis and their use has now declined. The technique is relatively straightforward and does not require a craniotomy or stereotactic equipment. The electrodes are inserted percutaneously through the face via the foramen ovale and then passed around the brainstem, lying medial to the hippocampi. There is a significant complication rate, including facial pain, meningitis and vascular damage to the brainstem. Further, the recordings are subdural and can give results that are subsequently contradicted by depth EEG recordings.

## 10.3 SURGICAL APPROACHES

### 10.3.1 Focal resections

Focal cerebral resections can be considered in patients with:

- Foreign tissue lesions
- Hippocampal sclerosis
- Non-lesional cases
- Dual pathology

*Foreign tissue lesions*

The nature of the underlying pathology is a key determinant of outcome for epilepsy surgery. Small indolent lesions such as low-grade gliomas, dysembryoplastic neuroepithelial tumours (DNT) and small cryptic vascular malformations carry the best prognosis for epilepsy surgery, with about 70–80% of cases being rendered seizure-free following adequate resection (Cascino et al 1993). Large or complex vascular malformations, particularly if they have bled and resulted in a deposition of haemosiderin, or traumatic injuries, have a less good prognosis for epilepsy surgery, with considerably less than 50% of cases being rendered seizure-free. Unfortunately, cortical dysplasia (other than tumoural forms such as DNT), one of the commonest aetiologies of medically intractable epilepsy, carries a poor prognosis for surgery (Raymond et al 1995). Presumably this is because such abnormalities represent a more diffuse process than is usually apparent. Only a small percentage of patients with gross cortical dysplasia become seizure-free following epilepsy surgery (Fig. 10.5).

For the most part, temporal lobe epilepsy surgery carries the most favourable prognosis. However, with certain small indolent lesions in the temporal lobe (especially DNT) an excellent outcome often necessitates additional removal of the mesial temporal structures (Raymond et al 1995) (Table 10.4). Extratemporal resection carries a less good prognosis, particularly if there is no identifiable pathology removed or if the abnormality is diffuse and not all resected (Table 10.4). Further research work needs to be carried out in order to determine which parameters can identify those patients who require this approach.

In evaluating potential candidates for epilepsy surgery, therefore, it is crucial to determine as much as possible about the nature and extent of any underlying foreign-tissue lesions. Virtually no patient with medically intractable partial epilepsy should be totally excluded from initial

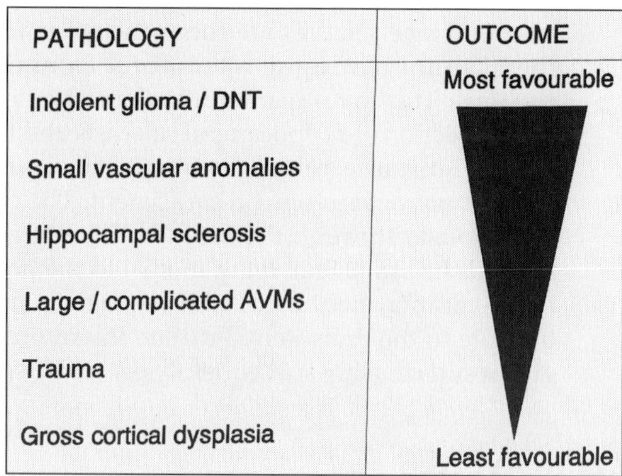


**Fig. 10.5** The importance of pathology in determining postoperative seizure control

**Table 10. 4** Approximate surgical outcomes, according to pathology

*Outcome after temporal resection*

- Best with anterior temporal lobectomy, if focal pathology removed
  70% seizure free, 25% > 90% seizure reduction
- DNT* > cavernoma* > hippocampal sclerosis > trauma > cortical dysplasia
- < 20% seizure free if no pathology removed

*Outcome after extratemporal resection*

- 60% seizure free, 20% > 90% seizure reduction, if focal pathology removed: DNT, indolent glioma, cavernoma
- < 20% seizure free if no pathology removed, cortical dysplasia

* If medial structures of temporal lobe also removed

consideration as a potential surgical candidate until the underlying aetiology and structural basis of the seizure disorder has been established, irrespective of the routine EEG findings. Occasionally patients with apparently widespread/multifocal scalp EEG recordings are found to harbour discrete surgically remedial lesions, the removal of which renders the patient seizure-free.

*Hippocampal sclerosis*

This is the commonest pathological substrate in patients undergoing epilepsy surgery. The optimum outcome appears to occur in those patients with severe diffuse hippocampal sclerosis associated with a history of a prolonged febrile convulsion in early childhood (Duncan & Sagar 1987, Williamson et al 1993). The chances of a good outcome are further enhanced if the patient has suffered only rare secondary generalized convulsions (Williamson et al 1993). Earlier studies suggest that overall approximately two-thirds of patients with hippocampal sclerosis treated surgically will become seizure-free on long-term follow-up. In a recent MRI-based series, 62% of patients with hippocampal sclerosis became seizure-free (Berkovic et al 1995). These figures are likely to improve when the impact of modern neuroimaging becomes fully apparent, and become more sophisticated as various subcategories are recognized (e.g. unilateral/bilateral atrophy, focal anterior, posterior or diffuse atrophy, isolated hippocampal damage or dual pathology). Although in the past most operations were guided by the EEG findings it is evident that in the presence of hippocampal sclerosis (and other factors leading to selection for surgery) these results are of little prognostic significance (Williamson et al 1993). Potential candidates with MRI-defined hippocampal atrophy/-sclerosis (Ch. 3, 3.3.4) should not be excluded from surgical evaluation because of bilateral independent interictal spikes on EEG recordings.

*Non-lesional cases*

In the era of electroclinical assessment without adequate neuroimaging a substantial proportion of patients were found in whom the resected surgical specimen showed no significant pathological change. This is becoming increasingly rare. Earlier studies had established that there was a poor outcome to epilepsy surgery if the pathological specimen was normal (Engel et al 1975, Duncan & Sagar 1987) and these cases are likely to be selected out of surgical programmes, especially if the clinical pattern suggests an extratemporal epilepsy.

*Dual pathology*

With increasing sophistication of MRI techniques it is becoming apparent that a significant proportion of patients harbour more than one cerebral abnormality. Raymond et al (1994) reported that 15 of 100 patients with hippocampal sclerosis had areas of cortical dysgenesis (usually outside the area of a standard temporal lobe resection) demonstrated on MRI. Occasionally other abnormalities have been associated with hippocampal sclerosis (Fish et al 1991, Cendes et al 1995). In patients with dual pathology it is of fundamental importance to establish the characteristics of the epileptogenic zone and in particular determine which (or both) of the lesions is responsible for the seizure disorder. This is likely to become an increasingly important area for clinical neurophysiology (Fish & Spencer 1995). In the past, the majority of invasive EEG studies were directed towards the problem of right versus left temporal lobe epilepsy. In the future, they may instead be more directed towards resolving the problems of patients with dual or extensive pathology.

## 10.3.2 Temporal lobectomy and amygdalo-hippocampectomy

*Temporal lobectomy*

The anatomical temporal lobe resection extends for 4–5 cm behind the temporal pole, sparing the posterior part of the superior temporal gyrus, and can be more extensive in the non-dominant hemisphere. This operation has the advantage of removing pathology that may be widespread within the temporal lobe, such as an infiltrating glioma. The main disadvantage is the risk of a superior quadrantanopia, which in up to 3% of patients extends to an hemianopia, as a result of damage to the optic radiation. A crucial point in this operation is to preserve the pia—

arachnoid that overlies the midbrain and associated blood vessels, such as the anterior choroidal artery. Damage to this artery results in an infarct in the internal capsule and a contralateral hemiparesis. A mild and transient mild dysphasia may develop with dominant temporal lobe resections; the risk of this being permanent and severe is of the order of 1% in a specialized unit.

*Amygdalo-hippocampectomy* A selective operation should be considered for patients with pathology such as hippocampal sclerosis or a DNT confined to the region of the amygdala or hippocampus, but is not suitable if there is widespread pathology in the temporal lobe. Recovery from surgery is generally quicker than after a full temporal lobectomy and the risk of dysphasia and a visual field defect is less. It is not yet established, however, whether there is less memory impairment. The results in terms of relief of seizures do not appear to be quite so good as after an anatomical temporal lobe resection.

This operation is done in two principal ways. The transcortical approach, via an incision in the middle temporal gyrus (Niemeyer 1958) and a pterional approach (Yasargil et al 1985). An advantage of the latter approach is that neocortex is spared and there should be no visual field defect. The disadvantages are that exposure is limited, it is not easy to obtain a good pathological specimen and there is a risk of damaging the optic tract and the anterior choroidal, middle and posterior cerebral arteries. The benefits of the transcortical approach is better exposure and fact that the amygdala, hippocampus and parahippocampal gyrus can be removed intact. Further, there is the option to extend the operation to carry out a more extensive resection or lobectomy if need be.

An intermediate approach is to carry out a resection of the temporal pole and then a removal of the medial temporal lobe structures, sparing the greater part of the neocortex. At present the anatomical temporal lobe resection is commonly used for the non-dominant temporal lobe, and for the dominant temporal lobe when the pathology is not confined to the amygdala and hippocampus. The selective amygdalo-hippocampectomy is often used for the dominant temporal lobe if the pathology is confined to the amygdala, hippocampus or parahippocampal gyrus.

### 10.3.3 Extratemporal resections

*Surgical technique*

Extratemporal foci are often close to eloquent areas of brain. In such cases mapping of cortical function is necessary. This can be carried out prior to surgery using functional MRI techniques (Turner 1994, Pritchard & Rosen 1994) and with electrophysiological recordings carried out during the course of chronic subdural grid monitoring. A further option is for the operation to be carried out under local anaesthetic, with corticography and cortical stimulation during surgery to identify the relationship of the planned resection to functionally important gyri. In the future, functional MRI is likely to be used increasingly to identify the location of specific cerebral functions non-invasively in relation to areas of planned resection and this data to be available in the operating theatre, with feedback of the site of the operative field being provided from a stereotactic surgical 'wand' that relays its position in space to a linked computer that contains the 3D dataset of the patient's MRI. As noted by Horsley in 1908, a subpial dissection should be carried out whenever possible in order to preserve the vascular supply to adjacent gyri.

*Lesional resection*

If a well defined lesion is identified there are a range of options:

- To resect the lesion only
- To resect the lesion with surrounding brain tissue
- To remove the lesion and any apparent remote epileptogenic focus

It is generally appropriate initially at least, to excise the lesion, with surrounding tissues whenever possible. Stereotactic techniques or peroperative ultrasound may be necessary to localize the lesion accurately during surgery.

## 10.3.4 Risks of focal epilepsy surgery

It is important to evaluate not only the chances of the patient becoming seizure-free but also any individual hazards with regard to epilepsy surgery. These may be divided into the following categories:

- Neurological deficit
- Neuropsychological deficit
- Psychosocial problems
- Psychiatric problems

The risks of particular neurological deficits are dependent upon the site of surgery. In patients with lesions close to eloquent areas such as the primary sensorimotor cortex, there may be a substantial risk of major neurological deficit. These can be reduced by preoperative functional mapping (using functional MRI or stimulation studies if seizure monitoring is performed with implanted electrodes) as well as peroperative mapping under local anaesthesia.

In patients undergoing routine temporal lobe epilepsy surgery the risks of a major neurological deficit (stroke with hemiplegia, hemianopia) is of the order of 1%. With anatomical or extensive temporal lobe excisions a homonymous upper quadrantanopia is common. This visual field deficit is usually asymptomatic but may prevent the patient from gaining a driving licence if the deficit extends to within 15° of the meridian. Alternative surgical strategies to resect the mesial temporal structures (amygdalo-hippocampectomy, anterior temporal corticectomy with more extensive mesial resection) have been developed to minimize these risks and with the intention of having less adverse effects on memory. The precise operation performed is likely to vary between centres, depending upon local surgical expertise. Operations on the dominant temporal lobe carry the added risk of language impairment if the resection is carried too far posteriorly.

A large non-dominant frontal lobectomy can be carried out with no deficit, with an approximately 3% risk of hemiparesis. The inferior part of the central area, over the face area, both motor and sensory, can be resected without permanent deficit. A resection that involves the hand or leg areas of cortex will produce a mono- or hemiparesis. Resection of the non-dominant parietal lobe can be carried out, with some sensory loss, but dominant parietal lobe resections usually result in profound loss and dyspraxias. Occipital lobe resections are very likely to cause congruent visual field defects. These risks need to be borne in mind when advising the patient and planning surgery.

It is important that patients are aware that the prime aim of epilepsy surgery is to control seizures and not to improve memory function or reverse other deficits. Many patients with temporal lobe epilepsy complain bitterly of difficulties with memory. This is unlikely to improve following epilepsy surgery and, especially with dominant temporal lobe surgery, may be made worse. In this regard there are double winners and double losers. If surgery controls the seizure disorder then the effects on memory may be much less significant than if the seizures continue.

The psychosocial outcome is very dependent upon the premorbid situation, those with better social support already in place having a more favourable result. It is important for patients and their families to be extensively counselled about changes that may occur following surgery, as they often have unrealistic expectations that their social situation, relationships and employment prospects will immediately improve. If someone has been socially isolated and unemployed for many years because of the seizure disorder, or has failed to receive an adequate education as a consequence of the seizures, change may not be effected for many years even if the seizures stop. This is a major reason for considering early epilepsy surgery, before secondary social or learning deficits become manifest. As a result, there is now a growing tendency towards offering operations in childhood or early adolescence. It is crucial, however, that paediatric cases are evaluated and operated on in specialized children's units with the necessary support facilities.

There is a significant psychiatric morbidity associated with epilepsy surgery. Many patients undergo mood swings following neurosurgery for several months. This risk seems to be greater after epilepsy surgery than other types of neurosurgery. In addition there is a small but definite risk of postoperative psychosis (see below, 10.4.1).

### 10.3.5 Hemispherectomy

Hemispherectomy should be considered in a child or adolescent with medically intractable epilepsy due to severe unilateral hemisphere damage. This can occur, for example, following pre- or perinatal injuries, cerebrovascular accidents, prolonged early childhood convulsions, large congenital malformations of one hemisphere (e.g. hemimegalencephaly, Sturge–Weber syndrome) or Rasmussen's encephalitis.

It is important to establish that the seizures arise in the affected hemisphere. However, it should be remembered that a severely damaged hemisphere may be incapable of generating electrical signals that are detectable on a scalp EEG, and that the finding of interictal and ictal epileptiform abnormalities over the other hemisphere is not necessarily an adverse prognostic factor (Smith et al 1991).

Patients will only be suitable for hemispherectomy if they have a severe fixed neurological deficit, with no useful fine finger movement on the hemiplegic side. Following surgery the gait may become more spastic, although ability to walk should not be affected, and the patients will lose any fine finger movement. Clearly if this operation is performed on the language-dominant hemisphere and language has not transferred to the other side of the brain, then there will be the risk of permanent aphasia. In children under 8 years of age it may be worthwhile considering an operation on the speech-dominant hemisphere, as language functions can subsequently develop in the previously non-dominant hemisphere. In older age groups, however, this becomes less likely and in such patients the operation is largely restricted to the non-dominant hemisphere. The chances of appropriately selected patients being rendered seizure-free by a hemsipherectomy are approximately 75%. In addition there is often a marked improvement in behaviour.

In the past there have been considerable problems with long-term complications following anatomical hemispherectomy as a result of a haemorrhagic membrane forming in the hemispherectomy cavity which bled intermittently into the ventricular system, resulting in haemosiderin deposits, ependymitis and consequent obstructive hydrocephalus. A variety of procedures have been devised to overcome this problem. Many centres now undertake what is termed a functional hemispherectomy (Rasmussen 1983) in which the affected hemisphere is disconnected from the rest of the neuraxis, without the removal of the whole cerebral hemisphere and with the occipital and frontal lobes remaining in situ.

An alternative procedure is for the diseased hemisphere to be removed, leaving the basal ganglia in situ, with the dura being stitched down to the falx and tentorium, so that there is only a small surface area of dura and the cavity created is extradural and not in contact with the ventricular system (Adams 1983, Beardsworth & Adams 1988). Very careful haemostasis at the time of surgery is necessary to minimize the chance of a subdural haematoma forming. Isolation of the subdural cavity from the ventricular system is achieved by obliterating the ipsilateral foramen of Monro with a plug of muscle and the occlusion of any defect in the septum pellucidum. The overall operative mortality of hemispherectomy, which is often carried out in very small children, is 1–2%.

### 10.3.6 Corpus callosal section

This is an operation that disconnects cortex rather than resecting abnormal brain. The rationale is that section of the corpus callosum will prevent the rapid spread of epileptic activity from one hemisphere to the other. In consequence patients in whom there are sudden falls due to rapid seizure propagation may have less severe seizures, manifest by slower or less sudden drop attacks. The operation is not intended to stop epileptic seizures occurring, although it may do so in rare cases, but to reduce their severity and in particular to reduce injuries due to falls. It is important that patients and their relatives realize that the procedure is palliative and not curative.

The indications for corpus callosal section are medically intractable epilepsy with severe frequent drop attacks and injuries, in the absence of localized resectable pathology. The procedure should be considered in patients with tonic or atonic seizures. In such patients, there is an approximately 70% chance of a corpus callosotomy resulting in control of seizures causing injury (Spencer et al 1993). Other indications are less clear, and include generalized tonic-clonic seizures and secondary generalized seizures in which no resectable focus can be identified.

There are hazards to corpus callosal section. In addition to the risks of the neurosurgical procedure (e.g. hemiparesis, resulting from traction on the hemisphere or damage to the pericallosal artery), a transient disconnection syndrome with mutism, urinary incontinence and bilateral leg weakness may develop. The risks of the latter may be reduced by carrying out an anterior two-thirds rather than a complete callosal section. The extent of the section can be subsequently determined by a sagittal MRI. If troublesome seizures continue consideration may be given to completing the posterior third of the callosal section, although in published series the results of this are generally rather disappointing.

Overall the risks of severe sequelae to corpus callosal section, either neurological or neuropsychological, are of the order of 5–10%. The outcome from this procedure appears to vary considerably between centres and its exact role still requires further evaluation.

### 10.3.7 Multiple subpial transection

This operation is also referred to as Morrell's procedure (Morrell et al 1989). It is designed to be used when the epileptogenic zone involves eloquent brain cortex, which cannot be resected without resulting in a significant neurological deficit, and has been particularly applied to patients with lesions in language, or primary sensory or motor cortex. It has been suggested that seizures may come under control by making multiple incisions throughout the epileptogenic zone and therefore reducing the lateral recruitment of neurones to the epileptogenic process while preserving functionally important, vertically-oriented afferent and efferent connections. Limited evaluation of the procedure has been performed.

The best results have been seen in seizure disorders which may improve spontaneously e.g. the Landau–Kleffner syndrome, and in other cases the subpial transection has been combined with removal of a lesion, so that the effect of the subpial transection itself is uncertain. The only role of multiple subpial transection is likely to be in patients with very severe, frequent seizures arising from eloquent cortex in whom all alternative strategies have been exhausted.

## 10.4 FOLLOW-UP OF PATIENTS UNDERGOING EPILEPSY SURGERY

Patients undergoing epilepsy surgery need to have detailed post-operative outcome assessments performed to identify not only the effect of the procedure on the seizures but also the neuropsychological, social and neuropsychiatric outcome. A minimum follow-up schedule is necessary for an epilepsy surgery programme. This needs to involve neurological, surgical, psychological, ophthalmological specialists and

MRI (Table 10.5). This protocol should be regarded as a minimum, and if there is clinical need the patient and their family may need more intensive follow-up.

**Table 10. 5** Minimum epilepsy surgery follow-up strategy

| | | | |
|---|---|---|---|
| • *Neurosurgery:* | 6 weeks, | 1 year, | 2 years |
| • *Psychiatry:* | 1 month, | 3 months, | 1 year |
| • *Neurology:* | 3 months, | 1 year, | then annual |
| • *Psychology:* | 3 months, | 1 year, | 5 years |
| • *Ophthalmology:* | 6 months | | |
| • *Imaging:* | MRI at 3 months | | |

Consider AED reduction at 6–12 months if significant adverse effects from drugs

Consider AED withdrawal at 2 years if seizure-free (c. 30% risk of relapse)

## 10.4.1 Outcome

Patients who become seizure-free may require psychological counselling or other social support in order to gain the most advantage from their new situation. It is crucial to follow-up patients who do not become seizure-free as psychiatric disturbances, neuropsychological difficulties and psychosocial problems may follow a failed operation.

In both practical and biological terms it is necessary to consider those who are seizure-free separately from those who are not. Becoming seizure-free allows the patient to drive and to lead a much more normal social life than someone who has even a small number of seizures per year. However the type of seizure following surgery is also relevant. If secondary generalized tonic-clonic seizures are replaced by less severe partial seizures then this may be considered to be a worthwhile improvement. Many centres use the outcome scales proposed by Engel (1993) (Table 10.6).

**Table 10. 6** Classification of seizure outcome following epilepsy surgery (Engel 1993)

*Class 1: Free of disabling seizures (excludes early postoperative seizures)*

A. Completely seizure-free since surgery
B. Non-disabling simple partial seizures only
C. Some disabling seizures after surgery, but seizure-free for 2 years
D. Generalized convulsions on antiepileptic drug withdrawal only

*Class 2: Rare disabling seizures (almost seizure-free)*

A. Initially free of disabling seizures, but has rare seizures now
B. Rare disabling seizures since surgery
C. More than rare disabling seizures after surgery, but rare seizures for 2 years
D. Nocturnal seizures only

*Class 3*

A. Worthwhile seizure reduction
B. Prolonged seizure-free intervals, amounting to greater than half the follow-up period, but less than 2 years

*Class 4: No worthwhile improvement*

A. Significant seizure reduction
B. No appreciable change
C. Seizures worse

Seizures, including generalized tonic-clonic seizures in the first few days, occurring in the first few weeks after surgery are generally considered to be of little prognostic significance to the long-term outcome, and may reflect the acute trauma of surgery.

Occasionally patients subsequently develop recurrent generalized tonic-clonic seizures following epilepsy surgery when these were not present previously. These tend to occur as a late phenomenon, several years after surgery. Usually these seizures are more readily controlled but it is important that patients are warned about this rare possibility prior to surgery. Similarly, some patients display a so-called running-down phenomenon whereby the frequency and or severity of seizures does not change immediately after surgery but progressively improves over several months, sometimes to the extent of the patient becoming seizure-free, without any changes in medication.

The outcome with respect to seizures is predictable, with 90% reliability at 1 year following surgery. If a patient is having seizures at that time, there is only an approximately 10% chance that they will enter remission over the subsequent 5 years. Conversely, if they are seizure-free at 1 year following the operation there is a 10% chance of seizures relapsing over the next 5 years.

*Reducing AEDs after surgery for epilepsy*

If the patient is seizure-free or had a marked improvement in seizures following surgery and has side-effects from medication, it is reasonable to reduce the AEDs in the months following the operation, so that the adverse features resolve. Otherwise the drugs would generally be left unchanged until 1 year after the surgery, and then reduced to a single agent. If a patient is seizure-free 2 years after surgery, the complete withdrawal of the AEDs over several months may be contemplated, recognizing that this is associated with an approximately 30% risk of seizure recurrence.

*Reoperation*

Any patient who does not have a satisfactory outcome following epilepsy surgery should have an MRI scan to determine the extent of the surgical resection, and the presence of any residual pathology, in order to consider the possibility of a further surgical procedure (Germano et al 1994). About 15% of patients who have hippocampal sclerosis also have evidence of another pathology, and this may be amenable to further surgery. If a patient has had a lesionectomy and continues to have seizures, a second more extensive operation, to remove surrounding cortex, should be considered. The patient should be informed of this possibility during the initial evaluation stage.

*Postoperative psychological deficit*

Following temporal lobectomy, the most predictable concern is impairment of memory. The presurgical evaluation is directed towards identifying patients who are at risk of such a complication (Ch. 3, 3.5.5). In general, if a patient has a resection of a non-dominant temporal lobe they do not usually note any postoperative memory impairment and often note an improvement. If a sclerotic hippocampus is removed from a dominant temporal lobe there is usually an impairment of verbal memory preoperatively and little change seen after surgery. The situation in which there is most likely to be a noticeable worsening of memory following surgery is if a relatively normal hippocampus is removed, as may occur in operations to remove a foreign-tissue lesion adjacent to the hippocampus.

*Psychosocial outcome and rehabilitation*

It should not be assumed that, if a patient with epilepsy ceases to have seizures, their life will be automatically transformed for the better. Patients and their families need to be prepared for a sense of anticlimax after surgery and to be aware that, if seizures do cease, they need to make a complete readjustment and rebuild their lives without epilepsy being present as a reason or explanation for any hardship or disappointment that may occur. Many patients say afterwards that the adjustment to life without epilepsy was as traumatic as the initial adjustment to life with the condition. Those who continue to have seizures are often keenly disappointed, particularly if obtaining a driving licence was a major goal for them.

The most important factors for determining the psychosocial outcome following epilepsy surgery are: the age of the patient at surgery; duration of epilepsy; whether they become completely free of seizures or not; and the existence of a supportive family or carer. At one extreme, the best outcome may be expected in the child or young teenager with supportive siblings and parents, who had seizures for 2–3 years and became totally seizure-free. In this case, the epilepsy was a brief episode in their early life, and education and normal interactions with a peer group can be soon made up.

At the other extreme, a patient in their 40s with a 30-year history of epilepsy who lives alone and does not become totally seizure-free would not be expected to derive significant psychosocial benefits. Even if they became seizure-free, it is commonly the case that they will have become socially isolated, missed out on educational, career and social opportunities and developed a defensive attitude that can be very difficult to modify. Becoming seizure-free may also have a profound effect on interpersonal relationships, as a person who was once dependent seeks independence and to cast off the well meaning attentions of others. In some cases this leads to the break-up of a long-term relationship and to divorce.

Preoperative counselling on these issues helps to prepare patients and their families, minimizes subsequent problems and increases the chances of a satisfactory psychosocial outcome. In addition, for some patients, a proactive rehabilitation programme may be helpful. This needs to be individualized to each patient's needs. In general, attainable goals of activity and social achievement are set and regularly reviewed by the rehabilitationist, who would usually be a clinical psychologist. In some cases, the patient may have been very protected and could benefit from an intensive residential rehabilitation programme that covers activities of daily living including use of public transport and budgeting, as well as social skills and vocational training.

*Postoperative psychiatric morbidity*

Anxiety and depression are very common in the first 6 months after epilepsy surgery. If further seizures have occurred, there is inevitable disappointment. If there have been no seizures, there may be great anxiety lest they reappear. Depression may develop in response to the anticlimax after surgery, the realization of the impending adjustment that may be needed, and biological factors (Devinsky & Bear 1991) (Ch. 9, 9.3.2). Psychosis develops in about 3% of patients following epilepsy surgery (Ch. 9, 9.4.4), more commonly occurring after right temporal lobectomy than other procedures (Mace & Trimble 1991). Preoperative psychiatric assessment and follow-up after surgery are necessary to identify persons at risk from these problems and to deal with them effectively, although the preoperative psychiatric factors that identify patients who are at high risk of postoperative psychiatric morbidity are not yet fully defined. Specific pharmacological treatment may be necessary for psychiatric complications and in addition, the patient and their family will require a considerable amount of professional support and counselling.

## REFERENCES


Adams CBT 1983 Hemispherectomy – a modification. J Neurol Neurosurg Psychiat 46; 617–619

Beardsworth ED, Adams CBT 1988 Modified hemispherectomy for epilepsy: early results in ten cases. Br J Neurosurg 2; 73–84

Berkovic SF, McIntosh AM, Kalnins RM et al 1995 Pre-operative MRI predicts outcome of temporal lobectomy: an actuarial analysis. Neurology: 45: 1358-1363

Cascino GD, Boon PAJM, Fish DR 1993 Surgically remedial lesional syndromes. In: Engel J (ed) Surgical treatment of the epilepsies, 2nd edn. Raven Press, New York., p 77–86

Cendes F, Cook MJ, Watson C et al 1995 The frequency and characteristics of dual pathology in patients with lesional epilepsy. Neurology: in press

Devinsky O, Bear D M 1991 Varieties of depression in epilepsy. Neuropsychiat Neuropsychol Behav Neurol 4: 49–61

Duncan JS, Sagar HJ 1987 Seizure characteristics, pathology and outcome after temporal lobectomy. Neurology 37: 405–409

Engel J (ed) 1993 Surgical treatment of the epilepsies, 2nd edn. Raven Press, New York

Engel J, Driver MV, Falconer MA 1975 Electrophsyiological correlates of pathology and surgical results in temporal lobe epilepsy, Brain 98: 129–156

Fish DR, Spencer SS 1995 Clinical correlations: MRI and EEG. Magnetic Res Imaging: in press

Fish DR, Andermann F, Olivier A 1991 Complex partial seizures and posterior temporal or extratemporal lesions: surgical strategies. Neurology 41: 1781–1784

Fish DR, Smith SJM, Quesney LF, Andermann F, Rasmussen T 1993 Epilepsy surgery in children with medically refractory temporal or frontal lobe epilepsy: highlights and results of 40 years experience. Epilepsia 34: 244–247

Germano IM, Poulin N, Olivier A 1994 Reoperation for recurrent temporal lobe epilepsy. J Neurosurg 81: 31–36

Mace C, Trimble M R l991 Psychosis following temporal lobe surgery: a report of six cases. J Neurol Neurosurg Psychiat 54: 639–644

Morrell F, Whisler WW, Bleck TP 1989 Multiple subpial transection: A new approach to the surgical treatment of focal epilepsy. J Neurosurg 70; 231–239

Niemeyer P 1958 The transventricular amygdalohippocampectomy in temporal lobe epilepsy. In: Baldwin et al (eds) Temporal lobe epilepsy. Charles C Thomas, Springfield, IL, p 461–482

Pritchard JW, Rosen BR 1994 Functional study of the brain by NMR. J Cereb Blood Flow Metab 14: 365–372

Rasmussen T 1983 Hemispherectomy resvisited. Can J Neurol Sci 10: 71–78

Raymond AA, Fish DR, Stevens JM, Sisodiya SM, Shorvon SD 1994 Association of hippocampal sclerosis with cortical dysgenesis in patients with epilepsy. Neurology 44: 1841–1845

Raymond AA, Fish DR, Sisodiya SM, Alsanjari N, Stevens JM, Shorvon SD 1995 Abnormalities of gyration, heterotopias, tuberous sclerosis, focal cortical dysplasia, microdysgenesis, dysembryoplastic neuroepithelial tumour and dysgenesis of the

archicortex in epilepsy: Clinical, electroencephalographic and neuroimaging features in 100 adult patients. Brain: Vol 118: Part 3, 629-660
Smith SJM, Andermann F, Villemure JG, Rasmussen TB, Quesney LF 1991 Functional hemispherectomy: EEG findings, spiking from isolated brain postoperatively, and prediction of outcome. Neurology 41: 1790–1794
Spencer SS, Gates JR, Reeves AR et al 1993 Corpus callosum section. In: Engel J (ed). Surgical treatment of the epilepsies, 2nd edn. Raven Press, New York., p 637–648
Todorov AB, Lesser RP, Uematsu SS, Yankov YA, Todorov AA 1994 Distribution in time of seizures during presurgical EEG monitoring. Neurology 44: 1060–1064
Turner R 1994 Magnetic resonance imaging of brain function. Ann Neurol 35: 637–638
Wieser HG, Elger CE, Stodieck SRG 1985 The 'foramen ovale electrode': a new recording method for the preoperative evaluation of patients suffering from mesio-basal temporal lobe epilepsy. Electroenceph Clin Neurophysiol 61: 314–322
Williamson PD, French JA, Thadani VM et al 1993 Characteristics of medial temporal lobe epilepsy: interictal and ictal scalp electroencephalography, neuropsychological testing, neuroimaging, surgical results and pathology. Ann Neurol 34: 781–787
Yasargil MG, Teddy PJ, Roth P 1985 Selective amygdalo-hippocampectomy operative anatomy and surgical techniques. In: Symon L (ed) Advances and technical standards in neurosurgery, vol 12. Springer-Verlag, Berlin

# 11 Delivery of care

The medical care provided for patients with any illness is dependent on three principal factors:

- The epidemiology of the condition in the population
- The funding available for health care provision
- The priority given the management of that condition, in competition with other demands

In the UK, over 90% of health care is delivered by the National Health Service (NHS). Funding of the NHS amounts to 6.7% of the gross national product (Central Statistical Office 1992), considerably less than other western European countries and the USA.

## 11.1 EPIDEMIOLOGY

The annual incidence of new cases of epilepsy is 50/100 000 and that of non-febrile single seizures is 20/100 000. The cumulative lifetime incidence of a seizure, i.e. the risk of a person having a non-febrile seizure at some time in their life, is approximately 20/1000 of the population. The point prevalence of active epilepsy, with epilepsy being considered active if a seizure occurred in the last 2 years, is however about 5/1000. The difference between the cumulative lifetime incidence of a seizure and prevalence of active epilepsy underlines the fact that, in about 75% of people who develop seizures at some time, the condition remits and they do not continue to have active epilepsy (Hauser & Kurland 1975, Goodridge & Shorvon 1983). Table 11.1 summarizes the approximate incidence and prevalence figures for a typical population of 1 000 000, and the medical care requirements for these people with epilepsy.

## 11.2 CURRENT PROVISION OF CARE

The treatment of people with epilepsy involves many different professionals and specialists, working in hospitals and the community. In the UK, the general practitioner provides the primary level of care and coordinates the patient's management, involving specialists when appropriate, counselling, prescribing AEDs and giving emergency care and long-term follow-up. Hospital consultants, usually neurologists in the case of adults and paediatricians in the case of children, assess the

**Table 11.1** Epidemiology of epilepsy in a population of 1 000 000

| | |
|---|---|
| *Incidence and prevalence* | |
| Annual incidence of febrile seizures (50/100 000) | 500 |
| Annual incidence of single seizures (20/100 000) | 200 |
| Annual incidence of new cases of epilepsy (50/100 000) | 500 |
| Prevalence of active epilepsy (500/100 000) | 5000 |
| Cumulative lifetime incidence of a seizure (2000/100 000) | 20000 |
| *Medical care required* | |
| Institutional care | 400 |
| Residential care | 300 |
| Ongoing medical attention | 3300 |
| Occasional medical attention | 2600 |

majority of patients at the onset of the epilepsy and may participate in the long-term follow-up of patients whose epilepsy is refractory. Some patients, for example those with psychiatric problems or learning difficulties, may also require referral to psychiatrists, specialists in mental handicap and clinical psychologists. In other developed countries in which there are many more neurologists per head of population, these practitioners undertake a lot more of the 'primary care' for patients with epilepsy. In all countries, there is scope for epilepsy nurse practitioners to take on an increasing role in the follow-up of patients with epilepsy. For patients with concomitant psychosocial problems, counsellors and social workers may also have a very important role.

### 11.2.1 Primary care

In most European countries the general practitioner is responsible for the primary care of patients with epilepsy (Table 11.2). A general practitioner with an average practice size of 2000 patients may expect to have 10–12 patients with active epilepsy, and one or two new cases of epilepsy developing each year. He will often be the first doctor to see patients developing seizures and refer the majority of them to hospital for specialist evaluation. Subsequently, the general practitioner, with their knowledge of the patient's background and social situation, will have a major role to play in the education and counselling of the patient and their family, school or employers. Areas that need to be discussed include the characteristics and causes of epilepsy, the investigations performed, the nature of AED treatment, reasonable expectations of efficacy, side-effects, restrictions on driving and other occupations, inheritance, prognosis, contraception and pregnancy.

The general practitioner may be responsible for initiating AED therapy, particularly if a treatment strategy has been agreed with a specialist. He is likely to see the patient with acute drug-related problems, and to need to adjust medication even in the case of those patients who remain under hospital supervision. The general practitioner will often be called upon to deal with serial seizures and status epilepticus. Patients whose epilepsy responds to AED therapy will remain under the supervision of their

**Table 11.2** Role of the primary care physician in the management of epilepsy

*Initial diagnosis*

*Referral to specialist*
- Investigation
- Clarification of diagnosis
- Management plan
- Re-evaluation, change of therapy

*Continued follow-up of patient*
- Monitoring of efficacy and adverse effects
- Repeat prescriptions
- Monitoring of medical developments
- Re-referral of complicated patients to specialist
- Consideration of treatment withdrawal

*Counselling*
- Nature and aetiology of epilepsy
- Practical management of seizures
- Results and implications of investigations
- Treatment aims, limitations, adverse effects
- Prognosis
- Driving and employment
- Potentially hazardous activity; particularly bathing, cooking
- Education, employment, leisure
- Inheritance
- Contraception and pregnancy

general practitioner after initial assessment and initiation of treatment by a specialist and he is likely to be consulted for advice on when to discontinue medication. Even when patients remain under the review of a hospital clinic the general practitioner will generally be responsible for issuing prescriptions. In view of the shortage of epilepsy specialists, particularly in the UK, a practical way of improving the management of patients with epilepsy would be by improved education of primary care physicians at an undergraduate and postgraduate level.

Clinical nurse specialists or practitioners, modelled on diabetes nurse specialists, are beginning to take an increasing role in the routine monitoring, support and counselling of patients with epilepsy and their families (Table 11.2). These nurses may be attached to a group of general practitioners and alternatively or also to a hospital clinic. In many countries there are formal training programmes for clinical nurse specialists, organized by various bodies; for example, in the UK one such course is run by the National Society for Epilepsy.

Other community-based practitioners may also play an important part in the management of the patient with epilepsy, including the school medical service, occupational health departments, community mental handicap teams and social workers.

### 11.2.2 Secondary care

The diagnosis of epileptic seizures and syndrome, identification of aetiology, formulation of a treatment strategy and initial counselling should be by the neurologist, paediatrician or other specialist to whom the patient is referred by the primary care physician. In practice, referral to and care by consultant specialists is inevitably limited by their availability. In the UK there is the equivalent of one whole-time neurologist for 373 000 persons (range 157 000–626 000) (Langton-Hewer & Wood 1990) (Table 11.3). If every adult developing epilepsy was assessed by a consultant neurologist, each consultant would see 160 patients developing epilepsy each year. In addition a number of children with refractory epilepsy are referred from paediatric to adult neurology clinics. A recent community-based study in the UK found that 98% of children under 16 years, 94% of those between 16 and 59 years and 82% of the over 60s were referred for specialist evaluation (Hart YM, personal communication).

**Table 11.3** Medical manpower in England and Wales (1987). WTE = whole time equivalents

| Personnel | Approximate mean population per practitioner |
|---|---|
| General practitioner | 1800 |
| Consultant neurologist (WTE) | 373 000 |
| Consultant physician | 39 000 |
| Consultant paediatrician | 14 000* |
| Consultant paediatric neurologist | 738 000* |
| Consultant psychiatrist (mental handicap) | 293 000 |
| Consultant psychiatrist (mental illness) | 40 000 |
| Consultant neurosurgeon | 512 000 |
| Consultant clinical neurophysiologist | 966 000 |
| Clinical neuropsychologist | 837 000 |

* Children under age of 15 years

For 70–80% of people who develop epilepsy, seizures are controlled and follow-up will normally be with the patient's general practitioner. These patients would only be referred back to the specialist if further problems occurred or advice was sought, for example on whether to continue or taper medication. There are good arguments for patients who continue to have seizures remaining under hospital supervision. The follow-up of patients with established epilepsy, however, generates a significant workload. The hypothetical average population of 373 000 served by one neurologist in the UK will include 1865 patients with active epilepsy. If all patients with active epilepsy were reviewed every 6 months by a neurologist, they would see 75 such patients for follow-up each week. In countries with 10 times more neurologists per capita, such as the Netherlands and the USA, such a follow-up strategy is feasible. In a recent study in the UK 28% of people with active epilepsy were continuing to attend a hospital clinic (Hart YM, personal communication). As the problems for patients with epilepsy are often multifactorial, and have strong social and domestic implications, the provision of general-practitioner-based primary care carries many advantages for simple cases of epilepsy. For severe or chronic cases, however, specialist liaison is essential.

Even with the increases in the numbers of consultant neurologists in the UK (Department of Health, Medical Manpower and Education Division 1989) it is inevitable that a large proportion of the follow-up of patients with epilepsy will devolve to the primary care level. The situation in the UK is in contrast to that in the USA, in which there are many more neurologists per head of population (1/32 400) (Menken et al 1989). Other key differences are that, in the USA, care is not free at the point of service, upwards of 30 million people are not covered by health insurance, there is no comprehensive network of primary care physicians and direct or self-referral to specialists is the norm. In consequence, neurologists in the USA provide considerably more neurological primary care than do their counterparts in the UK. In the case of children, primary care is almost entirely provided by paediatricians, who commonly refer children with epilepsy to a paediatric neurologist.

Services for epilepsy are probably at their most developed in the Netherlands. There are 407 neurologists for a population of 15 000 000, or 1:37 000. The care of patients with epilepsy is shared between general practitioners, neurologists and paediatricians. There are also specialist epileptologists, assessment centres and a comprehensive network of epilepsy clinics. However, the relative costs and benefits to patients of medical services for epilepsy being provided mainly by specialists, rather than by general practitioners, has yet to be proven.

There is a shortfall in the provision of paediatric neurological services in the UK. Cumulative incidence figures indicate that about 25% of cases of epilepsy begin before the age of 15 years. There is one consultant paediatrician for 14 000 children and, with general practitioners, these consultants will take on the bulk of the management of epilepsy in children. Paediatric neurologists serve an average population of 738 000 children (Department of Health, Medical Manpower and Education Division 1989).

Geriatricians also play an important part in the management of epilepsy; in a recent community-based study, 25% of those presenting with seizures were aged 60 years or more (Sander et al 1990). Many of these patients also have non-neurological problems and referral to a geriatrician, who has the facilities to oversee patients' medical care and attendant social difficulties, is often appropriate.

The prevalence of mental handicap and epilepsy has been estimated at 0.07%, with just over half of these being cared for in institutions (Table 11.1) (Commission for the Control of Epilepsy and its Consequences 1978). Extrapolation to the UK suggests that there are approximately 35 000 people with epilepsy and mental handicap for whom, in 1977, there were 170 consultants in mental handicap.

### 11.2.3 Facilities for investigation

There has been a rapid increase in the provision of X-ray CT and MRI scanners in recent years. Most district hospitals in the UK, USA and in western Europe have X-ray CT scan instruments. There is no doubt about the superiority of MRI over X-ray CT for imaging the brains of patients with epilepsy in the majority of circumstances (Ch. 3, 3.3). The provision of MRI is also increasing rapidly, being available in all regional centres and university hospitals and an increasing number of district hospitals. In view of the operator-dependent nature of optimal MRI a greater problem in many areas is the shortage of skilled personnel to obtain and interpret images optimally.

Basic electroencephalography (EEG) facilities are generally widely available in developed countries. Specialized EEG facilities such as ambulatory monitoring and EEG-video telemetry are generally much more limited, and are mainly available in centres with specialist epilepsy clinics.

Serum AED concentration monitoring should be widely available in district hospital clinical biochemistry laboratories. Analyses are often carried out on a 'batch' basis once or twice a week, reducing its benefits to the clinical management of epilepsy. Monitoring of serum AED concentrations is of most benefit when results are available on the same day, so that the patient may be reviewed with the current result (Ch. 4, 4.3.1). Specialist neuropsychological assessment of people with epilepsy is of value in those patients whose seizures appear to be accompanied by a deficit of cognitive function or memory (Ch. 3, 3.5). Specialist psychometric assessments, however, can be difficult to obtain because of limitations of the number of clinical neuropsychologists.

### 11.2.4 Developing countries

In many developing countries the numbers of physicians per head of population is much less than in the West and one neurologist per 5 000 000 population would not be unexpected. Investigatory facilities such as CT and EEG may also be very limited. In Kenya and Nigeria, for example, CT was available in only one centre in each country in 1990. A further problem is that medication for epilepsy may be in short and irregular supply. In Pakistan, for example, it is estimated that 95% of patients with epilepsy are not receiving AEDs (Shorvon & Bharucha 1993). Contributory reasons for this shortfall include failure to identify patients needing treatment, an inadequate health care delivery infrastructure, failure to prescribe appropriate therapy and inadequate drug supply.

## 11.3 EPILEPSY CLINICS

### 11.3.1 The present situation

There is a consensus that epilepsy clinics should be established to improve the care of patients with epilepsy but there have been different views as to how comprehensive and widespread they should be. A contemporary opinion is that dedicated epilepsy clinics should be established nationwide for patients with difficult epilepsy and attendant problems, with a similar scope and role to diabetic clinics, which have been widely acknowledged to improve the care of patients with diabetes (MacFarlane 1990). A recent prospective, randomized study compared the care of patients with epilepsy in a neurology clinic with that provided by a dedicated epilepsy clinic. Patients attending the epilepsy clinic had better control of seizures, reported less side-effects from medication, received and retained more information and were more satisfied with the service provided than were those who were seen in the regular neurology clinic (Morrow 1990). At present there is no organized system of epilepsy clinics in the UK. Existing facilities have been arranged at a local level and vary enormously in their scope and facilities. At one extreme there are clinics with a full range of resources that have patients referred on a regional and supraregional basis. At the other extreme, a neurologist or paediatrician may arrange to see all of his referrals with epilepsy on one day a month, with no dedicated resources, and refer to this as an epilepsy clinic.

### 11.3.2 The way forward

It needs to be recognized that epilepsy clinics represent a concentration and more efficient use of resources, as well as improving the quality of care. Epilepsy clinics should be established in each health district, and be available for the management of patients with difficult epilepsy and associated problems, with referrals being made by general practitioners and hospital specialists for diagnostic evaluation and follow-up if necessary. The components and role of a specialized epilepsy clinic are summarized in Table 11.4. As well as the strictly medical aspects, an epilepsy clinic should have an epilepsy nurse specialist who, under the supervision of a consultant, can take on an important role in the counselling and education of patients and their families, schools and employers about epilepsy, and also act as a focus for education of the community as a whole and interact with voluntary agencies and local patient support groups. It would be desirable for epilepsy clinics to function under the auspices of a consultant neurologist and consultant paediatrician, with junior staff, to ease the transition of care in the mid-teens. Continuity of care for patients with refractory epilepsy is a major problem: with the other demands on their time it is not realistic for all clinical care to be delivered by one or two consultants. This is a particular problem in countries that have a paucity of consultant neurologists. Solutions that have been shown to function well in diabetes clinics include the use of long-term assistant medical staff in subconsultant grades, such as associate specialists, and specially trained general practitioners. Epilepsy nurse specialists may also provide useful continuity of care, act as a contact point, liaise between specialists and general practitioners and take on the important, time-consuming roles of monitoring of seizure control, adverse effects of medication and counselling (Table 11.2) (Ch. 7).

**Table 11.4** Components and role of epilepsy clinic

*Location*
- Hospital out-patient department
- Access to in-patient beds

*Staff*
- Supervision by consultant neurologist and consultant paediatrician
- Subconsultant grade specialists, junior medical staff
- Close liaison with clinical neurophysiologist and psychiatrist (mental handicap and mental illness)
- Clinical nurse specialist
- Administrative staff: receptionist, secretary
- Social worker

*Facilities*
- Serum AED concentration monitoring, EEG, CT and/or MRI
- Access to clinical neuropsychology and other hospital services

*Referrals*
- From general practitioners and hospital doctors

*Functions*
- Initial diagnostic evaluation and initiation of treatment
- Long-term follow-up of severe, refractory or complicated epilepsy
- Co-ordination of medical and non-medical services

*Counselling*
- Patient and family
- Liaison with schools, employers, social services

*Education*
- Medical and paramedical staff
- Non-medical staff, e.g. police, social workers, teachers
- Community at large
- Involvement with voluntary agencies

*Research*
- The clinic should act as a focus for clinical research

## 11.4 TERTIARY CARE

In addition to district epilepsy clinics, there is a clear need for regional epilepsy centres, referred to in the USA as 'comprehensive epilepsy programs'. These clinics will usually be located at a regional neurology and neurosurgery centre, often as a part of a university hospital. The principal function of such centres is to act as referral centres for difficult diagnostic and treatment problems. They need to have a full range of diagnostic facilities, including 24-h video-EEG telemetry and modern MRI, clinical psychologists and psychiatrists with a particular interest in epilepsy and related disorders and a clinical pharmacology unit.

Most tertiary referrals may be dealt with as out-patients with a small number of beds for patients having monitoring and invasive investigations. For a few patients, however, it is most helpful to have the facility for admission to a unit with low, but expert, nursing dependency. In the UK, such units are referred to as 'special assessment centres' and in the USA as 'quaternary centers'. The reasons for admission to such a unit would include: clarification of diagnosis of episodes that do not occur sufficiently frequently to make video-EEG telemetry feasible; optimization and rationalization of AED therapy; assessment of concomitant psychosocial difficulties and abilities for independent living; and consideration of a period of psychosocial rehabilitation or longer-term residential care. Further goals may include: initiation of treatment of non-epileptic attacks; and education of patient and carers about management of serial seizures and realistic expectations in terms of prognosis and independent living.

In-patient tertiary referral facilities or 'special assessment centres' are often ideally located outside a general hospital setting. A model that works well is to place such a unit next to an epilepsy unit that provides residential rehabilitation and care and to have very close links with an academic neuroscience centre that has all the invasive and neurosurgical facilities to hand. Close links are achieved by senior staff having joint appointments and junior staff rotating in their appointments. The components of such an arrangement will thus have a symbiotic relationship, be complementary, between them provide a complete spectrum of epilepsy care and also act as a research unit. Examples of this arrangement in the UK include: the National Society for Epilepsy–Chalfont Centre and the National Hospital for Neurology and Neurosurgery; the David Lewis Centre and the university hospitals in Manchester; Bootham Park Hospital, York and the regional neurology and neurosurgery centre in Leeds. Similar very successful arrangements exist in other European countries and as part of some 'comprehensive epilepsy programs' in the USA.

*Children*

Children with severe epilepsy and concomitant problems have the same range of needs as adults. They have the additional demands of education and growing up, and the need to develop satisfactory relationships with peers and family, the dynamics of which are likely to have been significantly disturbed by the occurrence of seizures. For the majority of circumstances, community services, district paediatricians and regional paediatric neurologists, child and family psychiatrists and supporting staff deal with the situation. In particularly difficult and complicated circumstances referral to a tertiary referral paediatric centre may be appropriate.

The trend has been to maintain children in mainstream education if at all possible. For some children with severe epilepsy and, often, concomitant difficulties with intellectual handicap and behaviour disorder, this is not possible and they benefit from being educated at a special residential school. In addition to an educational role, the residential schools provide close medical supervision and allow children to reach their maximum potential in an equal peer group. It is important that close links are maintained with the child's local school, and a return made to mainstream education, if possible.

## 11.5 EPILEPSY SURGERY

20–30% of patients who develop epilepsy will have seizures that continue despite optimal medical treatment (Goodridge & Shorvon 1983, Reynolds 1987). For some of these patients, surgical treatment may be an appropriate option (Ch. 10). The usual criteria for considering surgical treatment are: that the patient has seizures which have a focal onset, i.e. partial or secondarily generalized seizures, which have proved intractable to tolerated AED therapy; which are sufficiently frequent or severe to interfere with the patient's life; and the likelihood that the cessation of seizures would have an overall beneficial effect on the patient's quality of life. Elwes and Binnie (1990) estimated that approximately 7% of patients *developing* epilepsy would be suitable candidates for presurgical evaluation. It is likely that surgery would be appropriate in about 50% of those patients evaluated. On this basis it is estimated that in the UK, with a population of 56 000 000, there is an estimated backlog of 10 000 cases and an annual recurring need for 1000 operations. A consultant neurologist in the UK has an average referral population of about 300 000 and so would expect to have in that population 50 patients who were candidates for surgical treatment and an annual recurring need for 3–12 cases. A neurologist in the USA or some western European countries, with an average referral population of 30 000, may expect to have five potentially suitable patients, and a further patient becoming suitable every year.

At present, facilities for epilepsy surgery are limited and there is a significant shortfall of the necessary provision. In 1989 a survey of consultant neurosurgeons in the UK showed that 147 operations were performed for epilepsy (Hart & Shorvon 1990). A similar shortfall has been reported from other developed countries. There has been a considerable expansion of activity in recent years but there is still a marked underprovision. Limiting factors are primarily financial, with a need for intensive monitoring units, high-quality MRI and expert neuropsychology as well as skilled neurologists and neurosurgeons. The necessary facilities, skills and techniques for epilepsy surgery are demanding and highly specialized and there is no place for centres performing small numbers, e.g. five to ten operations per year. Centres should be established that perform at least 50–100 operations per year, implying five to ten centres in the UK carrying out a minimum of 25 operations per year so that skills are kept adequately sharp.

Epilepsy surgery units should be in close association with a tertiary referral epilepsy centre. A multidisciplinary team is essential, and should include: a neurosurgeon with a particular interest and expertise in epilepsy surgery and the time to carry out one to two operations per week; a clinical neurophysiologist; a neurologist; a neuropsychologist; a psychiatrist with expertise in this area; and the services of a paediatric neurologist. The facilities available should include high-quality MRI and CT scanning, 24 h video-EEG telemetry, facilities for invasive intracranial EEG monitoring, cerebral angiography, neuropsyc0hology (including carotid amytal testing), neuropathology, and laboratory facilities, including immediate access serum AED concentration monitoring (National Association of Epilepsy Centres 1990).

## 11.6 RESIDENTIAL CARE

The concept of residential care specifically for patients with poorly controlled epilepsy was established in the UK and other developed countries in the 1890s. At the time this represented a great advance over the previous situation. The initial concept was to set up 'colonies' that were largely independent and self-sufficient. Over the last 30 years there has been a decline in the numbers of patients with epilepsy in residential care. In the UK, for example, in 1962 there were 2246 persons in residential care primarily because of epilepsy, and in 1990 there were 1022. These figures exclude those patients who are in residential care primarily because of mental handicap but who also have epilepsy. The principal reasons for the reduction of numbers of patients with epilepsy in residential care include:

- Improved medical treatment
- Improved facilities for care and support in the community
- A swing in opinion, which started in the psychiatric sphere, against residential care and in favour of care in the community
- Greater public acceptance of epilepsy and the occurrence of seizures in public
- Increased financial demands on local health and social services authorities, who have the responsibility for funding care

While there is no doubt that care in the community is best for the vast majority of patients with epilepsy, provided there is an adequate support network, it is equally clear that, for a small proportion, residential care gives a better quality of life than living either alone, with ageing parents whose lives are dominated by anxiety about the next seizure (Thompson & Oxley 1988), or in inappropriate local facilities that may be primarily for those with mental handicap. Whereas in the past many patients admitted for residential care had epilepsy as their only major problem, most patients for whom this is considered at present have significant concomitant problems. Typically, these may include a degree of cognitive and physical handicap, a disorder of conduct and behaviour or mood. Other factors that need to be taken into account include the patient's family circumstances and the level of support that is available in the locality, such as supervised small group homes. In the UK at least, this provision is not uniform and the sophistication and adequacy of social and medical support available in the community varies enormously from area to area, with some of the greatest contrasts being between adjacent boroughs in large urban conurbations. Finally, the wishes of the person themself are paramount, particularly after a trial period at the proposed facility and regular reviews which involve the patient, carers, relatives and the care purchasers (usually the health and social security authorities of the patient's original domicile).

Residential care should be considered as one of a range of options for the patient with intractable epilepsy, after consideration of all the medical issues, with clarification of diagnosis and aetiology, optimization of treatment and assessment of the patient's psychosocial potential, and available family support and local facilities. It is generally best for such an in-depth review to be carried out at an assessment centre which has links with a residential facility. This has the added advantage that informal visits and trial periods may be easily arranged.

Persons with epilepsy who are admitted for residential care almost invariably have other problems and require a high degree of nursing and care. As a result of the more dependent population that they now care for, the residential centres for epilepsy are much less self-sufficient than was the case 20 years ago and in consequence require a higher level of funding.

The accent of residential care for patients with intractable epilepsy should not be on care and containment but on rehabilitation, with every individual achieving their maximum potential, moving on to live independently if possible, in a setting in which there is a peer group and a safety net of expert nursing, paramedical and medical care.

## 11.7 VOLUNTARY AGENCIES

The charitable sector and voluntary agencies play a considerable role in the provision of care for patients with epilepsy and their families. This is particularly important at a time of insufficient funding from central government. In the UK charities run the six residential epilepsy centres in the country. Other very important roles of the voluntary agencies, as exemplified by the Epilepsy Foundation of America, include:

- A comprehensive national network of local support and counselling groups for patients and their relatives
- Formation of pressure lobby groups, at local, national and parliamentary levels, to push for improved epilepsy services
- Provision of educational material about epilepsy for patients, their families, schools and employers and the public at large
- Education of medical and paramedical professionals
- Fund-raising and sponsoring of research

### REFERENCES

Central Statistical Office 1992 Key data 1992/1993. HMSO, London

Commission for the Control of Epilepsy and its Consequences 1978 Plan for nationwide action on epilepsy, vols 1–4. DHJEW publication no. (NIH) 78-279. US Department of Health, Education and Welfare, Bethesda, MD

Department of Health, Medical Manpower and Education Division 1989 Medical and dental staffing prospects in the NHS in England and Wales in 1988. Health Trends 21: 99–106

Elwes R, Binnie CD 1990 Assessing outcome following epilepsy surgery. In: Chadwick DW (ed) Quality of life and quality of care in epilepsy. Royal Society of Medicine, London, p 106–115

Goodridge DMG, Shorvon SD 1983 Epileptic seizures in a population of 6000. 1: Demography, diagnosis and role of the hospital services; 2: Treatment and prognosis. Br Med J 287: 641–647

Hart YM Shorvon SD 1990 Surgery for epilepsy in the United Kingdom. Acta Neurol Scand 82(suppl 133): 21

Hauser WA, Kurland LT 1975 The epidemiology of epilepsy in Rochester, Minnesota 1935 through 1967. Epilepsia 16: 1–66

Langton-Hewer R, Wood VA 1990 Neurology services in the United Kingdom. A report. Association of British Neurologists, London

MacFarlane I 1990 Quality of life and quality of care: the experience from diabetes. In: Chadwick DW (ed) Quality of life and quality of care in epilepsy. Royal Society of Medicine, London, p 50–58

Menken M, Hopkins A, Murray TJ, Vates TS 1989 The scope of neurologic practice and care in England, Canada and the United States. Arch Neurol 46: 210–213

Morrow J 1990 An assessment of an epilepsy clinic. In: Chadwick DW (ed) Quality of life and quality of care in epilepsy. Royal Society of Medicine, London, p 96–105

National Association of Epilepsy Centres 1990 Recommended guidelines for diagnosis and treatment in specialized epilepsy centres. Epilepsia 31(suppl 1): 1–12

Reynolds EH 1987 Early treatment and prognosis of epilepsy. Epilepsia 28: 97–106

Sander JWAS, Hart YM, Johnson AL, Shorvon SD 1990 National General Practice Study of Epilepsy: newly diagnosed epileptic seizures in a general population. Lancet 336: 1267–1271

Shorvon SD, Bharucha NE 1993 Epilepsy in developing countries: epidemiology, aetiology and health care. In: Laidlaw J, Richens A, Chadwick D (eds) A textbook of epilepsy, 4th edn. Churchill Livingstone, Edinburgh, p 613–630

Thompson PJ, Oxley JR 1988 Socioeconomic accompaniments of severe epilepsy. Epilepsia 29(suppl 1): S9–S18

# Appendix Addresses of International Bureau for Epilepsy Chapters and Friends

The IBE permits one voluntary organization to become a chapter (C) and additional organizations are awarded the status of 'friends' (F).

**IBE Head Office**
PO Box 21
2100 AA Heemstede
The Netherlands

**Argentina (C)**
Ass. de Lucha contre la Epilepsia
Tucuman 3261
1425 Buenos Aires

**Australia (C)**
Nat. Epilepsy Ass. of Australia
PO Box 224
Parramatta NSW 2150

**Austria (C)**
Elterninitiative für anfallskranke Kinder
Stumpergasse 1/15
1060 Wien

**Belgium (C)**
Les Amis de la Ligue Nat. Belge contre l'Epilepsie
135 Avenue Albert
Brussels 1060

**Brazil (C)**
Associacao Brasil de Epilepsia
Caixa Postal 20265
04034 Sao Paulo SP

**Canada (C)**
1470 Peel Street, suite 745
Montreal, Quebec
H3A 1T1

**Canada (F)**
Montreal Neurological Institute
3801 University Street
Montreal Quebec H3A 2B4

**Chile (C)**
Ass. Liga c.l. Epilepsia de Valparaiso
PO Box 705
Vina del Mar

**Columbia (C)**
Liga Colombiana contra la Epilepsia
PO Box 057751
Bogota DC

**Cuba (C)**
Cuban Chapter of IBE
Zona Postal 4, Apartado 4248
C. Habana 0400

**Denmark (C)**
Dansk Epilepsiforening
Dr. Sellsvej 28
DK 4293 Dianalund

**Denmark (F)**
Dianalund Epilepsy Hospital
DK 4293 Dianalund

**Ecuador (C)**
Asoc.de Padres de Ninos con Epilepsia
Casilla Postal 221
C Suc.15
Quito

**Ecuador (F)**
Liga Tung. de Control de la Epilepsia
Cevallos 6-09 Y Montalvo, officina 202
Segundo Piso Edificio Prof. 'Ambato'
Ambato

**Finland (C)**
Epilepsialiitto
Kalevankatu 61
00180 Helsinki 18

**France (C)**
AISPACE
11 Avenue Kennedy
F-59800 Lille

**Germany (C)**
Deutsche Epilepsie Vereinigung
Sulzaer Str. 5
1000 Berlin 33.

**Greece (C)**
Greek National Assoc. Against Epilepsy
Aghia Sophia Children's Hospital
Dept. Neurology/ Neurophysiology
Athens 11527

**Guatemala (C)**
Guatemalan Epilepsy Soc. Cagualice
Hospital Herera
6a Ave. 7-55, Zona 10
Guatemala City

**Indonesia (C)**
Jl. Jelita Utara no. 11
Rawamangun
Jakarta 13220

**India (C)**
Indian Epilepsy Association
1 Old Veterinary Hospital Road
Basavanagudi
Bangalore 560 004

**Ireland (C)**
249 Crumlin Road
Dublin 12

**Israel (C)**
Israel Epilepsy Association
PO Box 1598
Jerusalem

**Italy (C)**
Associazione Italiana contra l'Epilessia
Via Assarotti 44/4
16122 Genoa

**Japan (C)**
The Japanese Epilepsy Association
5F Zenkokuzaidan Building 2-2-8
Nishiwaseda Shinjuku-KU
Tokyo 162

**Japan (F)**
National Epilepsy Center
Shizuoka Higashi Hospital
886 Urushiyama
Shizuoka 420

**Kenya (C)**
Kenya Ass. f/t Welfare of Epileptics
Gertrude's Children's Hospital
PO Box 42325
Nairobi

**Korea (C)**
Korean Epilepsy Association
204-1 Yeonhi-dong, Seodaemun-ku
Seoul 120-112

**Mexico (C)**
Grupo Aceptacion de Epilepticos
Amsterdam 1928 L 19
Colonia Olimpica-Pedregal
Mexico 04710 D.F.

**The Netherlands (C)**
Epilepsie Vereniging Nederland
Hart. Nibbrigkade 71, flat 48
2597 XS Den Haag

**The Netherlands (F)**
Dr. Hans Berger Kliniek
Postbus 90108
4800 RA Breda

**The Netherlands (F)**
Federati voor Epilepsiebestrijding
PO Box 9587
3506 GN Utrecht

**The Netherlands (F)**
Instituut voor Epilepsiebestrijding
Meer & Bosch/Cruquiushoeve
PO Box 21
2100 AA Heemstede

**The Netherlands (F)**
Stichting Kempenhaeghe
Sterkselseweg 65
5591 VE Heeze

**New Zealand (C)**
New Zealand Epilepsy
Association Inc.
PO Box 1074
Hamilton

**Norway (C)**
Norsk Epilepsiforbund
Storgt. 39
0192 Oslo

**Pakistan (F)**
Epilepsy Advisory Clinic
Z-438 Ratta Road
Rawalpindi

**Poland (C)**
Polish Epilepsy Association
Ul. Fabryczna 57 (Xlp.pok.7)
15-482 Bialystok

**Portugal (C)**
Liga Nacional Portuguesa c.l.
Epilepsia
Rua Sa da Bandeira 162-1 o
4000 Oporto

**Slovenia (C)**
Liga Proti Epilepsiji
CIPD, Njegoseva 4/11
61 000 Ljubljana

**South Africa (C)**
South African National Epilepsy
League
PO Box 73
Observatory 7935

**South Africa (F)**
Epilepsy Care Centre, REEA
PO Box 41116, Craighall 2024
Johannesburg

**Spain (C)**
PENEPA
Calle Escuelas Pias n.89
08017 Barcelona

**Sri Lanka (C)**
Epilepsy Association of Sri Lanka
10 Austin Place
Colombo 8

**Sweden (C)**
Swedish Epilepsy Association
PO Box 9514
10274 Stockholm

**Switzerland (C)**
Schweizerische Liga gegen Epilepsie
c/o Pro Infirmis
Postfach 129
8032 Zurich

**Switzerland (F)**
Epicentre, c/o Dominique Ulku
30B Chemin de la Colombe
1231 Conches

**UK (C)**
British Epilepsy Association
Anstey House
40 Hanover Square
Leeds LS3 lBE

**UK (Scotland) (C)**
Epilepsy Association of Scotland
48 Govan Road
Glasgow G51 1JR

**UK (F)**
The National Society for Epilepsy
The Chalfont Centre
Chalfont St. Peter
Buckinghamshire SL9 0RJ

**UK (F)**
David Lewis Centre for Epilepsy
Near Alderley Edge
Cheshire, SK9 7UD

**UK (F)**
Quarrier's Homes
Bridge of Weir
Renfrewshire PA11 3SA

**UK (Wales) (F)**
Wales Epilepsy Association
Y pant teg Brynteg
Dolgellau, LL40 1RP
Gwynedd, Wales

**USA (C)**
Epilepsy Foundation of America
4351 Garden City Drive
Landover, Maryland 20785

**Zimbabwe (C)**
Epilepsy Support Foundation
PO Box A.104
Avondale, Harare

# Index